Introspective, richly l[
Emergency is a love lett
parts of her career.

For fifteen years, Joanna Sokol filled private notebooks with her confusion, humor, and anger toward the strange world of emergency street medicine. As her career on the ambulance progressed, she found herself taking notes on scraps of paper, the backs of gloves, and in the margins of EKG printouts. She listened to her patients' stories, left food out for their pets, and turned off the stove under their oxtail stews. Once, she read half a poem left in a dead woman's typewriter. She learned about the history that brought ambulances into their current role as the caretakers of society's forgotten and spoke to her colleagues about their own experiences and perspectives.

Those reflections are collected here, in a series of raw, powerful essays about the state modern healthcare.

Sokol's life as a paramedic took her to three different counties: the casinos and trailer parks of the Nevada desert, the cozy beach town of Santa Cruz, and, eventually, the crowded tenements of San Francisco's Tenderloin district. There are no clear villains or heroes in Sokol's world, only a group of patients and medics who are doing their best in a deeply broken system.

Combining impactful research, compassionate reflections on her most memorable patients, and the strong voices of her fellow paramedics, Sokol takes readers deep into the everyday reality of 911 first responders, offering insight, empathy, and a reminder of both the power and limitations of care.

Praise for *A Real Emergency*

"*A Real Emergency* deserves a place among the great work memoirs. Compassionate, humorous, a flat-out fantastic book."
—**Caitlin Doughty, Bestselling author of** *Smoke Gets in Your Eyes, From Here to Eternity,* **and** *Will My Cat Eat My Eyeballs?*

"I would read Joanna Sokol's grocery lists, her texts, her musings on anything. Her work is raw, poignant, and funny. She drops you into the rarely seen world of street medicine—Narcan and mending tools at the ready—in a way few other writers can. At a time when paramedics increasingly serve as safety-net bridges to care, *A Real Emergency* is a gift of understanding and, ultimately, hope."
—**Beth Macy, author of** *Dopesick* **and** *Raising Lazarus*

"*A Real Emergency* is a five-alarm firestorm of a book that every American must swerve over to read. Keenly observed and gorgeously composed, it is a testament to both the brutality of our medical industrial complex and the humanity of the paramedics frantically trying to save us from it. A page-turning, soul-enraging act of narrative justice that will haunt you to the core."
—**Stephanie Elizondo Griest, author of** *All the Agents and Saints*

"Hilarious, horrifying, and poetic. In *A Real Emergency*, Joanna Sokol perfectly delivers the chaotic world of street medicine in all its tarnished glory. Sokol's account of fractured lives in San Francisco is both timely and riveting and is filled with moments of genuine grace."
—**Kevin Hazzard, author of** *A Thousand Naked Strangers* **and** *American Sirens*

"After a decade on the frontlines of a very broken system, Joanna Sokol has let loose one hell of a memoir: compelling, shocking, funny, galling, urgent, and beautiful. The best I've read in quite some time."
—**Mary Roach**, *New York Times* **bestselling author**

"For those of us who want our journalism unvarnished and direct, with no hint of sugar-coating, this book is a pinnacle of the craft. Joanna's journey into the heartbreaking, shocking, hilarious, inspiring, and draining world of paramedic work is so unflinching and detailed it leaves you exhausted—and in awe of her and her colleagues as they strap in for their brutal day-to-day dash from one emergency to another. There's nothing pretty about their world, but through Joanna's eyes it is brutally, grittily elegant. Read it and learn."
—**Kevin Fagan, author of** *The Lost and the Found*

"Reading Joanna Sokol's *A Real Emergency* often feels like hurtling down the freeway without a windshield, or riding in a helicopter with the hatch open. There's a sense of turbulence and unpredictability to it, a frantic, propulsive energy that makes for an exhilarating read. But underneath the tense, unnerving anecdotes and the people's lives hanging in the balance, Sokol also unpacks the quiet importance of paramedics in today's society, their unheralded role as nonjudgmental, supportive figures for Americans toiling on the invisible margins. There is real sincerity and compassion lying beneath Sokol's breakneck prose—and a larger point about what America chooses to pay attention to, and what it wilfully ignores and neglects."
—**Mike Mariani, author of** *What Doesn't Kill Us Makes Us*

A REAL EMERGENCY

A REAL EMERGENCY

JOANNA SOKOL

STRANGE
LIGHT

Strange Light is a registered trademark of Penguin Random House Canada Limited.

The authorized representative in the EU for product safety and compliance is Penguin Random House Ireland, Morrison Chambers, 32 Nassau Street, Dublin D02 YH68, Ireland, https://eu-contact.penguin.ie

Library and Archives Canada Cataloguing in Publication Data is available upon request.

ISBN: 978-0-7710-0657-9
ebook ISBN: 978-0-7710-0658-6

Cover design: Kate Sinclair
Cover art: Kate Sinclair
Printed in the United States of America

Strange Light
Penguin Random House Canada
320 Front Street West, Suite 1400
Toronto, Ontario, M5V 3B6, Canada
penguinrandomhouse.ca

1st Printing

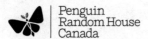

Penguin
Random House
Canada

For my grandfather, the surgeon, who would always say:
"When are you going to quit screwing around with this
ambulance shit and go to medical school?"

When you're running, it's five in the morning, it's you and the rats and the hookers and you're seeing things no one's supposed to see, I call it the Poo Show. And it'll take you right down with it if you don't have your head right. I've seen good medics, great medics broken out there.

This job is the dirt and the shit and you've got to find a higher power to come home to if you don't want to end your career at the bottom of a bottle or the end of a barrel.

San Francisco Fire Department EMS chief Jeff Myers

Every day people were dying there because of some small detail that they couldn't be bothered to observe. Imagine being too tired to snap a flak jacket closed, too tired to clean your rifle, too tired to guard a light, too tired to deal with the half-inch margins of safety that moving through the war often demanded, just too tired to give a fuck and then dying behind that exhaustion.

Michael Herr, *Dispatches*

Talkin' this leprechaun talk

They been chasing me for almost two years

Runnin' and screaming

They watching my every fucking move

Bella, high on meth in San Francisco

CONTENTS

AUTHOR'S NOTE

ON ACCURACY

Like all medical writing, this work contains a balancing act between protecting patient privacy and telling a truthful story. I have changed names and identifying details of all of my patients and most of my co-workers. I have also adjusted the timeline of events; for example, in certain instances I suggest that a particular call took place earlier or later in my career than was the case. I have used fake names for various hospitals for legal reasons.

Like many paramedics, I always carried a notebook and a Sharpie on the ambulance to write down vital signs, medication lists, and patient information during the call. Long before I began writing formally, I found myself jotting down interesting quotes from patients or details of a run that stuck with me. After a particularly challenging situation, I would pour my feelings and impressions into a journal. In this way I have managed to keep some of the exact wording from calls I ran ten or fifteen years ago. Other pieces of dialogue have been reconstructed from memory to the best of my ability. It is true that the traumatized brain can change or erase certain types of experiences, so I have done what I can to allow the reader to understand my relationship with my own memories. Sometimes the tape gets blurry on the replay, and that confusion is also part of my story.

Language is a continually evolving entity. When I became a first responder, we were taught to use the word *homeless* instead of *bum* or *hobo*. This was to indicate a respect for the human in their circumstance. At the time of this book's publication, some institutions have moved on to use the phrase *unhoused individual* or *person experiencing homelessness* instead. The rationale is exactly the same: to highlight the person instead of their condition. Likewise, many academic institutions have swapped *alcohol use disorder* or *opiate use disorder* for *alcoholism* or *opiate addiction*.

I have chosen my words carefully to best reflect the truth of my own experience as a paramedic. While I admire the medical institution's constant effort to revise our understanding of addiction and social welfare, I have found some of the newer vocabulary to be both grammatically unwieldy and emotionally distancing. I have sometimes used the language that my patients and my colleagues use to describe ourselves, rather than that which is recommended by current academia. My hope is that if some of my phrasing is unfashionable, my respect for the humanity of each patient is found instead in both my storytelling and my actions.

PROLOGUE: A REAL EMERGENCY

The Tow Truck in the Tree is a fun one. The beginning doesn't matter, but it ends with me and my partner staring like slack-jawed idiots at a full-sized commercial tow truck hanging twenty feet in the air, suspended impossibly from the branches of a large tree. The driver is limp in the front seat. The radio crackles, requesting an update.

Or the Undead Sparkle Panties Jump Scare: We point flashlights into a dark corner of a cheap weekly-rate motel, kicking through broken furniture and piles of clothes. I hear a sound and raise my light to see a woman rearing up out of the bathroom, covered in so much blood that it swings off her breasts and elbows in goopy stalactites. She groans and reaches for us, spraying coagulated drops onto the wall. We both shriek like cartoon characters. She is naked but for high heels and a red-sequined thong. When I am moved to a different ambulance shift a few months later, my partner buys me a small rubber zombie as a going-away present.

Another fan favorite is the kid who finishes off a handle of whiskey with his friends, then accepts a dare to pour Dave's Gourmet Insanity hot sauce all over his softest bits. I pull into a cute cul-de-sac to find a buck-naked teenager writhing and screaming in the middle of the street while a neighbor sprays him down with a hose. On the way to the hospital, I try to ask him about his allergies and medical history, but he can only gasp and cry. "It went in the hole!" he sobs. "It went in the hole!"

Moments like these make for great anecdotes when trying to impress a stranger. Exciting, entertaining, gruesome enough to inspire sympathy but not so tragic as to be depressing. They grab the reader and promise a gripping memoir full of wacky medical hijinks, sprinkled with humor and tenderness and lots of good trauma porn. Yes, I am fun at parties. No, this is not my real personality.

I've worked on a 911 ambulance for ten years in three different counties. My job isn't really what people think it is.

"I think it's encephalitis," she tells me. "Because it hurts back here, in my neck." The woman motions to the back of her hairline, which is grayed and dry.

Susan is seventy years old and called 911 today for a runny nose and some neck pain. She's been sick for several days but hasn't seen a doctor. She lives in a "single room occupancy" government-assistance high-rise downtown, where she shares a small room with a younger woman she tells me is her friend. We're in San Francisco, where ancient tenement-style hotels are crammed next to new-money high-rises, condos, and row houses. A tipsy young couple might walk an extra few blocks to avoid a neighborhood like Susan's.

She wears an oversized orange sweater and unravels one sleeve with her thumbs as we talk. The sweater isn't as dirty as a lot of clothes worn by the people we treat, but it's not clean. I take Susan's vital signs and hook her up to the cardiac monitor. I turn the heat up in the ambulance.

Susan is like most of my patients: lonely, destitute, and nursing a minor medical complaint.

On a TV screen, paramedics are always rushing to try to save a woman crushed under a building, a man bleeding out, or a baby taking its last breath. There are a lot of sirens, a lot of shouting, an occasional goofy drunk for comic relief, but the bulk of the job is invariably depicted as an adrenaline rush.

The truth of my work is both less and more interesting. A paramedic today exists in a poorly defined gray area, some combination of field doctor, social worker, and street sweeper. We answer many of our calls without sirens at all, and sit with people nursing complicated problems that only distantly relate to actual medicine. When we arrive at a hospital, we are rarely ushered straight to a room. We often wait with our patients for hours until a nurse has time to take over.

As a street medic, I'm never going to see most patients' lab values. But I'll see the inside of their bedroom, and their neighbors' bedrooms. I'll see the photos stacked in the dark corner of a closet before I'll ever see a chest X-ray. I climb my bags up three flights of stairs, past potted plants, framed certificates, and family photos. I know which houses have illegal back units, which have meth labs, which have a beautiful rooftop deck. I look in the fridge for insulin. A patient directs me into her closet to pick out a jacket to wear to the emergency room; she doesn't like the yellow one, grab the blue behind it. A Vietnam infantry hat falls as I reach for the hanger. She tells me to put it back; it was her husband's once. The edges of the hat are worn thin.

I see moldy kitchens, rotted attics. I leave food out for pets, switch off lights, turn down the stove under a pot of oxtails. Once I read half a poem left in a dead woman's typewriter. We call it the "scene." What was the scene like? Is the scene safe? Are we at a house, a clinic, an alleyway behind a row of dumpsters?

Ambulance services, at their core, are about transportation. We do a lot of assessment and a little bit of intervention, but our main function is to get people from wherever they are over to the hospital.

In a normal month I run on, roughly, between seventy and one hundred patients. Usually two or three of those are lights and sirens, step-on-the-gas, "Johnny, get the paddles"-type emergencies. Your car wrecks, your heart attacks. The rest are people like Susan: poor, homeless, old, drunk—people who have stepped away from or been kicked out of society and don't know where else to turn for help. Overdoses always go up on the first and fifteenth. I know more about social security checks than I do about cancer for sure. And people who have run out of resources, who are lost and scared and alone, will always vastly outnumber people who happen to be bleeding to death or having a stroke. There's just more of them. In poor communities, stable access to medicine is rare. Frequent moves mean frequent changes in insurance, Medicare eligibility, and transportation ability to a new doctor. When the food runs out, when the housing runs out, when the relationships break, we are the last resource. As long as 911 remains easy to access, and fast, the bulk of our work will never be about life-threatening emergencies.

I usually see each patient for an hour or two, street to hospital. We have some frequent flyers, but we only catch them on their bad days. When we don't see someone for a while it usually means they sobered up, went to jail, or died. We arrive at the crisis point of a story and we almost never witness its resolution.

We have a regular patient in my city named Leena. Her temperament reminds me of a hungry child. She flips a switch in an instant between happy and angry, laughing and crying, co-operative or spitting at us. She calls us in the middle of the night because she ran out of vodka or her bus driver looked at her the wrong way. She likes to describe her sexual escapades in uncomfortable detail and has thrown punches at paramedics with little warning.

A strong series of laws prevents me from "patient abandonment," which is what it's legally called if I were to sit down with her and say, "No." If I told her, "Honey, you've called us nine times in the last four days. You got kicked out of the emergency room this morning for spitting on a nurse. You got ejected from your last shelter for fighting a guard. You don't even have a medical complaint, you're just tired. I get it, the sun's going down, and the sidewalk is cracked, and the rats come out soon and that sucks, I hear you. I wish there was something I could do. But the emergency room is supposed to be for medical emergencies, for people who are dying, you know, faster than you. And the ambulance is supposed to be for driving fast, for people who are so close to the reaper that they can't wait at a red light because they might not make it until the light turns green. And there could be someone like that trying to call us right now, but we can't help them because we're here with you. Again."

I wish I could be the person who got Leena into a long-term care facility, who got her therapy, who single-handedly lifted her from the darkness. But all I can do is put her on the gurney and take her back to the hospital.

I was trained in school to react in a matter of seconds to life-or-death situations. Open the airway, stop the bleeding. Save the heart that hangs precariously on the edge of death, reach out and grasp the last slim chance at life. Emergencies. But, for someone like Leena, being tired and alone is an emergency. Her life has gotten so far outside of her control that she can't see more than an hour from now. And in the next hour, the sun's going to set and the night fog's coming in. Instead of leaving her on the street, I try to talk some sense into her, and give her a blanket and a ride back to the ER. Maybe this time something will change.

Three hours later Leena calls again, about a block away from the hospital where we left her. A different crew runs on her this time.

In the United States, we have this thing. We have this phone number you can call when you need help. The idea seems mundane until you stop to think about it. It turns out that it doesn't actually matter what kind of help you need—there's a guy with a gun; my dad's having a stroke; I'm stuck behind the washing machine; there is a sea monster coming after me with a flamethrower—no matter who you are, where you are, or what your problem is, you dial a three-digit phone number and a group of trained professionals will show up at your current location, right now, and do their very best to help you with whatever is going on. When you take the time to stop for a moment and consider what that means, it is astonishing. For most of human history, the world did not have anything like it.

To me the most incredible thing about this phone number is that anyone can call. Absolutely anyone, any time of day or night, whether from a penthouse or from the inside of a dumpster; you call and we will show up just the same. You don't have to present money or justification or reasonable cause. You just call the number, say you need help, and there we are. This means that a massive amount of our call volume isn't made up of the four or five sexy medical emergencies they like to show on TV. Because you don't actually require a true "emergency" to dial the phone. All you need, really, is a situation that you can't handle by yourself. Sometimes this is due to the nature of the problem, but more often it's about the patient and their way of life. Most of the calls we run are the everyday difficulties of people who are simply too old, too poor, too sick, or too mean to have anyone else willing to help them out. A huge portion of our workload is incredibly repetitive and frustrating; we become exhausted by the redundancy of it all. But here's the thing: these people are calling us with their "BS" because they literally have no one else to call. When you are too old, too lost, too alone, when you have burned every other bridge in your life and no one will help you with your empty prescription or your toe pain, you call us. And we come. Every time, no matter what, we come. And what an astounding, unspeakable honor that is. What indescribable virtue it is to be the guy who shows up when no one else will. That's what I tell myself, anyway.

Susan, the woman in the orange sweater, tells me she takes medicines for high blood pressure, psychological issues, and pain management. She's had one heart attack. She ran out of most of her medications about a week ago and hasn't been able to make it to Safeway to refill. She says she usually wheelchairs down there but it's been cold this week. She looks up at me, a little embarrassed. "I didn't think they do anything anyway."

She tells me she has some Haldol left—a common antipsychotic medication—but she doesn't always take that one because she doesn't like it. Her knees rock back and forth on the gurney, which is probably a side effect from the drug. Patients on lifelong psych meds are often a little twitchy. She tells me the blood pressure cuff feels too tight.

She's been receiving disability since she was twenty-four or twenty-five for hallucinations. She was living down south back then. She spent a year in Tulsa, two years in Sacramento. She bounces around. She gets disability payments and welfare sometimes. I look her up on our computer system; she's been transported by us four times this month.

As we're pulling away from her hotel I ask her, if she has been sick all week, what was it that changed tonight to make her call 911?

"I keep blowing my nose but it's still runny."

When we drop Susan at the emergency room, my partner and I both compliment her sweater. We say it looks nice on her, and cozy in the winter air. She smiles broadly. "I've had it for so many years," she says. "It's my favorite." She pulls at the sleeves and sets her chin in the knitted bundle of cloth. I tuck in her blanket and wish her the best. I hope she gets to feeling better, gets her prescriptions sorted, and stays out of the hospital for a while. In other words, I hope I never see her again.

Part I

"THE COOLEST JOB IN THE WORLD"

THE BEST EIGHT BUCKS
I'VE EVER SPENT

My partner for the day is Dustin, a new EMT who had shown up to his first shift bright-eyed and ready to save lives. Over the last few months of working together in Reno, Nevada, I have watched his attitude shake and crumple as he sees more and more of the realities of the job. We have just walked out of some awful call, and feel coated in a thick layer of grief. Almost choked by it. We hike our gear out of the stifled house and into the heat of the desert day.

We find ourselves in the back corner of an industrial neighborhood, barbed wire and cracked pavement. My paramedic uniform hangs heavier than usual, and my joints are sticky with sweat. I feel like the hot disease cloud from the house is still trapped inside my clothes. We trudge back towards the rig, looking for some shade to sit in and chart. A few blocks away a large warehouse looks like it might block out some sun, but I know if I move the wheels on the rig, dispatch will see the movement and assign us another call. I need a break. We are both dirty, exhausted, hungry, dehydrated, and behind in our charts. The radio whines and cries, dispatchers interrupting each other to send out calls or move ambulances around the city. *Please*, I think to myself. *Just five minutes.*

I crawl into the rig and Dustin starts the engine. The dashboard burns to the touch and the air conditioning coughs dust towards my chest. I wipe sweat off my forehead.

"Hey man, fuck this," I tell Dustin. "I'm gonna find some shade and at least write half this chart before we clear. If they hassle us just tell them we're working a refusal or something."

"Yeah, I got you." Dustin leans his face towards the warm puff of air leaking out of the dash. He sends dispatch a message telling them that we will be delayed on scene helping a patient who does not want to go to the hospital. "Shitty old-ass rigs. If we're going to run fourteen calls in a shift at least they could get us some air conditioning."

"Right?"

I grab the laptop and step back into the sun. Heat radiates off the cement like an oil slick, making my vision seem blurred. I walk about half a block towards a little awning over a closed storefront, thinking if I sit on the ground and lean against the wall, I can at least get my face out of the sun.

As I trudge closer I hear some tinny music from the direction of the shop. At first I curse, thinking if they are open I really can't lean against their wall in uniform without attracting some attention. But the store looks closed. There's nothing on this block but fences, empty buildings, and trash. No cars even.

The music is coming from behind the storefront, down an alleyway I hadn't noticed. It feels inappropriately joyful for the mood of the day. Is that a ukulele?

I pass the shop awning and crane my neck down the alley now, bouncing the laptop against my knees.

The alley opens into a wide parking lot, still empty but for some sort of brightly colored food truck.

Dispatch asks after us over my radio, wondering when we will be available to cover a different neighborhood. There are no runs pending, but they would like us to start driving south just in case one comes up. I put my finger on the button but hear my partner's voice saying we are working our call and will clear as soon as we can. Good man.

The food cart is closer now, the sound of Hawaiian folk music louder and even more incongruous with the industrial desert landscape. A brightly painted sandwich board comes into focus, advertising "Island Shave Ice" in bubbly print. Strawberry, pineapple, guava, lime. Four dollars a scoop.

He could have charged me a hundred.

I wonder if the cart is real or if I finally have severe enough heatstroke to have collapsed into some animated Disney-oasis fantasy hallucination, but I order two rainbow scoops, one for me and one for Dustin, and ask the man if he has always been here. Which is the most polite way I can think to say, "What the hell are you doing in the middle of an alleyway behind a crack house in Reno, of all places?"

He says, "Oh, hey, it's a new business, thank you so much for ordering, glad to be here," in either a real Hawaiian accent or the best fake one I've heard in my life. He calls me "sistah" and pours syrup onto two fat scoops. I hand him a ten and scuttle back to the ambulance, the ice already dripping cold sticky syrup down my fingers.

When I get to the rig I open the door, throw the laptop in, and yell, "Dustin! Get the fuck up!"

"What?!" Dustin pulls his headphones out. "What are you holding?"

"Get up, dude! We're tailgating!"

He follows me to the back of the ambulance, still confused. I hand him his cup and spoon.

"What? Where did you . . . what is this?"

"It's shave ice, dude. It's a tropical thing. You ever go to Hawaii?"

"No, what? It's ice? Where did you even get this?"

"Just try it."

He crunches into a bite and smiles. So do I. Holy shit. For five sweet minutes we close our eyes and smack our mouths on the coldest, sweetest illegal rest break ever taken. Dispatch asks after us again, twice, sounding more irritated. We've been attached to this call for thirty-eight minutes, and they need us to clear. By my count it was twenty-seven minutes of patient care, six minutes of trying to complete documentation, and five minutes of ice-cold bliss. If a 911 call goes out, we will answer the radio and do our jobs. But we've been running non-stop for seven hours, and we're guaranteed another five or six more before being allowed to rest. No one has gotten a lunch break or gone home on time in weeks. I figure they owe me at least until the end of this cup. I lean over the tailgate, dangle my feet below me, and look at Dustin. I tell him "this job will eat you alive, friend, you have to take it when you can get it." We both squint and smile into our spoons.

FOUR ON THE FLOOR

A young couple runs into the medic tent shouting. Something about his eyes. He's grabbing his face; she's pointing at him. Both are dressed in neon underwear, with glow-in-the-dark paint splashed all over their bodies. They've got to be underage, sixteen maybe. She tries to explain but he's screaming too loud for me to catch the story. They were playing with glowsticks, she says; I mean, it's a rave, everybody is playing with glowsticks. She points to the bright streaks all over their bodies and holds up a handful of plastic shards. "Wait, what? Were you guys, what did you, did you break a glowstick open?" "My eyes, my eyes," he's screaming.

We tell the kid to lie on his back on a cot, and then we throw a plastic basin underneath. We use an old trick where you connect a length of oxygen tubing to a saline bag and then slide it onto the bridge of the nose so that it drips liquid into both eyes at the same time. The saltwater blends together with tears and colored paint to pour cloudy rivers down the sides of his cheeks. When he opens his eyes, you can see tiny green splatters all over his sclera like the most delicate miniature neon Holstein cow print. His pupils are still huge from the molly. I look at my partner and then the patient and say, "Hey, you mind if I try something real quick?"

We turn out the lights for a second. Sure enough, his eyes glow.

I turn the lights back on and keep washing out his eyes, but it's hard to keep him still and hold his head at the right angle. We dump two liters of saline onto his eyeballs but the spots are still there and he's still gasping from the pain. Eventually we say, "Look, there's not a lot else we can do out here, do you have anybody in your group who can drive?" The girlfriend says they can call someone sober to get him to an ER. They thank us for trying. I ask before she leaves, "What were you thinking, breaking those open? Who knows what the fuck they put in those?" She points at the lights, the thumping music, the costumes. "I don't know," she says. "We got caught up in the moment."

My parents were both academics. As a kid growing up in the Bay Area, if I wanted a bowl of cereal I would clear a space on the table by pushing away piles of books, magazines, and five daily newspaper subscriptions. If something significant happened in either of their professional fields, it wasn't unusual for the local news to call our house for a quote. I fell in love with science early in life and assumed I would follow their lead—working my way up through medicine and research until I was eventually an Important Person just like them.

I was accepted into a rigorous biology program at a competitive university. I loved the idea of spending hours buried in books, watching rain fall out the library window as I learned the intricacies of cellular interactions or evolutionary pathways. But the reality was claustrophobic and lonely. The material was dense. I could only read for fifteen minutes before my attention span would dissolve and frustration would overwhelm my curiosity. I got anxious before projects were due and cried in bathrooms during midterms. I cut class to go snowboarding. The weather was depressing instead of romantic, and I hated being trapped indoors all the time. I dropped out and spent a year working odd jobs and drinking too much. I met ski patrollers and wildland firefighters with EMT training and began to daydream about broken limbs and rescue operations. I returned to school for what should have been my third year, but halfway through the semester I felt like I was falling apart. I stayed up nights, crying and homesick, and late one Tuesday found myself staring at the registration page of a community college back home. I'd found a night class offering an Emergency Medical Technician certification for $272. There were three spots left.

I didn't know much about the details, only that the class taught basic medical skills and emergency operations. I thought I could move home, get the license and then, I don't know, get paid to lean out of a helicopter and say, "Don't worry, ma'am, we've got you now."

I stared at the open spots, wondering what my life might be like in ten years, and if this would be one of those defining moments I'd look back on with gratitude or regret. I would have to withdraw from school, break my rental lease, and most likely break up with my boyfriend. I could probably still finish a degree somehow, but there was no way I was coming back to this particular school for a third time if I left again. I put the course fee on my debit card and signed up for the class.

Two months later, I sat in a classroom in Aptos, California, listening to a stern blonde firefighter with curling-iron bangs tell me how to hold open an airway in case of a choking. She told us to keep things simple, focus on the basics, and don't get distracted by "what-if" scenarios. It was the opposite of university. As an EMT, no one would ever care what grade I had gotten on a test or where I had placed in my class. They wanted to know if I could do the skill. I spent four months learning to perform CPR and a handful of basic medical interventions, passed the exams, and got my certification in the mail.

During the class I was embarrassed to admit how little I knew about the career options ahead of me, but I eavesdropped and googled and figured out what I could. The EMT certification allowed me to perform simple lifesaving skills and was useful for a number of different jobs. It seemed that most EMTs got their feet wet working for inter-facility transport companies, which until I took the class I had never even heard of. I learned that these were a whole category of ambulances that do not answer 911 calls at all; instead, they are paid to take Grandma to dialysis, transfer a stroke victim to a specialty facility upstate, or pick up a bedbound senior from a care home. After a year or two on an "IFT" rig, I could get bumped up to answering emergency calls on a 911 unit. If I wanted to make a living out of it, I could look into becoming a paramedic: two more years of school, and a lot more responsibility. I got a crash course in firefighting also—many of my classmates didn't seem particularly interested in medicine, but were tolerating the class so that they could get hired as local firefighters. I also found out that EMTs could be hired to provide medical support for theme parks, cruise ships, and ski resorts. After some digging, I realized I could even work at music festivals. That sounded fun.

I knew something about the festival scene. I had reveled in the energy of it in my teens and in college: a perfect antidote to the high expectations I placed on myself during the rest of the year. Before camera phones and social media gained popularity, large campouts provided a near total escape from the default world. For a few summers I wore tie-dye, built theme camps, fought with my college boyfriend, ate piles of drugs, and danced until late morning. I had thrown myself into those parties with all of the energy that I could never figure out how to focus in school.

Now I had ended up back where I started, in a different uniform. In the midst of all that chaos, in a place designed to lose yourself, to not know whether it's day or night, a place made out of colors and blinking lights and fire and music, I suddenly had to bring a watch and a schedule. I had to stay sober. I had to pack clean underwear and socks.

I spent the first few events shadowing more experienced members of the team. We worked in pairs, taking turns covering the medical tent or posting around the venue. Some of the gigs were only one night, a concert or rave at an arena in the Bay Area. Others were multi-day campouts spread around California, with dozens of stages and shifts broken up around the clock. My co-workers were EMTs, nurses, paramedics, and even a couple of doctors. Some were young and looking for experience like me; others were older and kept the job as a fun side gig or a source of free concert tickets. Some seemed to just be friends with the boss.

We supported anywhere from a couple hundred to twenty thousand attendees. During the day, we saw bee stings, skinned knees, dehydration, and food poisoning. Industrial accidents from setting up stages. Infections, asthma. In rural areas patients without insurance would come to us for a blood pressure check or a rash, having heard there would be a doctor at the party. At one event a nearby rancher pulled his truck sideways into the parking lot, slammed on the brakes, and ran to us carrying a large black dog. My partner was an older guy, a longtime ER nurse who had actually grown up on a farm. He gave the dog a once-over, checked for signs of concussion, and patched up the wound on her head like it was no big deal.

At night, it was drugs, and alcohol, and more drugs, and more alcohol. I found out that all of the experiences I'd had fighting with my own brain actually gave me a good understanding of how to talk to people who were having a bad time. I chugged energy drinks to stay up all night, which made me feel like I always had to pee. I still hadn't seen anything that was particularly life-threatening, but over a few months I started to get more comfortable talking to people and anticipating how quickly I'd need to grab the stethoscope or the barf bucket.

I'm posted backstage a little after eleven. I've been a part-time EMT for six months or so, and still haven't cracked the smooth leather exterior of my first pair of boots. It's me and one other guy, Ron. A lot of this job is standing around. I wear a blue company T-shirt tucked into my work pants, with duty boots and a belt. My shirt says "medical" on the back and I feel important and fraudulent.

At 11:18 p.m. we receive a call on the radio that there is someone bleeding on the stairs, a possible fall. We weave our way through the crowd to find a young teen on the floor of the hallway. Her body is still but her arms and legs move awkwardly, like they are batting at imaginary flies. Is this what a seizure looks like? I've never actually seen one. Ron jumps down and gently holds the patient's neck in place while I'm still frozen. *Right*, I think. *Stabilize the cervical spine.* I grab a pulse at her wrist. It's weak and rapid but palpable. She's breathing but the breaths don't look quite right. *Skin signs*, I think to myself, running down the assessment I've practiced a thousand times in school. Her skin is warm and moist. *Trauma*, I think, *rapid trauma assessment.* I start at the top with her head.

Some ravers tell us she fell and came down straight onto her face, didn't hit anywhere else, no other injuries. She's got a deep laceration on the side of her head, which I clap a gloved hand on, thinking I should stop the bleeding, but it's not actually bleeding that much. *Why isn't your scalp bleeding? Scalps are supposed to bleed.* I think, *Okay, ABCs: airway, breathing, circulation. Bleeding and pulse are okay, airway's okay, breathing is okay. Wait, is her breathing okay?* I look at her pupils. The right one is reactive, but the left is blown wide open and doesn't move when I shine my flashlight into it. *Okay. Bad.* I get on the radio. I tell them where we are, we have a patient, I say "head trauma, request an ambulance immediately."

The radio is busy. I hear voices talking over each other and requesting backup for seizures. I can't even get through at first. I break in a couple times, saying: "Need help right now, rapid pulses, blown pupil." Until now I have only ever seen patients who were mostly okay, and I can't understand why this obviously critical scene hasn't made the entire world stop moving. I get a security guard to walk up the hall and tell him to find anyone wearing a uniform with a blue shirt and lead them to us.

The music is still blasting out of the doors at us and the hall is packed with thousands of candy kids half-dressed and sweaty and high as hell, tracing rainbows and dancing and shouting. They see us and suck in their breath when they pass us by. The floor and walls are wet with sweat.

I hover over the body on the floor trying to remember what I can from my training. I hear my EMT teacher's voice saying, "Go back to the beginning, do the assessment. Run your call." My partner and I lock eyes through the noise. He holds the neck, I grab the head. He moves his arms to let me feel behind the girl's neck.

I feel around the rest of the head and cervical spine, the collarbones. I try to get lung sounds, a detail I remember practicing in class, but I give up quickly because the music is still so loud that it makes the floor vibrate and I obviously can't hear anything.

We cut the girl's outer shirt off. Her whole chest rises and falls with every breath. Her ribs heave dramatically, like someone breathing intensely on purpose. But the rhythm is perfect, unnaturally perfect. I try to figure out how to describe what I'm seeing, but I won't remember the phrase "tidal volume" until much later that night.

We strap her to a hard plastic backboard and carry her out to meet an ambulance at the nearest exit. When the paramedics arrive, they are relaxed and efficient. They get her loaded onto their gurney and start an IV. As they buckle her in and wave us on our way I feel as though I have turned in a homework assignment. Ron and I lean back, exhausted, and he gives me a fist pound. I tear off my gloves, noticing for the first time that they are covered in sweat and ripped in multiple places. Oops.

I check in on the radio, expecting to head back to the main tent and have some time to recover and think for a second about the first real emergency of my career. Instead, our dispatcher tells me to get to the backstage area as soon as I can. I take one last look towards the ambulance, then pull myself away and follow the instructions. We find a panicked security guard, who leads us to a tiny teenage boy leaned against a trash can, slick with sweat. His whole body shakes like a machine gun, as though every muscle is contracting at once. I realize: okay, that is definitely what a seizure looks like. We throw him onto a canvas tarp and make our way back to the medical tent, his body in spasm the whole time.

The building is a swamp. We find out months later that the venue was packed way past capacity and there was some kind of ventilation problem. In the moment, we don't know how or why but the air is such a thick miasma of heat and fog machine vapor and sweat that it is condensing on the ceiling and raining back down onto us, thick hot drops of chemical tears splashing on our shoulders. You can barely breathe. There are two- and three-inch puddles on the ground.

When we arrive at the tent for the first time we stop in our tracks. There are firefighters and paramedics everywhere. Many are wearing bright orange Incident Command vests, and the cots are backed up with patients. Cardstock triage tags are looped around wrists and ankles. I see uniforms from three different counties. We walk outside to meet another ambulance and it's the goddamn apocalypse. There are ambulances, fire engines, police cars, and mass casualty transport buses. Two helicopters are circling. Red and white and blue lights flash so bright all over the parking lot that you can't tell where the rave ends and the disaster scene begins.

I do laps back and forth from the dance floor, helping to carry more seizing bodies. One of them wakes up as soon as we get back there, one gets transported in an ambulance. Everyone in uniform is passing looks back and forth with raised eyebrows. As I walk one girl back to the tent the guards have cleared a path through the crowd down the entire hall and back to the door. It saves time but it means we're walking a gauntlet of wide-eyed ravers staring at us.

The weirdest part of any mass casualty incident is that, usually, just as quickly as they explode, they melt away. You get that last patient transported, the non-criticals mill around looking freaked out, the radios quiet down again. A couple more patients sometimes emerge out of the crowd, but sooner or later, the hyper-focused cyclone of activity blows itself out and you're left with an empty clinic and a lot of personnel. We slowly clean up, packing up cellophane and bloodstained gauze, and then stand around twitching as the adrenaline cycles through our bodies.

The story unfolds in confusing layers, and we never really get a clear picture of events. A "bad batch" of something, the building was too hot, the ventilation was wrong, something about imported designer pharmaceuticals from New Zealand. I never find out exactly how many people survive or what condition they end up in. News segments from that night keep changing the details and the total number of people involved. We hear that two or three or maybe four people died, but I never learn the whole truth.

The weird part is, about fifteen thousand people had a beautiful, amazing night of partying and probably didn't even notice the ambulances parked out front for a couple hours. Couples fell in love, broke up, got in fights about the carpool, and waited for each other outside bathrooms. Someone's drugs didn't hit right and they ended up bored; someone else's hit too strong and they ended up dead.

In the end they tell us we had fourteen total transports, half of whom were critical. Somehow it seems like more. The next morning I sit at my parents' kitchen table and chew on some breakfast, still shaky from the caffeine and the energy of it all. I've only slept a few hours. I watch TV with them as images of my night splatter across the news. One program plays an emotional news segment with the parents of one of the dead teens, begging viewers not to judge their son. "He was a good kid," they say. "A good person, with good grades, he wasn't a . . . drug user. This is not what you think. Have compassion for our son." I choke when I see a photo and realize their kid could have been one of my patients.

I'll never know the whole story of that night, only my pinpoint perspective. Our team did the best we could. I did the best I could. The old guys tell me that's exactly what this job is: you didn't create the emergency, but it fell to you and you did what you could with what you had.

I kept showing up for events. The truth was, I loved it. I loved having somewhere to be, feeling like I was part of the thing. I loved knowing the inside scoop and what was going on behind the curtains. A radio unlocks a whole second layer of reality. With a speaker microphone near my ear I know that while you are high out of your mind on ecstasy, dancing, drinking, fucking, losing touch, there's a guy about to run out of fuel for the generator at the main stage. He's running out to the back side to try to get some restock but fucking Daniel's still got the keys. I know there's a girl getting evacuated from an orgy tent for going into anaphylaxis right now. I know the lighting guys are still setting up at the next camp over, I know the dispatch tent is going for dinner soon, I know who is where and what is happening. But I also learned how heavy it could feel to carry everyone's grief around all the time. To look over a raucous celebration and know exactly how many of them would end up sedated or hospitalized by the end of the night. Once I kept a guy company for three hours telling him we would keep an eye out for his lost friend, writing down a description, while the chatter in my right ear told me that the CPR wasn't working and they were calling a helicopter to evacuate the body. I wasn't allowed to tell the friend because they hadn't officially ID'd him, but he fit the description and was lost in the same place. I kept my face steady and chatted while I listened to a stream of death chaos pouring into my ear piece. Above the surface, polite and calm. Below, bedlam.

I was surprised by how much I loved being part of the team. We worked around the clock, taking naps here and there on a cot and passing around energy drinks and beef jerky. We would stand around the medical tent telling stupider and stupider jokes as the patient load dwindled. The hours from 6:00 a.m. to 8:00 a.m. were the hardest, the coldest, the achiest. There were moments when I missed being in the middle of the throng, but even when I did have time off I soon found myself hanging around the medical tent, chatting with people in uniforms and trading bits of gossip about the inner workings of the event.

The job somehow broke me away from the dopamine rush of music and drugs and forced me to focus on the task in front of me. I loved having to use my hands to open an airway or compress a chest. I loved that my pants had extra material sewn into the knees, for when I had to get down on the ground to help a patient. I took the information I'd memorized in class and used it to help live humans in real time. I did eventually finish a university degree, barely, from a less prestigious school and without a graduate research plan or any publications to brag about. I kept working part-time for music events and tried a handful of other EMT jobs over the next couple of years. Eventually I realized that it was time to apply to paramedic school. Unlike an EMT, a paramedic could start an IV, intubate, and employ a wide range of procedures and medications. The program would provide a deeper understanding of anatomy and physiology, and if I completed all of my testing I would emerge as a licensed medical clinician. If I took this step I would be committing myself to emergency work in a very real way.

I would earn a modest wage punching a time clock, in a world I knew nothing about. Most of my colleagues would not hold college degrees. My name would not be published on any lists of contributors. But I had a badge. And boots. And a radio. And people called me when they needed help. There was no denying that I had somehow become an Important Person after all. My parents were confused by but pleased with the development—they worried about the risks of the job but liked to see me sober and focused. My mom asked if I would be making decisions about people who were dying and then looked suddenly concerned, saying, "That's going to be intense."

I laughed. "Yeah, Ma, I mean . . . That's the idea."

MOSTLY ADRENALINE

Tonight began yesterday and tomorrow begins tonight, and the days become one rolling night.
EDWARD CONLON, *Blue Blood*

Scared finally shitless, purged and purified, he is now at last too tired for fear, too exhausted to think of surrender.
 . . . The naked desert is no place for little secrets.
EDWARD ABBEY, *The Monkey Wrench Gang*

After four years as an EMT, I am accepted into paramedic school. The program is two years long, and includes classroom, hospital clinicals, and a six-hundred-hour unpaid paramedic internship. When I get my license, I apply to every position I can find. An old ski patrol friend offers to put me in touch with the hiring manager for an ambulance company in Reno, Nevada—a place I have driven through a couple of times but otherwise know only as a desert gambling town somewhere east of Lake Tahoe. It seems barren and intimidating. Travis has been working in Reno for about a year and says they are busy, progressive, and hiring like crazy. He tells me earlier that week he'd run on a hatchet murder.

"A what?"

"Yeah, this dude hacked up his sister with a hatchet and then slit his own throat. It was nuts, man. You should call, I bet you get picked up by next month."

I have enough experience by then, both as an EMT and as a field intern, to know that a single violent call is not a good description of a 911 system. That is the overly dramatic trauma-boner bullshit they put on TV, the stuff we all pretend we are too cool to get worked up about. I want to be a Real Paramedic, ready to help folks in need whether their wounds are exciting or not. But still, I mean, a hatchet murder. And he did say they were hiring.

I get the job. I have to pass a six-week academy, with written tests and in-person field shifts. My training officer is a woman named Julia. She is five-three, maybe 130 pounds and, according to the guys, anyway, held her own on a Hotshots wildland fire crew for a few summers before getting into paramedic school. That is their way of telling me to do what the fuck she says.

My field training period is terrifying. I am expected to waltz into an unfamiliar system and run every call, and I am dumbfounded by Julia's competence. She seems to know more medicine than a doctor, talks fast, and has no embarrassment in telling a patient what to do when she believes they are full of it. The radio never stops beeping. The paramedics are young, loud, aggressive, and full of bravado. There is one other Californian in my academy, a kid from Sacramento who says "fuck" so many times per sentence that we start a tally.

The culture shock is violent. At home in lawsuit-happy California, paramedics are kept on a much tighter leash. In Nevada, I am suddenly allowed to give treatments and perform skills that I never learned in paramedic school at all. I watch a YouTube video about how to complete a surgical cricothyrotomy, a difficult airway procedure that in California is reserved for doctors. I practice the hand motions with a kitchen knife and a paper napkin. I spent weeks in my internship memorizing indications, dosages, and counter-indications for every medication on my list, only to open my red bag in Reno and see bottles of drugs I've never even heard of. When I waffle about whether to give a breathing treatment to a woman with a history of asthma, Julia glares at me, then writes YOU ARE THE PARAMEDIC in Sharpie on her gloved hand and holds it up behind the woman's head.

My training period is capped by two testing scenarios completed in the classroom back at the main campus. If I pass, I will be released onto the streets alone. If I fail, I'm welcome to reapply for the job in six months. The first dummy has a drug overdose, then dies of septic shock on the way to the imaginary hospital. I am sitting on top of the table doing chest compressions when the proctor says the time is up. My second scene is worse. I find a pediatric mannequin on the floor underneath a desk lamp, which I am told to pretend is a fallen-down Christmas tree. The child was crushed by the branches and electrocuted by the string of festive lights. I try to remove him from danger and treat his injuries, but when I give medication, he has an anaphylactic reaction to my choice of drug. I verbalize treating the anaphylaxis, and listen to his plastic chest for pre-recorded sounds, desperate to keep this fake little boy alive. The proctor finally brings me into the break room and after a tense minute tells me that I have passed. I collapse onto my knees, leaning against the wall behind me as he and Julia laugh and high-five. They tell me the test was designed not just to measure my medical skills but to see how I would react when everything goes wrong. "This was nothing compared to how crazy it's going to get out there," he says with a smile. "You did okay." He points me down the hall to talk to scheduling, where a nice lady behind a computer says I will start work at 0400 tomorrow morning. Welcome to Reno.

———

We don't always use the lights and sirens. On the way to a call, the dispatch center will indicate whether to drive "code two" or "code three." A code two call requires a response within twenty minutes: I have time to pee, follow traffic laws, and stop at stoplights. Code three means go. Now. When I arrive and assess the patient, one of the most basic decisions I will make is how quickly I believe they need to be seen by a doctor. Driving code three is dangerous, and loud, and distracting, so we only actually use the sirens on the way to the hospital for a small fraction of cases when we think extra speed is worth the risk.

I'm in the bathroom when we get dispatched out to a two-week-old in cardiac arrest. Code three. I look up from the toilet, knowing I have time to either wipe my ass or put in a new tampon, so I reach for the toilet paper and hope I don't bleed through my pants. Halfway to the call I'm blasting through intersections and forcing my breathing to slow down and ripping through infant code protocols in my head and we get a second page on the radio. "Never mind, it was a doll . . . We think . . . Please continue priority to a possible psych . . . Um . . . Let us know when you get there." So now I'm at the homeless shelter at 9:00 a.m. on a Saturday with my heart still jacked and we're all staring at this lady pushing a stroller. She's telling me how he died in her arms and she's sick of people telling her it's not a real baby because that's disrespectful to her and her son, the security guards are all hyperventilating on the sides of the room, and I'm just standing there staring blanky and wondering how much blood is dripping down my leg. The plastic doll looking up at us is surprisingly realistic.

We almost make it to coffee but get called back to the homeless shelter. Code two this time, for one of our usual guys. He's got a big dent in the side of his head from some kind of motorcycle wreck and a speech impediment that makes him slur his words. The drinking also makes him slur. It's hard to tell with Billy. He called today because his feet are itchy. He smells like leather and vodka.

My partner's pissed because he's already down a few charts and the radio's still sending out calls non-stop. We are not allowed to refuse transport to anyone, ever, even if their medical complaint is, well, itchy feet. In fact, as a paramedic I am not even allowed to *recommend* that the patient visit an urgent care instead of the emergency room, as ambulance companies do not believe our training prepares us to accept that kind of liability. Instead I am taught to encourage every single patient to be taken to the nearest hospital, and if they do not accept I will write that they "declined" or "refused transportation" in my chart. Even if it is painfully clear to me that my patient does not need an expensive ambulance ride to an over-crowded ER, my protocols require me to try my best to convince them that they do. This policy, set on a county level, is true in most but not all parts of the United States. Over time I learn to watch for cameras and tiptoe through my language. Sometimes I will say that while I am not a doctor and cannot authoritatively diagnose a condition, I have never personally seen a case of itchy feet lead to immediate death. Or I might explain that I am happy to transport to the emergency room but that the bill may be quite high, and I believe that they will be waiting for several hours upon their arrival, and have they thought of trying an urgent care or a foot cream?

I can tell from Billy's attitude today that no part of this conversation will be worth the time. He seems determined to get to a hospital. I should probably just start driving, but we have been running non-stop all day and I want to breathe for just one second. I ask Billy a few questions to buy time. So how long have your feet been itching?

Is it one foot more than the other? Any pain? What about your legs? I lean back onto the bench seat. He gazes at me and tilts his head. He starts to pee.

After a couple of months in a short-term apartment, I find an empty single-wide in a small trailer park in Truckee, California, just across the state line from work. The town is blanketed in snow when I move in, but I'm told that come spring I will have about three feet of dirt next to my driveway in which I'm free to plant a garden. I've always wanted a garden.

The propane heater is loud but warms the trailer well enough. My schedule consists of four twelve-hour shifts per week, back-to-back. Some weeks I buy an eight pack of chicken thighs at Safeway, smother them in cheap teriyaki sauce, and split them into Tupperware, two per shift. I find a cheerful pink tray to help marinate, but accidentally leave it in the oven drawer one night while I cook. I scream when a chemical burning smell fills the trailer and pull two pieces of drooping, melted plastic off of a cookie sheet.

When I have enough time I cook pork stew in the Crock-Pot, dumping all the ingredients in the night before. My alarm wakes me up at 2:35 a.m. to the smell of garlic and pepper and fat steaming up the whole trailer. The windows are fogged. I pour the stew into four portions, placing three in the fridge and one in the seat of my truck. Once it cools I stuff it into my lunch box with a couple of ice packs, hopeful that later in the shift I might have time to heat it up in a hospital microwave instead of eating it cold on the way to a call.

My commute is about forty minutes. During the day it is a stunning drive; a fast four-lane highway that cuts through the mountains along the Truckee River. Green trees, blue sky, rich brown earth. Sparkling gray and white granite. As the road winds east, the trees spread thinner. The ridges of the mountains open out wide and shallow, and granite turns to clay. The road weaves through lighter brown, khaki, and ash, until alpine peaks give way to desert.

But I mostly drive in the dark. I'm expected at work at about 3:30 a.m., so for now my mornings are black sky and silhouettes. On a lucky night I race the lights of a passenger train, feeling like a hero in an old Western. When I come down over the pass the view widens and I see the Washoe Valley, a huge bowl carved into the mountains with city filling the bottom and buildings splashing up the sides. The casinos stand in tall neon clusters. The lights on the Circus Circus casino blink like they're making fun of me. I swallow my fear, look straight back at them, and say out loud, "Good morning, Reno. You're looking beautiful today."

Our dispatch office holds a wall-sized display of television and computer screens that color the city in red, yellow, and green, depending on where the computer thinks the calls might come in. The algorithm has been compiling data for the last ten years or so to try to predict where to post our ambulances. The system is complicated and full of errors, and 911 is inherently unpredictable, so the ambulances usually end up bouncing back and forth across the city all night like a herd of cats at a laser show.

Depending on system levels, time of day, day of the week, and weather, we have anywhere from four to twenty-five ambulances on. We use "ambulance levels" to describe the number of ambulances available at any given moment. "Level three" means there are three ambulances in the whole county that are not currently attached to calls or stuck at a hospital. "Level zero" means no ambulances are available. I do not know the actual statistics, but it feels as though we usually spend a quarter of our day at level zero or one. On a busy summer weekend sometimes we're there all night. The phrase "status six" means no one is available and we have calls waiting to be answered. If it gets really bad and stays there for really long, sometimes a supervisor will come round the hospitals with Costco pizzas for the crews. Which is their way of saying: you will not have time for dinner tonight.

One way we blow off steam on shift is by screaming at the radio. "You *fucking* cunts!! You shit-guzzling, cock-gobbling cunts!" my partner yells with his thumb hovering on the trigger. He presses the button, and in a calm voice says, "Medic thirty-six, ten-four. Show us en route." Thumb lifts. "You motherfucking *whoooooores*."

We were *this close* to getting to eat. It's nine hours into a twelve and the sandwich had actually made it up out of the lunchbox into his hands this time. I've thrown a laptop at the radio before; we all have.

The guy's drunk as nuts and we're trying to figure out what protocol we could possibly run this under so that we can do the least amount of paperwork and make his day the easiest. We're bullshitting with him. He's laughing and hitting on me and saying weird, dirty shit. "Tell me a joke!" he yells. "I want a joke!"

My partner, Miller, leans in conspiratorially. Okay.

"Danny. What's the difference between jam and jelly?"

No, Miller, you fucker. I put my head in my hands.

"I do not think that this is an ambulance-appropriate joke," I say slowly, trying to be serious.

"I'm not about to jelly my cock up your ass!!!"

The patient's eyes widen, and he opens his mouth and rips up with laughter. He is howling. His head rocks backwards and you can count all five of the guy's teeth, his mouth is open so wide. He almost falls off the gurney. I laugh with him for about five minutes, muttering,

"Oh my god, we're getting so fired." I stand up to pick up the radio and the patient tells the one about Kermit's fingers smelling like pork and I lose my shit all over again. My radio report to the hospital is terrible. I tell them I honestly don't know his medical complaint, security thinks he had a seizure, he's drunk, whatever. He knows his name but not what day it is. We'll see you in a minute.

We're still silly when we get to St. Joseph's, but starting to get it together. As soon as we walk in the ER doors the charge nurse takes one look at us and his face turns to stone.

"This guy? This *fucking* guy? NO. Fucking nope! Get security. I'm not doing this shit again."

Five minutes later I'm pulling out his IV and fending off security long enough to get some gauze taped down where we stuck him. They pick him up by his shirt collar and haul him out. Everyone is yelling. Turns out it's the third time the guy's been kicked out of the ER in the last four hours. Security chased him to Circus Circus last time, right where we picked him up. He's been faking all kinds of bullshit to get sandwiches. The charge nurse is beet red and cussing like a sailor, the guy who took our report is shaking his head at the whole scene. Me and Miller are just standing in the middle of it staring at each other whispering about Kermit and jelly and trying not to piss our pants.

I stare out at the skyline. On a given summer night there are roughly half a million people in our response area. Twice that on a big weekend. If any single one of those blinking buildings has something go horribly wrong inside, I'm the person who's expected to show up and fix it. The next time my radio beeps, chances are it will be something I can handle, a drunk or a tummy ache. But on the off chance that something absolutely insane happens, literally anywhere in the city, it's on me.

Level one coverage means you are it. No other ambulances available. We are posted downtown, and if a call goes out anywhere from Mt. Rose to the Oregon border, we light up and go. It's a little over two hours to drive from one end of our coverage area to the other. We are level one so often that I don't usually think about it much, but every once in a while on a late night I look around at the city and remember what that really means.

"You know, we're it right now. If anyone, anywhere in this county, needs *anything*, it's on us. Nobody else is coming."

My partner laughs.

"You mean it's on *you*, Jo. I'm an EMT. They don't pay me enough for that kind of responsibility."

I stare out the windshield and remember what I can from my childhood. Fighting with my brother, building dirt forts in the forest. Stuffing books behind my shin guards at soccer camp so I wouldn't have to make friends. How did this strange, moody little child wind up driving back and forth across Reno, Nevada, at four in the morning? I have an arsenal of cardiac drugs in the back, some sedatives in my knee pocket. There are restraints on the gurney and oxygen in the bags. I think of my crazier calls, and more mundane. I don't have time to get too philosophical, though. The radio's already beeping.

My brother asks me, "So what do you do on, like, a Saturday night?"

He is visiting for the weekend, on a ski trip with friends. He stands in my trailer, leaning his elbows on the small Formica countertop.

I raise my eyebrows. "I work on Saturday nights."

"Okay, no, like on a night off. You know what I mean."

I work weekends. I work nights, holidays.

"I guess I sleep. Watch Netflix, recover. During the day I like to get outside. Ride bikes or swim."

At night, the last thing I want to do is have to talk to people. I hide in my trailer and drink tea. Sometimes if I have the energy I go into town and get a beer with some guys from work.

"Mostly I just, I don't know, try to breathe a little."

My brother looks at me. He lives in an apartment in San Francisco and works at a startup. He goes to bars, and drinks, and goes on dates. He talks to people he's never met before and he enjoys making new friends. I don't even really remember what that's like. On a given work day I'm out of my house for about fifteen hours. I get home at five or six in the morning, shower, sleep until one. Sometimes I work out or eat a slow breakfast, but usually I just make lunch and go back to work. Do that four times in a row. By the time I get home from a week my bed looks foreign to me. I can't wait to make coffee and curl into the couch.

My partner for the summer of 2014 is named Michael Hamilton. He is my first real friend in Reno. He's a bull of a man: bald, emotional, self-destructive, and sweet. We stay up all night bullshitting and checking out girls, driving through alleyways looking for dark corners where he can sneak a cigarette in uniform. One of the first times we hang out outside of work he pulls up his right shirtsleeve to reveal a pipefitters union tattoo, says it's for his dead dad who was a mean, hard-drinkin', hard-lovin' son of a bitch. I take a sip of beer and know that I have found someone in Reno I can trust.

In a busy system, most paramedics spend more time with their work partner than with their actual spouse. You witness life and death and eat breakfast with this person. I know what my partner looks like when he wakes up from a nap. I know what time of day he poops. I know how he takes his coffee, when he's fighting with his wife, and what radio station he switches to when he thinks I'm asleep.

We work the 1630–0430 shift that summer, almost the exact opposite hours of my first assigned shift. My eyes get used to darkness. Hours and hours of dim lights and empty alleyways make the casino blare even more jarring.

We are in a car crash together. We're driving code three to a call and the big rig in front of us tries to get out of the way but doesn't see a tiny red sedan sneaking up its left side. We can see a little old lady bent over the wheel of the sedan as its hood and windshield crumple into the side of the big rig. Mike slams on the brakes of the ambulance and we hear metal snap and glass break. The whole thing plays out in slow motion—laptop flying, radios swinging from their cords. Everybody ends up okay, but I can see Mike's hand shaking in his pocket when we give our statements to the supervisor.

Journal, November 2013
   Saw my first incinerated patient today. It was kinda rough.

The firefighters are doing CPR when we arrive, but one walks out to meet me and shakes his head. He looks up at me and rubs a piece of charred skin off of his gloves.

"There were so many people watching us pull her out. We wanted it to look like we tried." He looks exhausted. "Jo," he says. "She's done."

They tell me she's lit fires before. That they've been here three times this year. She gets drunk and smokes cigarettes, then passes out. He's glad she didn't kill anyone else.

I put her on the monitor and watch the screen light up. The monitor beeps; some bumps appear in the glowing green line. Is that a rhythm? Oh, no, no. I suddenly wish that she was in a true flatline. It's hard to stomach the realization that inside this burnt husk of what used to be a human there is still a live heart trying to beat.

This means that now I have to call for orders to cease resuscitative efforts—that is, I need to ask a doctor for permission to stop CPR. I'm on the phone with our base physician, trying to describe what I'm looking at. About halfway through he interrupts me. "Christ, that sounds awful." Yeah, doc, it kinda is.

We put a blanket over her and wait for the fuss to die down. Fire standby always takes a while. Do you guys have any more of those Gatorades? It smells like dead people around here.

Journal, December 2013

I'm at a coffee bar, surrounded by the crowded energy of young athletic people. Laptops, flannels, shouts, friendly hugs, and clanking ceramic. Smiles and giggles and colorful scarves.

I feel like I'm sitting on the soft edge of a bubble, waiting for the membrane to burst. Anticipating this scene of bustling happy commerce will just crack open. A rift splits its way through the tastefully decorated ceiling of the café and all of the darkness and sickness and rotting disease pours through the widening cleft. The crack grows, large, jagged welts in the walls begin to splinter apart, bursting with piles of infected wounds and soggy trash. Heaps of weather-beaten, urine-soaked clothing and decaying newspapers pour through the breaking plaster. Well-dressed yuppies drop their coffees and stare in horror as stiff dead bodies and blood-soaked colostomy bags drop out through the mess. The landslide grows, a crushing weight of broken, stinking vestige of disease decimates the shop. Trash, filth, mucus, fluids, pain. The smell is overwhelming. A clinging woman, too weak to grip the oxygen mask on her face, is swallowed up in the storm. Her respirations get more rapid and shallow as she sinks. Tangled monitor wires, IV lines, Foley catheter tubing twist and braid themselves like sci-fi tentacles reaching towards you. The jolly coffee shop sounds are overwhelmed by the roaring, cracking, groaning avalanche crushing every bit of architecture in the room.

Outside, you can't see a thing. Truckee is beautiful; a light breeze rustles some leaves. A tourist couple notices closed doors on a shop and thinks, hmm . . . I guess we'll try back later. She smiles at him and squeezes his hand twice, a secret little signal they share. She flips a leaf pile towards him with a cute heel-scuff sort of kick and they stroll on down the street. It's their anniversary today.

One morning Mikey shows up looking tired, saying he was arguing with the wife. He tells me he hasn't slept well and he's worried he might be distracted on calls.

"I got you," I say. "No problem." God knows he's carried me through some tough shifts.

But then our first call of the day is a sick kid. Mike's always been great with kids. Before I even get our equipment off the gurney, he's down on one knee explaining everything to this angelic little six-year-old like it's the first day of a new school. He cracks a joke and gets a smile, and the kid is giggling by the time I get the treatment ready.

He works the rest of the shift like that: between calls, he is gruff and grumpy. But the moment we step on scene, a completely different human appears.

A few hours later we meet a drunk man with chronic shoulder pain. He is demanding and mean. He tells us that the paramedics never fix his shoulder, that we're all a bunch of greedy good-for-nothings who lie and cheat and steal. I ask the man why he called us exactly. He says we already know and we ought to be ashamed of ourselves. Mikey gives me a look.

I tell the patient that I'm not sure what I can do for a seven-year-old shoulder injury in the middle of a park. Would he like a ride to the hospital? Of course he wants to go to the fucking hospital, that's why he called us. What the fuck else would he want? We are useless sons of bitches, scam artists, liars.

We run the call, drop the dude off to plead his case at the emergency room, and try to find some coffee. Mikey takes an phone call from the wife, then hangs up and tells me he could use something stronger than coffee. We get another call.

Journal, January 2014

I don't know how to take notes about work anymore. There's just too much. The idea of trying to capture any of it is just so overwhelming. And . . . I don't feel like a tourist anymore. I feel like I live here. It's hard to write these shocking little stories about the experiences that you are professionally required not to react to.

I had four dead people last week. I don't want to write about that. I want to watch TV.

I guess the twenty-four-year-old was the first one I've had in a while who felt like a real person, who required me to access my emotions because of human connections rather than professional frustrations.

God, he just looked so young. So brutally, intimately young and completely dead. To see dry, rigored skin underneath some indie jeans and a band T-shirt. And the house looked like so many houses I lived in when I was twenty.

The lessons I learned in paramedic school are shockingly irrelevant to the field. Instead of asking a patient what they ate for breakfast this morning, I ask when they last ate any food at all. Instead of looking for medical bracelets, I learn to check patients' arms for hospital wristbands to tell us how many times they've been transported this week. Instead of asking a patient my memorized list of chest pain questions, I find myself arguing with a sick woman about whether I will drop her off at her favorite casino instead of the hospital.

I am surprised to find out that one of my favorite calls is a hypoglycemic event. This takes place when the blood sugar drops too low in a diabetic patient, often caused by an infection or an accident in diet or medication. It's usually a roommate or family member who finds the patient unconscious and calls us. We arrive to find someone unrousable, pale, and sweating. From across the room they look dramatically ill: what we learned in school to call "big sick." We check the blood to confirm a glucose level, start an IV if possible, and give medication to bring their sugar back to normal. The textbook advises that once the patient wakes up, they should be encouraged to eat a snack containing some protein or complex carbs so that they don't fall back into hypoglycemia once our medication wears off. What the protocols do not explain is where to find this snack: that is, the process of opening kitchen cupboards in a stranger's house at one in the morning, fixing a peanut butter sandwich, and washing the dishes. The patient leans up against the couch, IV dripping fluids into an arm, calling out instructions on where I can find a knife or some jelly.

Mikey fills me in on Reno history while we drive around the city. He tells me about silver mines, and the Rat Pack, and that time in the nineties when the punk rockers rounded up all the Nazis and kicked them out of town. He tells me about his own path into EMS, which began in his teens when he was offered a choice between community service or juvenile hall. If the conversation gets too personal, he switches to war stories from work, like the time he and his deeply conservative Christian partner were called to an overdose in the middle of a furry orgy at a nearby hotel.

Once a month I drive to Santa Cruz and surf. It's my main survival method the first year in Reno. I sometimes leave for these trips straight from a day shift, at nine or ten o'clock at night.

There's a montage in my memory of these weekends. Standing in dispatch turning in my paperwork at the end of my shift. The room is air-conditioned, administrative, and on the far wall hangs a bright digital clock which controls our lives.

"You're driving to *Santa Cruz? Now??*"

I shrug. "I gotta get in the water."

Next I'm pulling my bike from the back of the supply storage room, throwing it over the back of the truck. A spray of dust as I cruise into the night. The sound of an energy drink can cracking open.

This is when the music picks up, louder and heavier until a close-up shot of my speedometer at ninety-two miles per hour outside of Sacramento. I get pulled over. Sign the ticket and throw it in the glove compartment on top of two others. The air humidifies as I get closer to the coast until it begins to condense on the windshield.

Before I left for Reno, I had been getting to know a surfer named Kyle. I found him intriguing at the time but knew I would likely be leaving the state for work and kept him at a distance. Still, he takes me in on my trips home. I pull into his driveway at about 4:15 a.m.

I wash the ambulance off in an outdoor shower, inhale fog and salt spray and listen to muted ocean sounds from down the street. Kyle's room smells clean and sandy, and feels like the quietest place I have been all month. I crawl into bed at 4:40 or so. He rolls over and lays with me for a second, murmurs, "How was work?"

"I don't know. Work. How are the waves?"

"There's waves."

"Good."

The alarm wakes us both at 7:00. Kyle has to get to work at the shop. He doesn't say goodbye but our eyes meet as he laces his boots. I smile and he leaves.

In the next scene I am in a wetsuit, walking down the street to the break. Standing at the cliffs looking out over crashing waves and breathing. Paddling out, whitewater breaking over my head. The first session always feels like a dream. Even the cold sting of the ocean doesn't yet bring me back from wherever I've been. Reno still wraps me tightly, desert and ambulance and dark laughter and tragedy and caffeine and bedbugs and blood. My arms know how to paddle but I forget how to catch a wave, how to relax, what California sun even feels like.

A guy next to me tries to say something friendly but I still have that work look in my eyes, and after a quick glance he stays out of my way. The sun rises higher and I paddle until I can barely feel my arms.

Sometimes I don't even want to catch a wave; I just want to drop over the waterfall. I paddle for the biggest peak I can find and come in too steep, knowing I won't make the drop, slip a foot off my board and just jump. I fall so heavy that I have time to spread my arms while getting blasted from the white lip of a wave through the air into the churning bowl below me.

When I first hit the water, it's suddenly quiet. My leash grabs my leg and jerks me. Saltwater blasts through every pore in my body. I explode from the inside out. My legs tingle from lack of air. When I finally come up, whitewater spray clogging the gasp I try to take, it feels like being born. Wet, matted hair slaps me and I'm cleansed of all my sins.

———

It's about four in the afternoon on Labor Day. The day is hot. The desert sun overwhelms a crowded courtyard. The Porter Street homeless shelter will serve a full meal to hundreds of people today: some live at the shelter full-time; others travel across town just for the occasion. Our patient is seventy-one years old, and seated on a low brick wall among dozens of others in various states of poverty. He is faint, and coughs as he speaks. He says, "It's just all too much."

The man is tired, overheated, and wheezing. He has the papery skin of the elderly and it's hot to the touch. His lungs whistle and pop, full of pneumonia fluids and scarred from years of lung disease.

We learn our guy woke up at five that morning to get ready and took a bus all the way across town. The holiday itself holds some significance for him, and he was excited for a square meal served on a plate instead of from a can.

He waited all day for the food, but as the crowd grew and the heat intensified he became overwhelmed and dizzy. The air is thick with sweat and cigarette smoke, and desert dust sits heavy in still air. We listen to his lungs and take his temperature, shake our heads gently, and explain that he needs to come with us. I send my partner to ask if we can steal him a plate from inside, knowing the doctor probably won't let him eat until after a barrage of tests and a several-hour wait. The food's not ready anyway.

On the way to the hospital I ask him about his life, his day, and the last time he remembers eating a decent meal. He shrugs off the food question but tells me he is a veteran, and a lifelong train worker. He makes sure I know he is not homeless, that he does have a room on the other side of town, which he keeps "nice and clean." I give him some fluids, sugar, and a thiamine shot. I keep looking at his outfit, wondering what's in the rest of the closet and how carefully he saved this shirt for today. His lungs sound awful.

At the hospital I try to explain how brutal the scene was, how polite and kind our patient had been. I ask them if there's any way they can sneak him some food, something more special than the usual ER sandwich.

"He's been waiting for ten hours," I tell them. The nurses look tired. They are polite and dismissive with me and I feel suddenly lame. I'm not sure how to convey the difficulty of Porter Street on a busy day, the desperation, the smell. "It's . . . it's so hot out there."

Later that year I sit down to a Thanksgiving meal with my family. The plates overflow with rich food. Cousins are well-dressed and smiling, chattering about business and school, sipping wine as they take turns at the buffet. Bracelets bounce on an auntie's wrist as she lifts a glass. I stare at my plate: piles of meat, bread, and vegetables with gravy melting through the troughs. I think of the gentle starving man I left at St. Joseph's that day, and remember our goodbye. I shook his hand and thanked him for his service, told him I'd tried to sneak him a plate of food. "The nurses will take really good care of you," I said, "I told them you've had a rough go." I told him we'd stop back by if we could, knowing we wouldn't have time. He nodded and thanked me quietly and I sat next to him for a moment, wishing I could do more. When I got back to the rig I turned the radio up and my partner and I looked out the windshield for a minute before we cleared.

It was the clothes, I think now, that got me. He wore a faded blazer with folded cuffs. A belt. His shirt was threadbare, pale, and frayed, but tucked carefully into ill-fitting pants. His hands were worn and tired, and I imagined him running them along the seams to smooth what he could. Alone, in the pre-dawn light of a single-room apartment, this had taken place. He had dressed for the meal.

"More cranberry sauce?" My uncle smiles.

"What? Yes, sure."

"You okay, Jo?"

I blink.

"Of course."

The first time I meet Buck it is two weeks after his third heart attack. I guess he woke up in a hospital bed, threw away all of his medications, and walked home to get high. When I arrive at the house he is drunk, scorched on meth, and complaining of chest pain. Mike greets him like a familiar friend and introduces me.

"It hurts, guys, it hurts so bad. It feels like it did before last time." He looks up at me. "Do you think I'm having another heart attack?"

"Um." *I don't know, man. Probably.* "Let's get you on the monitor and take a look. I'll take care of you, okay? Take a few deep breaths and try to stay still while I get the stickers on."

There's something childlike about this man. It's hard to pinpoint. He's got an easy giggle; he's grateful for our help. When I ask him to move the meth needles out of my way he smiles sheepishly and apologizes.

"You know you're killing yourself, Buck. One of these days we're not going to get here in time."

A "wake accident" is when cars crash into each other trying to make way for an ambulance to pass. It's sort of a gray area in terms of responsibility. We will usually radio it in but proceed to our assigned call.

"Does it count as a wake accident if it's a . . . wake *fight*?"

One man had tried to step out in front of the ambulance, another grabbed his arm and pulled him back, yelling something I couldn't hear. Mikey is driving, and as we pull away I look through the rearview and see them coming to blows.

"Not if nobody calls about it."

The tires screech. We keep driving.

When the weather warms up in the spring a friend visits me from the Bay Area and we decide to be tourists for the day and drive over to the lake to rent paddleboards. The shop is clean and bright and smells like surf wax, and the owner seems wistful about living in landlocked Tahoe instead of Hawaii. We chat with him about waves, and Santa Cruz, and work. He rents us two boards and offers me a job in the shop on my days off. The last thing I need is another alarm clock, but I'm starved for friends and the surf video playing on a small TV in the corner of the shop makes me feel at home. I agree to come in once or twice a month to help rent boards and kayaks and teach tourists how to balance on the lake.

On days I work for Mitchell, I go straight from my night shift in Reno to the paddle shop. I jump in the lake itself instead of showering, my sense of time confused as the night's non-stop calls blur into a sunny day.

I take some girls out for a paddleboarding lesson and show them how to bend their knees and dip the paddle into the water. I tell them to use their core strength instead of their arms. They smile and I smile and the long dark night of blood and bricks and dust and sweat and laughter still feels much more real to me than this dreamlike summer day. We drift around the lake, and about fifteen minutes into an hour-long lesson I realize I've run out of things to say to them and feel suddenly incompetent. You'd think this would be the easier of my two jobs, but somehow coming up with a cute summery paddle-boarding anecdote for these sweet tourists seems much more challenging than my night shift of chaos. The last twelve hours were screaming sirens, driving over curbs, yelling, "Fuck you, get out of my way, I'm an ambulance!" "I'm sorry, ma'am, you put your crack pipe *where?*" "No, sir, I can't take you to dialysis right now, it's four in the goddamn morning." "Oh fuck, dude, he's bleeding like a motherfucker, give me a roller gauze, shit, can you hold this for me?" "Fuck it, yeah, let's go code three," and then again with the sirens and the wailing and the flashes of the top bar lighting up the sagebrush black and red in the night. But then a drive home, a quick splish-splash, and now here I am on a paddleboard, floating on glassy turquoise water. The girl in the pink tank top asks me how deep the lake is in the middle and I have no fucking idea. I smile awkwardly. I tell her I've seen birds here sometimes. She waits for me to answer her question. I feel bad that they've paid for a lesson and I'm just staring at them like an idiot. If only one of them would start choking or something, then I'd know what to do.

During our partnership, Mikey is finishing up his paramedic training but is still working as an EMT. Although I technically outrank him, he has a decade of experience on me. We learn to rely on each other: I defer to him for more complex medical issues, but he is energized by my new-kid enthusiasm and mediocre Spanish.

We run a call on a forty-three-year-old man who smoked weed with his secretary at the auto shop. The secretary leaves, the wife comes to pick him up and finds her usually strait-laced husband pale and fidgety. She worries it's a stroke or a heart attack, which honestly doesn't seem out of the question until we get her to step outside for a minute and Roberto gives us the real story. We run some tests to make sure that there's no cardiac involvement and tell the guy his heart won't kill him right now but we can't promise the same about his wife.

Mikey shows me his favorite coffee shop, a small brick building with a low platform in the back and flyers for open mic nights. He says this place is hip now, but when he was growing up it was dirty and crowded and raw. We read some flyers and see that they're doing their best to keep some of the old vibe alive. We order iced drinks and get called to an auto-versus-pedestrian accident. The drinks melt on the dashboard as we scoop up an elderly man crushed by a pickup truck and head straight for the trauma center. Then a drunk woman, so emaciated that her bones jut out like broken fenceposts. Then a giggling toddler with a rash. His parents shove a sunscreen bottle in my face and ask me if it could have caused the problem. It smells like coconuts.

Later that night I read a text from a friend back home and get so suddenly homesick that I feel my eyes well up and I remember one of the first things my paramedic field instructor ever told me: "If I see you cry on the clock, I will fail you." I tell Mike I need a minute and he sees the look on my face and nods silently. He pulls into a parking lot near Sparks Harbor and lets me out of the rig. I run behind a pile of boulders and sob into the darkness, wondering how it is that after living in two countries and three states, this is the farthest from home I have ever felt. I dig my boot toes into the desert dirt and look back towards the ambulance. After a couple of minutes I stand up and shake out my pants. When I get back to the rig, Mikey asks if I want to talk about it. I shake my head no and he nods again and turns up the radio.

Later that year I run on Buck again. He's still in a dirty motel room, still surrounded by random women, but he looks a little better today. More color on his skin, a little more filled out, I can't put my finger on it. He tells me he's been clean and sober for 104 days. Did some time in jail and they made him take urine tests afterwards. He says it's been working. He talked to his grandkids for the first time in years.

"You have grandkids, Buck?"

"Four! Usually they don't talk to me, because, you know," he shrugs. I nod. *I know, bud.* "But they're picking up the phone again since I got sober. I might go stay with my brother for a while."

He tells me he has family waiting for him a few hours from here, in a Bay Area neighborhood that I knew well as a kid. I tell him I grew up near there, some of my best friends are from right down the street. Can you imagine? Buck goddamn Baker, king of the Reno weekly motel circuit, St. Joseph's cardiology MVP, tattoos and junkie veins and Raiders beanie and all . . . as a younger guy back home. Before he ever found meth and wandered into Reno. Maybe he smoked a cigarette on a picnic table at the disc golf course we used to hang around. We probably asked him for a light.

Mike and I don't transport him that day. He'd called because he was finally trying to take his medications instead of shooting meth and it made him feel weird. I think he was just a little overwhelmed by it all. We stay with him for probably half an hour, chatting and helping sort his pills. At the end I finally let myself tear up a little and break my no-hugging rule.

I know Buck will probably relapse, probably won't go see his family, might be making the whole thing up. Maybe he's drunk right now. Maybe tomorrow he gets his fourth heart attack and a crew finally has to leave him dead on the floor of this very room. I know all of this. But I've had a shitty day, an even shittier week, and on just this one rainy desert afternoon I choose to believe in hope. The empty gurney splashes a few puddles on the way back to the rig and I picture Buck sitting on a porch in San Lorenzo, drinking coffee and smiling at awkward teenagers. The kids are untrusting of this strange new relative but they offer him some food and ask about

Reno. He puffs his smoke and says it was a mess. Who knows, man. Crazier things have happened.

I talk to dead bodies. Sometimes an urge arises to treat one as a small child or animal, pat it on the head, fold its arms together. I once find myself muttering, "Good night, dear" as I draw a sheet over a body on the floor. A firefighter helping clean up the scene gives me a sideways look and I realize I've said it out loud. The girl was in her twenties and had hanged herself in the bathroom. We'd worked her, got nothing back, husband is sobbing in the next room, and here I am kneeling on the cold tile floor and tucking her into bed like a parent on a stormy night.

Sometimes on a slow night you find yourself in a parking lot somewhere, staring out a dark windshield listening to your partner breathe. It's a bizarrely intimate moment to share with a co-worker, and the conversation can drift in any direction. Mikey and I talk about movies, then ghosts, then medicine. One of us mentions the uncomfortable overlap between the last two topics.

"So . . . have you ever gotten that feeling on a call?"

"Yeah . . . every once in a while."

The sky is black, and a wet breeze floats through the dashboard vents.

"Do you remember that bariatric lady at Meadow Lane? That awful arrest?"

"Yeah, that's who I was thinking of!"

"Seriously? You too? I thought it was medical. I kept checking to see if we'd missed something."

"Yup."

"She'd been in asystole like half an hour, we did everything, she just didn't . . . she didn't *feel* dead. I couldn't put my finger on it."

"Yeah, she was hanging on."

"Can you think of anything we missed? That one bugged me for a while . . ."

"Oh, no. Medically, clinically . . . You had to call it. Her body was long done. That was just the rest of her wouldn't let go."

"Damn."

"This job, man."

"Right?"

When things finally come apart in Mikey's marriage, he ends up on my couch for a few days. It's not that I am Mike's oldest friend, or even his closest; it's just that with our proximity on the ambulance, night after night, I am located right there to catch the fall. He shows up to a shift looking like a greasy shop rag and tells me he hasn't slept. He has a friend who will help him move all his stuff out over the weekend, but for the next few days he doesn't have much of a plan. I tell him he will stay in my trailer, obviously, until he gets back on his feet.

I wake up a few days later to the smell of shepherd's pie. Mike has cleaned the small kitchen and made us both some meals for the week. The blankets on my couch are folded. We split the food into Tupperware containers and drive to work together. On the ambulance, we settle into a quiet rhythm, switching seats to assess a patient or tossing a piece of equipment across the bench without needing to say anything out loud. The calls keep pelting in like a hailstorm, but I'm starting to learn how to withstand the onslaught.

Then Mikey bumps up from EMT to paramedic. We get split up because there aren't enough medics to let us work together. I get to know new partners, learn their idiosyncrasies and bathroom habits and family troubles.

Mike eventually gets through his divorce, finds his own place, and, a few years later, I introduce him to one of my best friends from Santa Cruz. When I give the maid of honor speech at their wedding, I leave out the blood-covered seventy-year-old in the red-sequinned thong, and the girl who swallowed a pile of ecstasy pills and slammed her car into a tree. I don't mention having to ask Mikey what the hell to do next on my first really sick baby, or the tears of laughter streaming down his face as he swerved into a gas station while I tried not to shit my uniform pants after picking up a stomach virus from a patient. Instead I say that this is the guy who's "talked me through some of the most complicated, overwhelming moments of my career and, honestly, my life," which I guess means the same thing. It's also something I could say about most of the people I've worked with in EMS, and it doesn't even begin to cover it.

Journal, September 2014

Life keeps moving . . . Getting into the rhythm of sleep depriva-tion, everything's just a little fuzzy all the time. You learn to fight through the tired and move on with your day. I had a great bike ride yesterday, the weather was perfect.

Fire is hiring soon. Everyone says, "Here comes the bleed." Once or twice a year we hemorrhage medics. Right as summer is ending, everyone is out on injury leave, and we're all exhausted. Here comes the bleed.

I've been here almost one year and I'm finally starting to feel like part of the crew.

One of my last calls last week there was a turtle floating in a thin layer of water in a big Rubbermaid bin. I saw her as we were wheeling out the gurney. Out of surprise I said, "There's a turtle in this tub!"

Daughter: "Oh, he's lived there for years. He loves it."

Tonight we've been on two cardiac arrests, a stabbing, and a high-speed car accident. It's been sirens and blood and paperwork and more sirens and more blood and more paperwork. Now I'm staring at a thirty-year-old female who needs a refill on her migraine medication. She called us because she didn't want to pay bus fare downtown. She hops into the ambulance and buckles herself into the gurney, saying, "I know you guys have to take me. You can't say no."

She's not wrong. I am still not allowed to refuse transport to anyone, even if they are mean about it, even if their reason is silly. No one is in the mood to argue, so we roll our eyes and start driving. When I get to the ER I tell the charge nurse the story and he silently points one finger towards the waiting room.

I walk our friend over and wait in line with her until she is registered. The girl at the desk looks overwhelmed today and pulls me in to ask a favor. She hands me a patient information wristband and asks if I wouldn't mind helping her get this over to the guy who just walked away without it.

"He cut off, like, two of his fingers, has them in a baggie. Just put this on the other wrist. Not the one that, you know . . ."

I smile and take the bracelet from her. There is a big blood smear on her desk and I ask if that was the guy, but she has already picked the phone back up and turned away from me. I play detective instead, following the dark red trail out into the middle of the waiting room, but lose it quickly under too many footprints. I'm sad I've lost my clue but look up to see a large cowboy type with a bloody towel wrapped around one hand. I walk over and read the name off the wristband.

"Terrence?"

"Yeah, that's me. Is it my turn?"

"No, sorry, not quite yet. Registration just wanted to make sure you got your wristband. I can help you put it on."

"I already got one of those."

"No, I have this—wait, what? Can I see that? Did she get your name wrong?"

"I'm Terrence."

"Yeah, but the last name is . . . are you Terrence Holt?"

"No, I'm Terrence Jackson."

"Did you cut your fingers off?"

"Just the one, but yeah, that's what I got here." He pushes a Starbucks cup towards me.

I walk back to the reg desk. She's positive she got the name right. I point towards Terrence Jackson, with his bloody towel and his cup. She shakes her head no as she answers the phone again. I throw my hands up, as in, *what the fuck*, but she has two more calls on hold and a line of people behind me.

I turn away from the desk and say loudly, "Okay, is there a DIFFERENT guy named Terrence who cut his fingers off tonight?"

Two rows back a man in a black hoodie shyly raises his hand. I walk over slowly, staring alternately at the wristband, the fingerless Terrence, and the other fingerless Terrence. I almost trip over my original ambulance patient, who is now on her phone complaining to someone that this bullshit hospital is making her wait for too long.

Terrence Two holds a Ziploc baggie with not one but two bloody lumps stacked inside. His wounded hand is wrapped in paper towels. I explain the mix-up, and he apologizes for forgetting his bracelet and thanks me for my trouble. I kneel down and meet his eyes. I'm not sure if I'm talking to him or myself or my ego or my dead grand-parents or what, but I tell him I want him to know that the ER is busy tonight and it might seem slow but I promise you, Terrence, other Terrence, and everyone else in here dealing with whatever you are dealing with, I swear to god we are doing the best we can.

"I JUST WANTED TO SAVE PEOPLE"

JODY GEARE, EMT/FIREFIGHTER;
TWENTY YEARS IN EMS AND FIREFIGHTING.
APTOS, CALIFORNIA

I just wanted to save people, I don't know.

I was in high school. I had been a lifeguard over the summer, but I felt like it was too easy. I wanted to join the military and become a rescue diver, or jump out of helicopters. My mom noticed that the community college offered law enforcement and firefighting classes and asked if I would be interested in trying one. I thought, *Yeah, let's try firefighting.* I took my first class when I was sixteen and I just fell in love with it.

Part of what fueled me was my kid brother. When I was in the EMT class, my brother had a seizure. It was just me and him at home; I was seventeen and he was sixteen years old. He was playing on the computer. And I'm older now; I've jumped out of helicopters, I've fought fire, but to this day it was still the scariest goddamn thing I've ever seen. He was sitting in a spinny chair, playing video games, and he made this awful noise. He fell out of his chair like he was in a fucking horror movie; his mouth was open and he was making a hellacious sound. I looked at him and said, "Carrie, what's wrong?"

When Aptos Fire showed up, they were great. They let me ride in the front of the ambulance. When I told them what had happened, they looked at me and said, "Hey, you did a pretty good pass-down."

I got my first job with Calfire when I was nineteen. We worked four days a week, twenty-fours, but we didn't get paid for the whole shift. We only got paid for nineteens, and if you got a call after midnight you'd get your full shift. When that happened we'd say you "got your nickel."

THE POO SHOW

For the last hundred years, physicists have searched in vain for a Grand Unified Theory of Everything: a mathematical description that unites all branches of physical force to accurately describe our existence in space. As I matured as a paramedic, I read more and more history of ambulances and EMS. The details swarmed my head like too many insects—overlapping, buzzing, twisting, and diving. I couldn't find a coherent narrative thread of how it all came together. I found myself fascinated with stories from turn-of-the-century ambulance work: horses and carriages, oil lamps, surgical interns sleeping in the hospital barracks and waking at midnight for a "hurry call." In the twenties and thirties, things were less romantic but still interesting. Large municipal hospitals shut down their programs for financial reasons and the gap was filled by private companies, police stations, or fire departments. Everything seemed slapped together, ragtag, barely functional. World War II pulled the last doctors from the ambulances, and in the forties and fifties emergency calls were answered by a wildly varied group of completely unregulated entities: private companies, volunteer departments, mortuaries, and funeral parlors. It's tough to say whether the "system" was working during this time, because there wasn't really a system at all to speak of—just individual cities and private or public companies doing the best they could.

In the 1960s everything changed. Every single book or article about emergency medical services describes the late 1960s and early 1970s as the beginning of the modern era of EMS. The completion of the transnational highway system, new trauma medicine from the Vietnam War, and the invention of CPR and the portable cardiac monitor completely reimagined emergency medicine. EMS would soon see sweeping public support, legislation changes, and a popular TV show. The government envisioned a nationwide network of rescue ambulances, ready to respond, based on a single phone call, to anywhere in the country. Urban or rural, rich or poor, all Americans would have access to lifesaving rescuers at their moments of greatest need. Sort of.

As I pored through books and articles, I almost always stopped when I got to the seventies. The last forty years of history are when my job as I know it was truly developed, and you'd think it would be the part I would find most interesting. And yet, every time I got to the standardization of CPR training, the federal grant money, the development of modern EMS protocols, I would stop reading and make a cup of tea. I couldn't focus on the last half of any of my books. It took me years to figure out why.

After a couple of years in Reno, I return home to a job in Santa Cruz. I spend a few months there and then receive word that I am in consideration for a paramedic position with the San Francisco Fire Department (SFFD), where I will eventually spend the bulk of my career.

One night in San Francisco I am paging through *Living Downtown*, a book by Paul Groth about the history of residential hotels in American cities. It's an amazingly told story about a largely unseen population that I may have personally spent more time with than any other single group. Groth describes long-term hotel residents as a "neglected" and "alien" population, largely ignored by policy and media. He describes walking through touristy North Beach in San

Francisco, passing under famous neon signs for Carol Doda's and Big Al's, "yet within three hundred feet of that sign, on the second and third floors of the buildings, are over three hundred hotel homes. Virtually no one passing on Broadway thinks about those seventy-year-old dwellings, or who lives in them." *Virtually no one?* I think, stumbling on his words. I mean, paramedics do. We think about those dwellings all the time. We haul our gear up their stairs. We lean over the patient for a peek out their windows onto the street. We search their cupboards for medications and their closets for a favorite sweater. We argue with the man in the wheelchair in the alleyway below.

This passage, for some reason, is where it strikes me. Perhaps I always cringe at the "legitimization" of EMS because somewhere deep down I don't really believe that EMS was ever supposed to be legitimized. Ours has always been the back alley, the dead of night, the forgotten soul. And while the expansion of our medical education has certainly helped us to establish ourselves as legitimate clinicians, I also believe that the intense focus on just a small sliver of our calls, on the "real emergencies," has distracted us from what it truly means to be a paramedic.

There is more to us than CPR.

We're behind a dumpster in North Beach in San Francisco. About two blocks from here, paleontologists once discovered the fossilized skeletons of three Columbian mammoths and a giant bison, a stunning relic of the ancient marshlands that once filled this peninsula. Today the neighborhood is mostly Italian food, overpriced apartments, and strip clubs. When we hear the location I wonder if we're going to be running a call on a rich person, maybe a tourist at a restaurant or a hipster in a fancy apartment. Maybe we will find another mammoth tusk. As we pull up to the address we are waved into a narrow alleyway with a few piles of blankets and some homeless people hanging out.

As we pull the gurney into the shadows we are approached by a middle-aged woman. She has expensive jewelry and scarves and long, dyed hair. She grabs my arm and cries, "No one will help him! I try and try but they won't help! They don't even listen!"

I peel my arm out of her grasp and shake off my sleeve, still thinking about dinosaur bones. We walk towards the alley. My partner squints, stops, and sighs. We know this guy.

Andrew starts the interaction, asks Randy how it's going. Randy says, "Get the fuck away from me."

Andrew says, "I know you, Randy. We're cool. It's okay. I know you."

They talk for a minute. The woman who called us is still crying but we make her wait at the top of the alley.

Randy lost both his feet from diabetes a few years back. He lives in his wheelchair. He's been kicked out of a bunch shelters and public housing in the last few years for breaking rules and using fentanyl. He asks if we're holding.

"No, man, we're not giving you any drugs. What's going on today? Do you know why this woman called us? Are you okay?"

He's been pooping his pants and falling out of his chair. There's a lot of flies. He keeps some belongings in plastic grocery bags tied to his chair handles, like many folks who live in wheelchairs, and today they're all tangled up and his leg stumps are caught in the mess. Everything's covered in shit.

He's angry with us at first, calling us names and throwing his drink on the ground, but after we talk to him for a minute he chills out. Andrew leans towards him. "Randy, let me shake your hand. How've you been? Can we talk?"

He lets us lift him into a more comfortable position in his chair and we scoot his bags around so that he can reach them better. We tie and untie some things, pick up his butt pillow and wipe some of the crud off, and generally set him up a little better. We tell him he looks terrible and ask if we can take him in and get him cleaned up? Get him to a doctor? Please? At least let us check him out in the ambulance a little? He gets agitated again and tells us to fuck off with that. He's not going.

Randy's what we call "alert and oriented." He knows what day it is and what's going on around him, which means he's allowed to refuse our help. He's also disabled, stoned, homeless, covered in his own feces, and living every moment of his life in horrific pain. He doesn't want to go to the hospital. There's a guy who comes around this corner sometimes with some stuff. He's fine, he says. Let me go.

We stay and chat with him for a while, take some vital signs, and let him move on with his day. Tell him to have someone call us if he falls out of his chair, or if he changes his mind about going. "Call us if you're ever ready to get cleaned up. We really would like to help you, man, if you'd let us." He mumbles and starts cussing again. "All right, Randy. Take it easy." He signs our release paperwork.

We hike our bags up, take a few steps towards the street, and hear a shriek. The lady with the scarves has seen our empty gurney. She panics. Starts yelling, grabbing at us, sobbing. Saying how awful it all is, how he needs help, what kind of monsters are we to leave someone like that? She says, "Why are you walking back? But what will you do for him? What are you doing to help him? Are you getting a different chair for him?"

Andrew and I swap a quick look, and he walks towards the ambulance, doesn't even look at her. I guess this one's on me.

"He doesn't want to go, ma'am. We can't force him."

"What?" She's shocked; her sobs grow louder. She tried calling the police but they left him here. She wants to know what will be done. That man needs our help. He's sick, he can't take care of himself. Who am I? She threatens to write down my name. She says I'm a monster. She says this city is all monsters. She wants to know what will be done.

"I know, ma'am. Yes, it's awful. I'm sorry. But there's nothing I can do. He doesn't want our help." She asks me what my badge is for.

"That's what they all say! I can't help, I can't help, well who can?" She moans. "Someone has to help him! Am I the only one who cares?" Her voice breaks on the last syllable.

I mean, I get it. She wants this to be someone's fault. Life sucks, you know? A homeless, sick, opiate-addicted amputee stuck out in the cold, night after night, trapped under a wet bag of his own bowel movements. It's awful. No one wants that type of suffering to exist in the world. But I'm trained as a paramedic: I can restart a heart; I can splint a broken arm. If I take Randy to the hospital, I'll be giving him a ride to an overcrowded emergency room. I'll measure his blood pressure, probably check a sugar. I'll lift him over into an ER bed where an overworked doctor will give him a three-minute once-over, maybe draw some labs, and tell a nurse to clean him up and kick him out. Then he'll be in a different neighborhood with a cleaner butt. To be fair, I think the clean butt would help prevent pain and infection, and that's why I tried so hard to talk him into going. But after that he's back out on his own.

We call ourselves the HRS sometimes, homeless relocation services. Don't want to think about Randy? Call an ambulance, we'll move him for you. Then someone else a few blocks away will have to be faced with the excruciating pain of human existence for a few days. Just do me a favor and admit you're doing it for you, not for Randy. You just want the world to be different than it is.

There is a big fight going on in California right now about human rights versus mental illness—about the point at which the state gets to decide that a person is no longer allowed to make their own medical decisions. At the time of the writing of this book, even if Randy were forced into the care of the system, we probably wouldn't have anywhere to house him anyway, so in all likelihood, after a many-week legal and medical battle, he would end up right back out in the alley where he started.

I give Screaming Woman the phone number for Adult Protective Services and tell her I understand that it's frustrating and I appreciate her compassion. She starts talking and sobbing again and I nod my head and take a step away. Tell her I've got to get back to other calls. She says, "How dare you walk away while I'm speaking?" Andrew honks. I nod again and turn my back. Her cries fade once I'm out of the alley.

After Randy we run on ten more Randys. By the end of the day I've written three refusals and transported six patients to local hospitals, all for minor complaints. I've started one IV on a gentleman who had been vomiting all night with a combination of flu and bottom-shelf gin. I've performed no other actual medical interventions in twelve hours on the clock. My uniform smells like piss and gin barf and I lean into the collapsed front seat of the ambulance and wonder if I'll hit traffic on the way home.

Overhead alerts buzz across the ER. Nurses scold their patients, chat with patients, lose their temper with patients. A doctor explains flu symptoms to someone, sounding tired. A patient coughs, cries, vomits, screams. The registration assistant slides over her computer caddy, one broken wheel scraping along the floor. Some cords yank on a suction cannister and the whole thing comes clattering down. An old man sits up and horks up some phlegm, bronchitis tight in his chest.

Every time the entrance door opens a cold wind sweeps in and rustles the flyers on the corkboard. The paramedics stand next to our gurneys in the wind. There are three pairs of us waiting for a bed at the moment, gurneys lined up near the ER doors like cars in a drive-thru. Our cellphones and radios tone on and off and our patients shout, complain, and talk to themselves. The charge nurse, Seth, has been presiding over night shifts at the downtown hospital for almost a decade. He is calm and omnipotent, the train conductor, the man behind the curtain.

Suddenly a new sound breaks through the fray. A big smash, followed by a loud, rhythmic *rattle, smack, rattle, smack, rattle, smack!* Plastic and metal against the floor, with a shaking sound and a rope sound slapping against something harder. There's a human voice too, talking quickly to himself in fast musical nonsense.

It takes quite a thing to make Seth say "holy shit." The man is unbreakable. And yet here it comes, a holy shit in the night, rattle-smacking down the hallway, knocking over vitals caddies and upending trays.

The patient has been restrained to a backboard, a common technique, so his wrists and ankles are tied to a heavy plastic rectangle behind him. He's naked save for the white straps of the restraints. He's sweaty and pale and bug-eyed, with long floppy greasy hair slapping against the board and pale pink parts slapping against his legs. He's so far beyond jacked up on whatever the fuck drug he's on that he's managed to jerk and jump the whole backboard-restraints-body aggregate off the edge of the bed and he's making a break for it, hopping the backboard side to side. He's a Red Queen's playing card; he's a straitjacket crucifixion. He's a full-speed, full-sized, full-noise blast of crazy, whack-waddling through the ER leaving a wake of sideways equipment and open mouths. The physics required to keep this guy upright and in forward motion are unimaginable but here he comes, down the hallway, around the corner, and no sooner do we hear the rattle-SMACK from Tweaker Jesus, the holy SHIT from Seth, then comes a guttural roar: our shortest security guard, head down, knees bent, full running-start football-tackles the guy and blasts him onto the floor and now the layers of backboard, naked guy, and security guard are all tied up and sliding across the ER with bits and pieces flying off like a cartoon cyclone, and that's all the medics need to abandon their patients and jump into the brawl.

One tired-looking EMT rolls her eyes and stays behind, guarding all three gurneys in the hallway while the other five medics pile onto the guy like dogs on a steak, everyone howling and grabbing limbs and doing their best to dodge the greasy hair and the floppy wiener flying around in the fight.

We get the guy re-tied, a little tighter this time, the nurses hit him with a heavier sedative, and he gets thrown back in his room. The commotion dies down a little and eventually everybody shuffles back to their own patients, each in their own little world of drunk and insane, orbiting their own universes, cruising through the hospital shitshow, just another San Francisco night.

Owner Given First
Jaunt in Ambulance

———oo———

DELAWARE, O., May 6. (U.P.)—
Saul Lewis of Detroit, an under-
taker, was the first passenger in
his new ambulance. While driving
from Piqua, O., where he bought
the ambulance, to Detroit, a passenger car driven by Lewis went
into a ditch when he swerved to
avoid hitting a dog. His partner,
Jack Snider, who was following
with the ambulance, brought Lewis
to the hospital here.

Imperial Valley Press, El Centro, CA, May 6, 1936

"SO WHAT'S, LIKE, THE CRAZIEST THING YOU'VE EVER SEEN?"

(Common Variations: "What's the weirdest/ grossest/worst thing you've ever seen?")

POTENTIAL ANSWERS:

The **"crowd pleaser"**: A funny/gross story, bonus points if it involves an injured penis (people love injured penises).

The **"camp counselor"**: "You know, that's actually a really uncomfortable question for paramedics. It's kind of like asking a veteran if they ever killed anyone—most of us don't love to relive the worst trauma of our lives on command in front of a stranger at a barbeque."

The **"sassy"**: A dramatic pause, raised eyebrows, then hit them with, "I once watched an entire season of *The Bachelorette* with an old roommate. It was, without a doubt, the strangest reflection of the human experience I have ever seen."

The **"conversation-ender"**: An honest description of a triple murder/ rape victim/dead child.

The **"sidestep"**: "Yeah, I'd actually love not to get into work stuff on my day off. You said you guys went for a hike at Wilder Ranch this morning? How was it? Still pretty muddy, or are the trails starting to dry off?"

The "I just got off shift from the worst fucking week, I really can't put on a show for your right now": "Um . . . I don't . . . I'm just not . . . excuse me please [spill drink/pretend to answer phone/ shuffle away]."

"POCKET MASK"

A.K., PARAMEDIC/EMS CAPTAIN, DISPATCH SUPERVISOR;
TWENTY-THREE YEARS IN EMS
CALIFORNIA

When I was thirteen, somebody at my church invited me to Red Cross Camp, over in the Marin Headlands. For the camp I had to take a CPR class, and I thought, *Man, this is really cool.* I used to carry around a little pocket mask on my keychain and everything.

When I first got hired at American Medical Response (AMR), I didn't have a car yet. I got a little bit of practice on my dad's Taurus, but most of my driving practice was actually in an ambulance. I got used to the dimensions and to driving something big. I got pretty good at it. Working for AMR actually helped me save up to buy my own car a couple of years later.

It's challenging driving code three in this city. There's a lot of hills and tricky intersections and one-way streets. Actually, there is a guy who is a battalion chief now; he and I would practice driving code three at nighttime. Totally unauthorized. In hindsight, that was pretty stupid. If we were to cause an accident or anything, that would have been really bad. But I was young! I was eighteen years old, you know? You're going to make those poor decisions.

I went to paramedic school and got bumped up to paramedic, then got hired with the fire department. I really just like helping people. I do really like the critical-thinking aspect of the job, trying to figure out what's wrong with somebody and how to fix them. I like using tools, like the cardiac monitor. I was a medic when we were working with a monitor that was really basic. I think that experience of working with fewer tools and less technology helped me become a better paramedic. It taught me problem solving, and how to look at the big picture of what is really going on.

When I explain this job to somebody relatively new, I always tell them we wear multiple hats. The paramedic hat comes every once in a while: the intubations and the bone drills and the needle decompressions. But I feel like we wear the social worker hat a lot more in general. People not taking care of themselves, people not knowing how a medicine works or the importance of it, or missing their hypertension medication for two months.

The job is a lot of switching gears and a lot of problem solving, which I really enjoy. Thinking about, *What does this person really need?* They don't always need to go to the hospital. I always found the job very interesting because you don't know what the next call is going to be. You could have somebody that just woke up from an overdose and they spit at you. And you took them to the hospital, and they walked out while you're still working on your paperwork and now they're cursing you out . . . and then go from that to taking care of somebody who is an eighty-year-old female with abdominal pain, the sweetest lady that reminds me of my grandma.

"THE COOLEST JOB IN THE WORLD"

MICHAEL HAMILTON, PARAMEDIC/RN;

TWENTY-FOUR YEARS AS EMT AND PARAMEDIC

RENO, NEVADA

I had just turned eighteen and dropped out of high school. My future looked pretty weak. I got my GED, got my first-responder certification, and then got my EMT basic. I remember going in for my first interview for an EMT position. I said something along the lines of, "It's a great gig. You get to save lives and be a hero and get paid a ton of money for it."

I had no idea. I had done some ride-alongs, but we'd never discussed the pay scale. I just figured that these guys do incredible work and put their asses on the line. Why wouldn't they get paid really good money? Needless to say, I did not get the job that first time around. The message was to come back when I knew what I was getting into.

Instead, I got two other jobs. I worked for the wheelchair transport van, and when I had downtime I would go help in the garage stocking ambulances. I worked my way up through the company until they let me reapply for the ambulance.

This is something that I haven't told a lot of people. It paints me in a less altruistic light, but I'm at a point in my life now where I'm comfortable talking about it. A lot of what fueled me to become an EMT was pride. Growing up, I was a deeply insecure person. I had a hard time navigating social situations or acting in a way that wasn't self-deprecating. I felt like I was worthless all the time. We can talk about the trauma, upon trauma, upon dysfunction that was my upbringing, but when I looked at paramedics, I thought, *There's something I can do and no one will ever question if I'm a good person or not.*

I thought it was the coolest job in the world.

Part Two

THE GRIND

DEATH

I smell the body before I see it . . . I start breathing through my mouth instead of my nose, but that transfers the sensation onto my tongue. Now I am eating death instead of smelling it.
STEPHANIE ELIZONDO GRIEST, *All the Agents and Saints: Dispatches from the U.S. Borderlands*

During my first experiment, a kind of enthusiastic frenzy had blinded me to the horror of my employment; my mind was intently fixed on the consummation of my labour, and my eyes shut to the horror of my proceedings. But now I went to it in cold blood, and my heart often sickened at the work of my hands.
DR. VICTOR FRANKENSTEIN, in Mary Shelley, *Frankenstein*

The teacher waves us over us to the cadaver on the far left, who was in her seventies when she died. I'm already working as a paramedic, but have signed up for a weekend anatomy lab at a local community college. The notecard tied to this body says she had a history of coronary artery disease and lists cause of death as cardiac arrest.

The chest cavity has already been dissected, so the two sides of her ribcage are split down the middle and resting on top of her chest like cabinet doors. The pectoral muscles hold them together, dried into tight jerky by heavy chemical preservatives. We flap them open to reveal the inside of her chest. When I pull on the muscle it collapses a little in my hand. The insides of the ribcage are stained like a gun has fired inside, a large black splatter across the inside of the ribcage doors. I pull the right side of her chest open and closed, open and closed, feeling the bones in my hand. All five are broken down the middle, violently; the black spreading out from them is dried blood. When you close the flap you realize that the stain and the fractures make a large round ring, like she had been hit in the chest with a heavy object. Something had pushed in the center of her chest hard enough to shatter almost every rib in her body.

Suddenly, all I can think is, *When did this woman die?* No, when *exactly?* The muscle and connective tissue holding the broken halves of each rib are attached so you can run your fingers along the splintered edge without actually separating the two pieces, and as I stare down at my gloved hands holding the blackened bone and the professor tells me when this body was donated, all I can think is, *I did this. I did this to her.*

The odds that this was me, of course, are quite low. I do chest compressions once or twice a month usually, and our county runs a couple thousand cardiac arrests a year, so the chance that she was mine is minuscule. Still, it's not zero. It may have been my hands that broke these ribs.

My voice that said, "You guys ready to call it?" My arms that pulled a blanket over her head on the kitchen floor.

I'm not the one who killed her, not technically. She would have died first, or almost died, and then someone would have called us, and I would have put down my sandwich and said, "Christ, dispatch, can we catch a break for five goddamn minutes," and then looked up the address on my phone and flashed the lights at my partner and held up my hand in the window with three fingers to tell him, hey, code three call, we gotta go, and then my partner would have said, "fucking seriously," and we would have driven to the wrong address, circled the block, found the house, headed upstairs, and done our very best to bring this woman back from the dead.

We're on the floor of a tiny bedroom in a house in San Francisco, stuffed into the narrow streak of carpet between the foot of a bed and the wall. The blanket hangs off the bed and tangles around arms and elbows until it is thrown towards the back of the room in frustration. The patient is an older Asian man, found in bed by his wife and dragged onto the floor by the first one of us to make it upstairs.

I'm kneeling over his face, in the airway management position, so I see straight down to his graying skin. There's vomit pooled in the sockets against his eyes, and with every chest compression it splashes up a bit, discolored wet puddles spattering down his cheeks. My job right now is to get a tube down towards his lungs so that we can oxygenate him, but his throat is so full of blood and vomit that it's spilling out down the sides of his face. My knees are soaked. There are five of us crammed around the body and it flops on the floor as we push and stab and tear at whatever's left of him.

"This carpet's never going to be the same again," I mutter to myself, trying to ignore what I'm really thinking, which is: *Stop. Just stop. Let this fluid-filled bag of death rest, you torturers, you pain-inflicting, misery-prolonging, protocol-following ignorant weapons of medical confusion, you paramedics, you ghouls.*

I pray sometimes that we don't get a pulse back, that we can leave the body to rest on the floor. That we don't have to package what's left of him, stuffed full of tubes and chemicals to keep his tired heart beating, drive him to a hospital where he will spend two weeks without brain activity in the ICU racking up half a million dollars in debt before his exhausted, agonized family finally makes a decision that was never really a decision at all. I know this guy's dead. I can see it in his graying, stiffening hands, in his unreactive pupils, in his angulated vomit-covered jaw. His ribs are broken, his white hair is torn, his foggy eyes are open and slack.

Don't make us do this to him, I beg silently as I drop the tube. I try not to think about decaying bodies hooked up to machines, the sound of beeping on an upstairs floor, the shuffle of tired nurses caring for glazed semi-humans.

In college I once pinned a chunk of a mouse's cardiac muscle into a petri dish of fluid and then injected a syringe full of chemical compound into the dish. I pushed down the plunger and watched the red patch of heart, lying like torn fabric in the dish, begin to quiver and spasm. It quickly found its rhythm and began to beat, *ka-thump, ka-thump, ka-thump*. The heart cell's ability to pump in rhythm with or without a heart to surround it is called automaticity, and it is a wonderful trick of biology, of myofilaments and gap junctions and ion differentials.

In the field, on a cardiac arrest, I often think of that shred of muscle, lying alone in a dish, the mouse's body sliced open on a lab table a few feet away. I've pushed so much epinephrine into so many bodies, on so many carpets and sidewalks and tile floors, in bathrooms and kitchens and alleys and bedrooms. I think a lot about how far those bodies were from human by the time we broke all their ribs and pumped their hearts full of adrenaline. On TV the neurologist will pull out a pen light and check the pupils to measure brain activity; they always seem so confident, so conclusive. "Pupils fixed and dilated," someone will say, and everyone will sigh. I have done the same thing, but without four years of medical school my penlight cannot make the same decision. I can look into foggy, stiff, open dead eyes and know we are torturing a corpse, but my job is to keep pushing until we either get a heartbeat back or we don't.

The word *code*, short for *code blue*, is a nickname referring to the moment when the human heart stops beating. It is used in emergency medicine the way that the word *fuck* is used by teenagers: as a noun, a verb, a descriptor, and an exclamation. A patient can code, be coded, or be a code. "Hey, get the pads out, this guy's about to code." "We coded her right there on the floor of the church!" "The paperwork says she's a full code." "Did you guys bring in that code yesterday?" A cardiac arrest is probably the most-rehearsed scenario in paramedic school. We were taught that the heart rhythm can change quickly and our reaction times must be within seconds. We spent months memorizing and practicing an algorithm of medications and electrical shocks depending on the presentation of the patient. We kneeled over dummies on the classroom floor, shouting at each other and fumbling with buttons on the portable cardiac monitor. Field interns ask each other, "Did you get a code yet?" as though it is the One True Test of official paramedic-hood.

Older medics will often tell you not to focus so much on these cases. "Look, an arrest is actually one of your simplest calls," says one of my teachers in a cardiology lecture. "Your patient doesn't talk, everyone works together, you just follow a simple formula and that's all it is." He's not wrong, but try telling that to a twenty-three-year-old who has just been given the power of resurrection.

For most of human history, death was seen as a permanent condition. Healers and families tried, mostly in vain, to bring back drowning and heart attack victims. They bent bodies over shipping barrels and rubbed their skin, hoping for a gasp of air. They wrote stories of vampires or zombies or ghosts, humans who stuck around this world despite their dead bodies and stopped hearts. A resuscitation protocol isn't this exactly, of course. After a couple hundred years of playing with electricity and heart surgery and oxygen tubes, doctors finally figured out that Miracle Max had it right after all in *The Princess Bride*: there is a big difference between *mostly dead* and *all dead*. Sometimes the heart wiggles for a little while before it sputters out, and if you can zap it hard enough, occasionally it will snap back into a rhythm and get back to work. These calls are a tiny fraction of our work, they are almost always futile, and yet they completely changed the role of the ambulance in America.

Resuscitation was not discovered all at once. Dozens of doctors over hundreds of years carved out small pieces of knowledge: rescue breathing works better if you do it like *this*; chest compressions seem more effective if you push like *this*. Young doctors applied electrical shocks to frog muscles and immersed patients in tubs of electrified water. They used fireplace bellows to blow air into dead mouths. For most of the 1700s, a common technique involved stuffing a thin rubber tube up a patient's anus and fumigating with tobacco smoke. When I try to review all the ways that a thousand-year medical history has led us to today, all I can remember is that they used to *literally* blow smoke up your ass.

Eventually, insanely, improbably, they figure it out. By the 1800s, researchers understand that applying electrical stimulation to human muscle can cause the tissue to contract. A series of gruesome experiments on recently executed prisoners (specifically, on their decapitated heads) proves that there is a short window after death in which applying electricity will still cause facial muscles to twitch—even if that face is attached to a head located in a guillotine catch basket a few yards from the rest of the body. In 1850, an equally ruthless investigation involving dogs reveals an odd phenomenon in which the heart loses its internal rhythm and instead gets stuck in a series of worm-like, undulating vibrations. They named this lack of rhythm *ventricular fibrillation* and observed that, left unattended, it will prove quickly fatal. Which is why on the ambulance we've been known to call its associated EKG printout "the death squiggles."

Rescue breathing, chest compressions, electrical stimulation: during the twentieth century all of the pieces of an arrest are refined by different groups of doctors in different time periods, and it takes decades to put it all together. For years the American cardiologist Dr. Claude Beck obsesses over the puzzle of how to restart a fibrillating heart. He tries manual massage, medication, and electricity. In 1947, a fourteen-year-old boy's heart begins to fibrillate in the middle of surgery right in front of Beck, and he uses the techniques he has been developing to restart it electrically—the first known case of a successful human defibrillation.

Meanwhile, scientists argue about the best way to perform rescue breathing for patients who are no longer moving air on their own. Techniques involve flapping a person's arms over their head, pushing up and down on their torso, or rolling them side to side. A young Austrian physician named Peter Safar becomes fascinated by this research.

As a teenager, Safar had just barely avoided conscription into the Nazi army by giving himself a life-threatening allergic reaction and hiding out in the hospital. After the war, he dedicated his career to protecting human life through medicine. By 1956, Safar has demonstrated that mouth-to-mouth resuscitation is far more effective than any of the other popular methods. He reads several papers explaining the usefulness of chest compressions to keep blood moving once the heart has stopped, and works with the authors to combine pushing on the chest and mouth-to-mouth breathing to create what we now know as cardiopulmonary resuscitation—CPR.

The movements we see in the movies—pushing on the ribs, blowing air in and out of the mouth—don't actually revive the heart. CPR is designed to keep the blood flowing to the brain and other organs until the heart can receive a jump-start. Those scenes on TV, where CPR alone revives the patient, without defibrillation? Bullshit. All of them. Of course, there are cases in which the heart restarts spontaneously, or never really lost pulses in the first place, but the act of CPR itself is not the reset button. You have to give a shock.

Which brings us to the ambulance. In 1966, a cardiologist in Belfast, Ireland, named Dr. Frank Pantridge reads an article detailing how quickly heart attack symptoms can lead to death and realizes that treating cardiac arrest inside the hospital isn't good enough. He understands that the faster a patient receives chest compressions and electricity, the greater the chance of survival. He wants to get to patients out in the field, in their kitchens and living rooms, right where they collapse. The conservative Irish medical establishment disagrees, and tells Dr. Pantridge to wait for further analysis. But Pantridge is not the type to sit down and shut up. Instead, he hooks a hospital defibrillator up to two twelve-volt car batteries and builds the world's first "Mobile Coronary Care Unit": a fully stocked medical van that will travel out to the homes of patients experiencing heart attack symptoms and attempt to resuscitate right there at the scene. After ten months, they get their first field save.

A true code save is vanishingly rare compared to what a good soap opera would have you believe, but it does happen. Small-town ambulance agencies have a "survivor's dinner" once a year where the paramedics can shake hands and pause for a photo with patients they brought back from death. Sometimes we hear from a nurse friend that a recent arrest survived, "walked out of the hospital," went on to live for years.

These are usually younger patients, with healthier bodies, who received early CPR and defibrillation. What Claude Beck and Dr. Mickey Eisenberg call "hearts too good to die." Forty-year-old guys who collapsed at work, got chest compressions right away, then popped back into a heartbeat after one shock. Their skin never got the chance to go gray, their pupils never dilated. I've run this call, more than once actually. A guy at a Greek restaurant drops right in front of his friend. We're parked fifty yards away waiting in line for coffee next door when the call comes out; we don't even bother to move the rig. My partner cranks on his chest with one arm while we slap on the pads, drop a simple airway, and give him some breaths. Within five minutes we've shocked him and he's wide awake, coughing, clutching his chest. He's angry and scared, his chest hurts, why are there so many people around? "You *died*, bro! It's cool, though, we got you back."

I parked the gurney right in the middle of a casino floor once, wedged between two rows of slot machines. The cameras caught the guy passing out. Within thirty seconds of his collapse two young security guards were by his side. One kneeled over the chest, counting out loud and giving compressions like he's closing in on the finish line at a race. The other is holding a clipboard and shouting directions nervously at the group. "Okay, we're doing chest compressions, got it. Jerry's got the AED, got it. Okay. Okay, he went down like five minutes ago, oh, shit, the paramedics are here. They're here!" He turned towards me, hands sweating and eyes wide. "Okay, here's what happened. He fainted at, um . . . 2:38. We started chest compressions. Jerry's getting the AED. He was playing the Lucky Lady

7 slot machine, that one there." I laughed, resisting the urge to pat the kid on the head. He was doing an amazing job, all things considered. The code was running smoother than anything I'd ever seen at a nursing home.

We switched the patient over onto our monitor, rhythm check, two shocks, and got a pulse back. His color was good, his oxygen and carbon dioxide numbers looked great. As we got him packaged, I tried to muster as much gravitas as I could and told security that they probably saved this man's life. The patient didn't wake up on the way to the hospital, but his pulse stuck around and his numbers stayed up and a few days later I sweet-talked the charge nurse into looking up his chart. "Full recovery."

My point is that it happens. Extreme measures do sometimes work. Code saves are *cool*. It's a good feeling, those calls. The adrenaline rush and the altruism can send you home smiling. But the older folks? The ninety-four-year-old grandmother with terminal cancer and dementia? Why am I pulling her dentures out of the way to shove a tube down her throat as my partner crushes her torso? Even if this woman does live another week, or month, or year, what will her life be like? Will her heart give out at the hospital? What kind of brain damage will she face? Will she succumb to pneumonia from the broken ribs? Or will she stagger home, alive, in pain and confused, to go on a little while longer?

There is a legal process in the United States to create "Do Not Resuscitate" paperwork ahead of time. DNRs are often used by those with terminal disease or severe disability, and can be put in place when a patient and their doctor can fill out forms requesting partial or total prevention of resuscitative efforts. In California, these forms are often printed on bright pink paper. The reason for the garish color is that as paramedics, we have about thirty seconds upon entering a house to decide whether or not to proceed with our efforts. If we cannot find appropriately signed and dated paperwork in a matter of moments, we are off to the races. Sometimes DNR forms are filled out incorrectly, or hidden in a file cabinet, or, much more frequently, don't exist at all.

There is no upper age cut-off in my cardiac arrest protocols. For better or for worse, paramedics are not allowed to make value judgments on the life a patient will live if they survive our efforts. To a certain extent this is simply logistics: we don't have time to gather a quorum and debate ethics while Granny is lying on the bathroom floor. But much of it is a function of the way that our protocols are determined. American paramedics technically work under a doctor's supervision. Each county reports to a single doctor who writes—like, literally *writes down*—a series of specific orders that paramedics follow like a recipe book. If this, then that. I am allowed to perform a limited number of interventions based on the exact situations and dosages that are printed in my protocols. Despite the breaks-the-rules-to-save-a-life scene in literally every medical drama, if I deviate too far from the book in real life I will definitely face consequences. I can be investigated, suspended, or fired. I can lose my license. I can even face criminal charges.

The rules in San Francisco, for example, allow me to withhold resuscitative efforts in cases of what they call "obvious death": decapitation, total incineration, a handful of other gory circumstances. There are similar rules in other counties, with the same end result: we occasionally burst into a room, bags swinging from our shoulders, ready to do our best, and find a body so decomposed that the smell alone tells us we will not be using our machines on this one. In these cases, we put our gear down and reach for a sheet to cover the corpse. But when faced with the elderly, the sick, the stroke victim who hasn't spoken or swallowed in years, unless we are met by a caregiver waving bright pink papers as soon as we walk in the house, paramedics are required to work every cardiac arrest we encounter.

Dr. Safar himself, the "father of CPR," once wrote: "Resuscitation applied without judgment and compassion is morally and economically unacceptable. The debilitated elderly patient or the otherwise terminally ill patient with incurable disease, particularly the one with irreversible coma or stupor, should be permitted to die without the imposition of costly and often dehumanizing efforts." Safar never intended for CPR to be used indiscriminately on every heart which has ceased to pump. A "moral injury," as described by psychiatrists and post-traumatic stress disorder (PTSD) research, is the distress that accompanies a professional "acting or witnessing behaviors that go against an individual's values and moral beliefs." In other words, it's the feeling of whispering, "I'm sorry, abuela. I'm so sorry," as I crack the ribs of an underfed Alzheimer's patient on a nursing home floor.

In recent years there has been an effort to educate patients and families about their options for end-of-life care. Writers like Atul Gawande and Caitlin Doughty have raised awareness in certain circles of the concept of death with dignity. But these changes trickle to the field slowly if at all. For the most part, we do the job we were trained to do—try to keep life flowing through every single human body, no matter who, no matter what.

I got in trouble with a partner once over a code on an ancient, fragile great-grandmother. It was my turn to lead the call and I did not intend to drag my feet but as I stared at her tiny, birdlike collarbones, I froze. The sounds of the emergency spun around me in a tornado. I heard the beeping of the monitor, the tearing open of plastic packaging, the phrases "ninety-six years old" and "lung cancer" and "can't find a DNR." Her face looked soft and wrinkled, her expression peaceful. I knew that it was my job to yank her lifeless body out of her wheelchair, throw her on the floor, and start breaking ribs, but I just couldn't make my arms move. I felt like I could see how brittle and porous her bones were through her translucent skin, and kept picturing them shattering under my hands. When I couldn't wait any longer, I pulled her to the floor and put my hands on her chest and felt her ribs, willing her to wake up. I looked around frantically, hoping to see a flash of pink paper in someone's hand. The engine crew stared at me expectantly. She was warm, her skeleton stiff and tiny. I winced and pushed down on her sternum, feeling her ribs pop out of the cartilage and crack one by one under my hands.

My partner yelled and elbowed me out of the way. He shouted orders, taking over the call and bringing us back to full speed. We had to get her on the cardiac monitor, insert a breathing tube, start giving drugs. A firefighter took over chest compressions. I tried to get myself together but was clearly frazzled and did badly with the rest of the call.

The next morning my partner pulled into a coffee shop parking area to rip me a new one. He was an old-school medic, with sixteen years of experience to my four. He took my poor reaction time as a sign of disorganization and inexperience. I nodded through the lecture and held back tears as he told me why my performance was so terrible and how unprofessional it was that he had been forced to take over. How I should have done a quicker assessment, been cleaner with my priorities, and delegated tasks to firefighters instead of getting sucked into doing them myself. The lead paramedic should never be the one doing chest compressions when there is help available. I swallowed and apologized and promised to do better. He was not the kind of guy you talked back to. He was extremely competent, purposeful in his actions, and ran each incident by the book. And more to the point, he wasn't wrong. No matter what games my head was playing with me that day, if something like that happened again I could be in serious trouble. I didn't cry that morning. I didn't tell him that I'd run dozens of codes like hers perfectly capably and each time it hurt a little worse. I didn't tell him that I felt tortured by the undeniable *wrongness* of what we were doing. Instead I took my licks, chugged half my coffee, and added some bricks to my internal wall. I refused to let him see me falter again.

I wish there was an easy protocol to follow: If a person has a green dot on their forehead, proceed with CPR. If the dot is red, let them die.

The nursing home smells acrid, and bitter, and cloying, and rotting, and sweet. Beds are lined up three per room, with stained curtains forming half-hearted partitions between patients. A janitor leans on his push-cart in the hallway, looking tired. A patient in a wheelchair in the hallway drools onto her chest, semi-conscious and confused.

We make our way to bed 78A, which contains a crumpled body that vaguely resembles a human. It's still alive, technically, and its eyes dart around as we approach.

"Hello, Mr. . . . anybody know his name? Anybody find any paperwork?"

I start checking the patient's vital signs and send my partner out into the hallway to try to find some staff. His name, it turns out, is Mr. Zanovitch. His packet says he has been at this facility for three years and has dementia and a page-long list of other medical conditions and disabilities. Infections, strokes, coronary artery disease, liver disease, antibiotic-resistant urinary tract infections, diarrhea. He's being "sent out" today because of some irregular lab values. He's baseline non-verbal, which means he hasn't spoken out loud in years, has just opened his eyes, closed them, and opened them again. His heart still pumps and his lungs still push air in and out. So he lays in bed in a feces-soaked diaper, rolling uncomfortably in cheap cotton sheets as buzzing overhead lights switch on and off to mark the passing of days.

There are floors full of these people, and buildings full of floors. Every city in the country has large, nondescript box buildings tucked into its corners called "The Meadows," or "Lakeside Manor," a boring name on a boring building with nothing to set it apart unless you notice a wheelchair ramp, or quietly marked ambulance parking space. Some extra electrical running in the wall for oxygen and machines. They are filled, on every floor, in every building, in every city, with our forgotten. The elderly, the confused, the gorked. Young folks with disabilities too overwhelming for their parents; older folks with lost memories and no families. A confused grandparent with children in another state. An uncle whose stroke took his ability to speak watches reruns all day and stares at an old Christmas card sometimes. People who used to be humans, who had childhoods and adolescences, and who from disease or accident or the unforgiving passage of time are now lying in a damp bed watching a fluorescent light flicker against a cracked ceiling.

The ambulance provides a shuttle service to bounce between all of these houses. Abnormal labs, infections, blood pressure changes. An Alzheimer's patient becomes too aggressive for the understaffed night shift; a developmentally delayed teenager spikes a fever. Maybe a nursing assistant doesn't know how to read the oxygen saturation or a nasogastric tube gets pulled out. Sometimes we are called for minor inconveniences that make us roll our eyes. Other times the patient has been neglected so severely they are on the verge of death by the time we walk in. Every paramedic I know has at least one story of arguing with a panicking orderly who insists that we transport a patient who was ignored for so long that their corpse has already started to stiffen.

I try not to blame the nurses. For every story I've seen or heard about patient neglect, I've heard equally terrible stories from their side: one nurse for every twenty, fifty, one hundred patients. Left alone with a whole floor of beds, with no one to call in an emergency but 911. Withheld paychecks, labor rights abuses.

Every single paramedic I know has lost their temper and shouted, "HOW LONG HAS HE BEEN LIKE THIS" to at least a dozen care home nurses in their career. Their answer is so well-rehearsed that it's become a running joke on the ambulance: "Not my patient. I don't know. I just got here."

Taking a patient home to begin hospice care sounds depressing but can be bittersweet. It's done by transport ambulances, which generally means young EMTs at the very start of their careers. We bring someone out of a smelly, loud, cold hospital room so that they can face death in peace at their house. We move them to the gurney as gently as we can, listen to some music on the drive home, and ask the family if they have a favorite nightgown or blanket. Then with two hands I pick them up, lift them over, and tuck them into the bed they will die in.

A lot of religions emphasize preservation of life at all costs. I wonder if the old prophets who first put ink to their visions knew that humans would someday invent a ventilator, a tracheostomy tube, a Foley catheter. When they said to let the Creator decide when it was Grandma's time, did they imagine a gray room with stained sheets, a stiff hose forcing air in and out of Nana's lungs, an electric pump shooting caustic chemicals into her veins to force her heart to beat, and a plastic tube shoved up her urethra and hooked to a bag of stale pee? I respect a person of faith, and I honestly love ancient religious texts. The exquisite bookbinding, the calligraphy, the smell of dust and tribal dreams. They make me think of deserts, and jungles, and clans of close-knit humans doing their best to stay together and survive. The directives given in these manuscripts on how to be a community seem to me to be the farthest possible thing from the tasks I perform at my job.

In a memoir about funeral home work, mortician Caitlin Doughty describes this feeling: she explains what it was like to work in a room filled with corpses, and how it forced her to face death and come to understand it as a connection to our animal past. "Corpses keep the living tethered to reality . . . We are all just future corpses." Doughty shares my revulsion at today's treatment of the elderly, at a society that values length of life over quality, and at placing humans who have long since lost their ability to think and communicate into rows of stinking beds in lonely rooms with poor care. She writes that she finds corpses with decubitus ulcers [severe bedsores] "more painful for me to care for than even babies or suicides." I don't blame her.

She goes on to propose an ambitious and refreshing upheaval of American attitudes towards death and dying. She describes a Buddhist meditation on the nine stages of decomposition that is designed to detach the monk from the desire for permanence: distension (*choso*), rupture (*kaiso*), exudation of blood (*ketsuzoso*), putrefaction (*noranso*), discoloration and desiccation (*seioso*), consumption by animals and birds (*lanso*), dismemberment (*sanso*), bones (*kosso*), and parched to dust (*shoso*). She argues that "a culture that denies death is a barrier to achieving a good death." She eventually opens an alternative funeral practice and devotes her career to educating and improving modern culture and legislation surrounding death.

I met a man once with an octopus tattoo who could barely breathe and begged me to let him die. He was in his thirties, nice house, nice girlfriend. He had epiglottitis, a respiratory infection that is common for children but incredibly rare in adults. So rare, he told me, that he had been studied at Hopkins. *Hopkins*, he rasped. His girlfriend had called us and as soon as we saw him, we jumped into the speed of what we assumed would be a load-and-go call. Epiglottitis causes swelling that squeezes the airway closed. This man's face was mottled, his skin pale and sweaty. His veins bulged with the effort of breathing. But when we got close to him with medication he swatted away the nebulizer and mumbled at us to back off. We thought he might be confused from the hypoxia, but after a few minutes it was clear that he was coherent: alert, sound of mind, and desperate not to return to a hospital. His girlfriend had called 911 against his wishes.

"I know!" he shouted, his voice a hoarse gasp. "I know it can kill me! And if that's how I go, that's how I go!" He ran away from us into the backyard, and used a garden hose to cool down the painful swelling in his mouth and throat. The stream of water splashed down his face and chest and onto the tile courtyard. He stopped to breathe between every two or three words. "This thing has gotten me five times. Five." Gasp. "Times!" Gasp. "I wake up in a hospital [gasp], tubes coming out of [gasp] every [gasp] part of me! A tube in my throat [gasp]. Tubes [gasp] in my arms [gasp]. A tube coming out of my dick!"

His eyes were red, his hair matted. His chest heaved like a sled dog after a sprint. He told us how horrifying it is to wake up like that, and to live in constant fear of the next time this disease would try to take his life. We stayed on scene for almost an hour with a man who I did not think would survive another fifteen minutes. We begged him to let us care for him, explained that without the proper paperwork, as soon as he passed out, we would be forced to intubate him.

My supervisor leaned over and said, quietly, "If we crich this guy, I'm doing it." Fine. All you. He is talking about a field cricothyrotomy—a dramatic but rarely-used procedure in which the neck is sliced open to force a tube into a closed airway. The man would wake up with a hole in his throat and a jagged, backyard-job scar on his neck. He might wake up on a vent. He might not wake up.

He was so young, though, this guy. And so alive. His house looked like the house of someone with hobbies, and dreams, and a favorite food. I tried to focus on the medicine, to see the man's respiratory rate and medical history instead of his life story, but pieces of his personality kept breaking through. His tattoos, his beard. I thought of all the tired bodies I had forced back to life over the years, too old and confused to tell me to stop. And this man, this young, otherwise healthy man who still had the agency to say these things and control his fate. This man who I could probably save.

He pushed through us like an NFL player, body-blocked my supervisor, and ran into the night. His torso heaved as he ran, and we expected him to stumble or lose consciousness before he got down the driveway. But I watched his outline disappear down the street and thought, *Goddamn, the human spirit can fight.* I'm not sure what was most astonishing, the man's strength to stay alive or his will to die. I never saw him again.

After a decade in EMS I begin to love talking to people about death. It's such a loaded subject, and one that those in our culture are inclined to sidestep around awkwardly. I enjoy helping people allow themselves to feel conflicted about grief. I learn to explain the scary parts and the gross parts in terms that are more comfortable and compassionate. I tell people that we pushed on her chest to keep blood moving to the brain, and we used a tube to breathe for her, but despite all our best efforts we weren't able to get her heart to pump on its own again. I say that I see so much sickness and death and how much of a difference it makes when a patient appears to have been loved and well cared for. How comfortable this home looks, and how I can see how much you helped her each week. I can't know for sure whether my words have any impact in the long run, but more often than not they seem to have a positive effect in the moment.

I actually find death itself grounding, a reminder that we are all of the earth and someday our bodies will die and decompose. Sometimes I sit with a dead body for a minute, feeling my breath move in and out of my chest and staring at their stillness. If I don't run a code for a long time I feel a little lost; life itself becomes a floating, dreamy experience with no tangible beginning and no end.

Usually, we will usher family out of the room. But not always. I worked a code just before dawn once, during my paramedic field internship in Santa Cruz, where the loved one stayed with us. We arrived to find a young couple who had been living in one of the dorm-style family rooms at the homeless shelter. They were surrounded by empty bottles and meth accessories and it would have been easy to judge. But the woman was dead and the man's pain was sincere.

The hallway was too small for the man to leave. He crouched in a corner and watched as we tried to revive his wife. At first, he was filled with panic, shouting to us and to her, begging her to stay alive. But as the code progressed he became more and more quiet. I saw something pass over his face after our third or fourth round of medication with no change to her flaccid heart. As we sweated over her, pounding her chest, pushing drugs, checking the monitor, pushing more drugs, pumping air, I saw his shoulders drop and his posture change. After twenty or thirty minutes his face seemed to register a level of understanding and acceptance that I don't get to see when family members wait outside. Spouses will ask the crew member keeping them company questions like "How's he doing?" and "Is he awake yet?" as, inside, we pull a sheet over the body and disconnect our gear. But by watching the whole process, by seeing our efforts and the anatomic contortions in his wife's face and torso, this man's frenzied desperation turned to still grief. I imagined that he had seen death before, or some version of it, because as we finally stopped compressions and began to explain he shook his head, waved us off and said, simply, "I know."

There's another call we ran, towards the end of my internship in Santa Cruz, which feels like a lifetime ago. It was in the latest part of a long shift, right before night becomes morning, way out on the east side of town by the ocean. There must have been waves that night because I remember smelling salt on the air as we trudged inside, half asleep in the dark. We walked up a narrow staircase lined with photos of sailboats and smiling moustached white men standing in the sun. I could feel the sea breezes whipping their seventies haircuts, broad shoulders, and salt-chafed hands.

A full engine and ambulance crew piled into an upstairs bedroom where a man lay in a large bed with a couple of family members. Thick quilts covered his legs and his back was propped up against dozens of pillows. His skin was pale and his breathing came in wheezes and rasps. He sucked air in and out and his eyes popped, the bug-eyed stare of someone who isn't getting enough oxygen. His hands clawed at the bedding. The firefighter closest to bedside rushed over and started to set up an oxygen mask as the family all began to speak at once.

"He's on hospice," they said. "He's supposed . . . he's supposed to stay home."

"We weren't supposed to call you."

"His breathing, I'm sorry, we just weren't expecting . . . we weren't . . . we didn't . . ."

We put the man on an oxygen mask and watched for a few minutes. He sounded like an athlete who had just finished a race, panting, sucking in air. His eyes started to relax, and over several minutes his skin pinked up. We got more of the story from the family. The man was on hospice for end-stage lung cancer, his family was gathered at bedside, a few minutes ago his breath had become wheezy and shallow.

There was a wife, a son, and a woman I assumed was the daughter-in-law. Everyone looked like they were about to cry. I took a moment to look around the room. More sailing photos, a painting of a crashing wave, old wallpaper with peeling corners. The room felt lived in but not cluttered. It was cozy in there, the thick warmth of an upstairs room filled with furniture and family. Only a few lights were on, so the wood-paneled walls appeared a deep yellow, as though seen through Tiffany glass.

The man's breathing started to slow back down. He was looking better and better. We called the hospice nurse. She said she could bring some oxygen over but she was about an hour away.

Everyone slowed their pace down, stopped pulling equipment around and settled in a little. We talked the family down for a few minutes, listened to the man's lungs, and checked his heart on the monitor. He looked okay now—he was doing much better with the oxygen mask. We told the family that we didn't have enough oxygen in our portable bottles to last until the nurse showed up. They seemed to understand the situation, and were clearly doing their best to stay calm. We told them it could get really bad.

"I know," said the son. He blinked. "I think I get it."

The family started to tell us about his life, and his disease. He'd been in decline for a few months now, and they'd decided to pull treatment and get ready. He wanted to die at home, in this bed, with these photos on the walls. They told us it had been going okay but when his breathing changed they panicked.

One of the firefighters was a larger guy who I worked with a lot during my internship. He was usually kind of mean and impatient with people, but on that call, even he seemed soft.

We explained that we could transport the man to the hospital if they'd like, where he could stay on oxygen. The patient shook his head. He knew that if he was taken to the hospital that night, he wasn't coming back home.

"I'll be okay," he told us between gasps. "I've got it." His hands stretched out against the quilt.

He said he wanted to stay home. He said he would try to breathe better so the family wasn't scared. They took turns holding his hand, sitting with him. The room was a good size, but with the family, the engine crew, and the medics all packed in against the bed, it felt small.

Our oxygen tank started to run low. We pulled the oxygen mask off and turned off the bottle. He started breathing harder almost immediately; the only noise in the room was his gasps. We called hospice again. His oxygen saturation dropped to 70 percent. He pulled in air with his chest, ribs, stomach, neck. His eyes were wet but determined. We made some small talk, we complimented his home. We chatted about who had run calls here before, earlier in his disease. The old man spoke in short, choppy sentences between breaths. Everyone was blown away by the detail of his memories of those earlier calls, which were more accurate than our own. The battalion chief near his head adjusted his pillow slightly and put a hand on his shoulder. We asked how he was feeling.

"Much . . ." he panted, "better." We watched his struggle, silent in the dim room. "Your oxygen . . . helped." His skin was growing pale again, his oxygen saturation slowly dropping. "It's already . . . beginning . . . to subside," he said, and then stopped trying to talk. Sixty-eight percent. Sixty-four. Sixty-one. His hands grasped and then released. He and his wife stared at each other, quiet. She nodded, slowly, and he nodded back.

"We're okay," she said to us. "We'll be okay."

She thanked us for coming out and apologized again. I often made fun of my Santa Cruz co-workers for all being from such similar backgrounds—it's such a small town—but there was something about this man, I thought, that reminded every guy in this room of his dad.

We packed up our gear, shook everyone's hands, and slowly filed back out of the room. We told them to call us back if they needed us. On the way down the stairs I saw the photos again of a smiling, broad-shouldered man on a boat. Younger days, brighter times. We took the beach road home and on the drive back I saw the first hint of sunrise against the water.

"UNTIL YOU START SEEING BODIES"

JODY GEARE, EMT/FIREFIGHTER,
TWENTY YEARS IN EMS AND FIREFIGHTING
APTOS, CALIFORNIA

I remember my first campaign fire; it was down south. Until then, I had only been on small fires. We drove old-ass engines back then with no air conditioning. I sat in the middle of a bench seat, between an operator and another fireman. You'd have your knees tucked into your chest every time you hit a bump. I was never scared back then. The thought of getting hurt or dying didn't even enter my brain. When you don't think about what it does, fire is awesome. I mean, fire at night is the most beautiful thing I've ever seen. We go on fires that are so big that they create their own weather systems. Where else in the world do you have a job like that?

But then I remember civilians running up to the engine screaming. Once you add the human element, that's what makes it feel real. Realizing that someone can get hurt, or someone's belongings are getting destroyed. Fire is awesome until you start seeing bodies, or dealing with the aftermath.

SEASONS PASS

The fog is thick and wet outside my bathroom window. It's June, the time of year when tourists arrive in Santa Cruz wearing flip-flops and board shorts, then head to the beach to shiver in the wind. I'm lying on the cool tile floor, recovering from ankle surgery. The narcotics have killed my appetite and constipated me, so I'm light-headed and full of cramping abdominal pain. I try to pull myself to the toilet but knock over my crutches and the noise wakes my roommate.

The whole time I'm lying there I've been thinking about work. I've probably been on hundreds of calls for constipation. Mostly old women, usually alone. *Is this what they felt like?* I ask myself, even though I know the answer. No. They felt much worse. You could see it in their eyes. They were fragile, and scared, and alone. They curled over the toilet like bass clefs, backs kyphotic and pale, thin fingers gripping the counter or the side of the bowl. Their bathrooms were decorated with dollar store shell soap or affirmations in cheap frames. Their translucent skin was pastry crust over bent bones.

Sometimes they dialed the phone themselves for the pain, or pressed their medical alert button. Maybe a caregiver found them and called. As I rest my cheek on the tile floor and hug my stomach, I think of a small woman who had called us in desperate pain. Her pills were scattered on the counter, and after a few minutes of conversation we discovered she had been taking Vicodin to control the pain of her constipation. Vicodin, like all narcotic painkillers, causes severe constipation. You can figure out the rest.

I look down at my stomach and think of hers. Mine is skinnier than usual from the injury but still muscular, with few stray hairs and mostly smooth skin. Old lady stomachs are frail, and sunken, and the skin gathers towards the bottom of the torso in thin folds. If the blockage is severe they pouch out a bit towards the pelvis, like the distended belly of a starving child. I think of starting IVs on these women, finding tiny spiderweb veins under cloudy skin. Even the smallest size of needle seems to rip the flesh apart.

Occasionally at the wealthier nursing homes you'll find a concerned family member, but usually the women wait alone. Often their eyes slowly track us into the room. Sometimes they are too faint or confused to look up. Sometimes they snap at us for stepping on the carpet. These women have survived wars, careers, good and bad marriages. Most have photos in the room, and souvenirs. Some rooms are sparse and we are left to make up our own stories. One aching woman had been a casino card dealer for twenty-five years. I asked her if the dealers ever hooked up with the pit bosses and she smiled and closed her eyes. "Oh, honey," she whispered. "You have no idea."

The memory of her thinning hair and fake nails brings me some comfort as I lie on the floor. I wonder how it will feel to have reached an age where my own bones will crack at a ground-level fall, where my knees will bulge awkwardly at the sides of frail legs. I glance at the ticking bathroom clock, think about how quickly seasons seem to pass, and figure I'll find out soon enough.

FORM C

TEXT OF INTERVIEW (UNEDITED)

FOLKLORE
——
NEW YORK

STATE   New York

NAME OF WORKER Clarence Weinstock

ADDRESS   43 Morton Street

DATE   June 5

SUBJECT   Ambulance Driver's Story

HARLEM AMBULANCE

Busy? Boy you ain't seen nothing. You got to come up for the weekend. It's a madhouse. Stabbings, g.y.'s and poison, in and out, in and out. Take 120th and Lenox. There's a bunch of night clubs around there. The stiffs start falling out of there after midnight. If they go west, they're all right; if they go east, god help 'em.FFFT!

When do we drive fastest? Well I couldn't say. Formerly we used to go like hell if we had an O.B.S. because of the kid dropped in the car, the doc and driver had to buy a keg a beer for all the boys on the shift.

You can't drive fast up here. People are so used to us they don't get out of the way any more like they do in other parts of town. Still I get em back as quick as I can; they're no different than any other people, though some of the guys thing, "I'M better than any of them, why should I risk my life they feel like killing one another." I don't figger that way. It's poverty that does it, four of five of them in one room, all of Harlem sleeps in one room. What the hell, here's a girl I just brought in. Lysol. Husband kicked her out. Where's she to go? You answer me that. Here's a call, So long.

****

Clarence Weinstock, "Ambulance Driver's Story," New York City, New York, 1939.

"YOU EVER SEEN A DEAD BODY?"

JAMIE PREDMORE, PARAMEDIC/FIREFIGHTER;

EIGHTEEN YEARS IN EMS

NINILCHIK, ALASKA

My first EMT job ever? Oh, boy. I found the job posting on Craigslist, you know, where everything reputable comes from [laughs]. I applied, and I got the interview. The owner of the company had been an EMT for nine years but had never worked as an EMT. He had applied to work for AMR but never got hired, and he had put his rejection letter up on the wall of the main office right next to his business license.

During the interview portion, he was asking the typical stuff, like why do you want to be an EMT, what got you interested in this field . . . And then he just leans in and says, "Have you ever seen a dead body?"

He gave me this look of intensity. Like he wanted to be the one to freak me out. And when I said that yeah, I had, he was disappointed. He wanted to fuck me up.

I believe a good term for the interview would be "awesomely bad."

I worked there for six months. It was nuts. Some parts of it were good. I think that a lot of people, myself included, when we go through EMT school we have this idea about working in a 911 system. But there is a very warm place in my heart for the inter-facility transport side of the business. It teaches you to work with a gurney, and move patients, and talk to nurses, and locate pertinent information in paperwork. Imagine one of your family members being hospitalized, and getting transported, and think about the people that you'd want to be there in that moment. What if it was a really kind, enthusiastic, compassionate individual? I think that's important. I think those guys don't get enough credit, especially the ones that stick it out for a little bit and try to learn as much as they can learn.

So those were the good elements. But as I said, the owner was out of his mind. The craziest part is that everyone I know in EMS has met a guy like this. We all have this story! What kind of psychos are we working with here?

I had to work a twenty-four with him on Thanksgiving, alone. He said all kinds of disgusting and inappropriate things to me, made creepy jokes. At one point I surprised him and he said, "Oh, you're lucky I didn't have my gun with me, I would have shot you in the face." I was like, okay, I feel real safe. As time progressed, he alienated almost every facility we worked with by either saying something offensive or sexually harassing the staff. My twenty-year-old brain was not ready to be in these awkward situations. But it did help me learn!

I eventually quit and went to a different inter-facility company, and I had a much better experience. They had procedures and standard operating guidelines. I wasn't afraid for my safety all the time.

Most people that have worked in IFT act like that is a part of their career that they want to forget. We say, "Oh, I don't do that anymore." But honestly, the calls that I ran there gave me a huge wealth of knowledge and a skill set for being able to deal with difficult situations.

There was one time when we transported this kid from a psychiatric facility, on a 5150 [the Californian term for an involuntary psychiatric hold]. He was my age, about twenty-one, I think. As soon as we pulled away from the hospital he just gets completely naked. He was not in restraints. My partner couldn't help me, because we were on the middle of the Bay Bridge. So I had to learn how to rely on myself. As stressful as it was for me, it helped me show myself a capacity to grow. You're always building on what you have done and coming up with new things that you can do, and your arsenal just keeps getting bigger and bigger in terms of tools for how to deal with chaos.

HOW TO WRITE A FILM SCENE
WITH AN AMBULANCE

(Inspiration stolen from Africa Is Not a Country:
Notes on a Bright Continent *by Dipo Faloyin, who stole it
from Binyavanga Wainaina's* How to Write About Africa.*)*

Sirens. Lots of sirens. Flashing lights. More sirens. All calls are code three, every time. We are always in a hurry. Do not under any circumstances ever depict paramedics running a non-emergent call.

If your television show or film requires the audience to know that a character has died, feel free to park an ambulance outside the house in question. We do not have anywhere else to be. When a dead body is found, we are happy to sit out of service flashing our lights dramatically for several hours while police, detectives, and CSI complete a full investigation and then eventually put the body on our medical gurney to be taken to the morgue. Our management is fine with this. Definitely do not call the coroner or the funeral home transport service. What even is a coroner anyway? Do they have a van? If they do, I bet it's boring and black and doesn't even have any flashing lights. Ugh. Lame.

If a patient has been rescued from a dramatic near-death experience—a fire, a terrorist attack, or a car sinking into a cold body of water (best)—do not lay them down on the gurney and turn the heat up in the ambulance. Hypothermia prevention is boring. These patients are to be sat on the tailgate and wrapped in a thin blanket to have meaningful conversations with their friends and loved ones while we medics stand around in uniform and . . . hold a clipboard, for some reason? We will stand to the side such that the blanketed character may freely achieve emotional resolution with their loved ones. Do not under any circumstances show paramedics packaging or treating or transporting these patients. During Tailgate Blanket Catharsis time, your medics may not perform any medical assessment or intervention other than the following: (1) blood pressure, and (2) gently patting an open wound with a piece of gauze.

If one of your main characters—say, a middle-aged anesthesiologist at a major Seattle hospital—wishes to become a first responder halfway through their season, tell them to go for it. They do not require any additional training or certification. They do not need to spend five or ten years getting their EMT certification, paramedic license, and Fire 1 certification. They absolutely do not need to wait two years for their local fire service to test, interview, complete background checks and medical exams, and schedule a new recruit academy. They can and should have several arguments with their spouse about their plans and then waltz easily into their closest local fire station to accept their new position. We are lucky to have them.

On a similar note, *paramedic* and *EMT* are totally interchangeable. They are the same word, and they describe the same thing: a uniform, a light bar, and a generalized sense of excitement and heroism. And lots of sirens. *Bee-do bee-do!*

If you would like to feature an actual medical emergency in your television or film, you have many options. All of them are traumas, heart attacks, deadly allergic reactions, and cardiac arrests. Paramedics do not run medical calls on patients with social issues, chronic diseases, or recurring symptoms. When you need to create tension, have the patient suffering from injury that is curable only by breaking a protocol to perform a dramatic procedure that will immediately save this patient's life. Do not take your patient to the hospital, where a doctor can perform this intervention. Definitely do not use any of the other skills or techniques that you have spent years learning to stabilize a patient exactly like this until they can receive appropriate treatment. Medical science is not a complicated, thoughtful process in which level-headed professionals try their best to use imperfect tools to improve a situation. On the contrary! It is binary. There is Saving a Life, and there is Not Saving a Life.

Important: have your medics make a lot of eye contact across the body during this tense moment of tension (remember: everyone is a medic because EMTs do not exist). When the Rebel Save a Life Paramedic decides to go against the advice of the Scaredy Pants Not Saving a Life Paramedic, the bravery will be rewarded. Sketchy, Hail Mary interventions without any previous training or practice always work the on the first try. They do not waste time, prove ineffective, and potentially cause further injury to the patient. The patient will definitely not deteriorate or die while the Rebel Save a Life Paramedic slashes blindly around the trachea, looking for an anatomical landmark that she read about in a textbook six years ago. The county medical director will not immediately pull her paramedic license, light it on fire, and then drop the ashes through a paper shredder. No. What will happen is the patient will gasp and open their eyes. Patients always gasp and open their eyes when they are cured; this is crucial. Now you may transport to the hospital. Not a moment sooner.

If you must, against your better instincts, use an EMT or paramedic as a character in your plot, know that we are hard-working and honest folk. We are the pure corporeal embodiment of the phrase "just doing my job, ma'am." When a character in your teen vampire romance needs a moment of self-reflection into what his life could have been if he had been "good" instead of complicated, make him a paramedic. When a surgeon needs a humble and honest fiancé that she can dump to run off with her challenging-but-passionate true love, make that guy a paramedic too.

Remember this, if nothing else: as a people, we are brave, kind, and stupid.

Also: sirens!

Author's Note: Notable exceptions to these instructions include but are not limited to: (1) Nic Cage in Bringing Out the Dead—*a New York City paramedic who burns out, does drugs, hallucinates, pursues a patient's daughter, and drinks on the clock (this movie is great), and (2) Chris Sullivan as the ambulance driver in* The Knick—*a brash, drunk, working-class Irishman who helps a nun perform covert abortions (this show is also great).*

NOT DEAD

We get called one afternoon to another cardiac arrest in a single-room occupancy in San Francisco. These buildings, called *SROs* by locals, are common downtown. They were built long before modern construction codes. They are tall and crowded, with ancient plumbing and rotting walls. The stairs are steep, the hallways skinny. The rooms are small boxes without kitchens or bathrooms; each floor shares a communal toilet down the hall.

The dispatch notes tell us a body was found by the janitor and it sounds as though we are going to an obvious death, unworkable, but we still bring all of our gear just in case. The red medical backpack, the oxygen bag, the cardiac monitor. A bone drill and a portable suction unit. The gurney is piled high when I wrench back the rusty iron elevator gate and push into the hallway. When we get to the room the fire engine crew is already there and one of the guys is rolling his eyes at me and sawing his hand at his neck to say "never mind."

"Guy's been here a while," he says. "All yours."

My partner nods, says he'll go get the laptop, and starts to leave. He gives me the portable monitor and turns the gurney around with the rest of the gear to take it downstairs in the elevator. I glance into the room. The three members of the fire engine crew are all climbing over each other to leave, one pinching his nose for the smell. They are a famously bedraggled engine, the busiest in the city, and the guys giving me this particular hand-off are as distracted as ever.

The room is small even for an SRO. The dead body lies on the bed, face down, with a big shit river sliding from the back pocket of his pants all the way down to his feet, where it drips slowly to the floor. His face is pressed into the stained sheets of a small twin bed. I see trash, empty bottles, a meth pipe—all the usual downtown decorations. I pick my way around dirty clothes and plastic bags towards the shit puddle and look at the corpse. It's pale, immobile, and smells a bit rotted. My supervisor is on his phone in the hallway but everyone else has left the floor. Just me and you, buddy.

For paperwork reasons we place the cardiac monitor leads on every patient who is found too dead for CPR, and confirm asystole. The monitor banks the data in case we ever get sued by a ghost. Which, today, might be more likely than I first realize.

I stand limp for a minute holding the monitor at my side. It's bulky, and heavy, and I have to figure out somewhere to set it down that's not covered in spilled alcohol, rotting food, or feces. I stare at the guy for a while. I don't even know where I'm going to place the leads. His T-shirt covers his back. Everything below his waist is covered in brown fluid. There's nowhere to put stickers on without either cutting his clothes or moving him or some other intervention that will both (a) piss off the coroner and (b) be super gross.

As I stare at the man's back I slowly realize that something about this scene isn't adding up. His back rises and falls just a little, slowly, rhythmically, maybe a centimeter at most. Up, pause. Down . . . pause. Up . . .

"Oh, FUCK me," I say out loud. "You've got to be FUCKING kidding me." I grab his shoulder and flip him over. The man groans and looks up at me. I shout at him. He mumbles a little. Not dead. So not dead.

My supervisor, Roberts, hears the commotion and sticks his head in the room. He's an old-timer with a faded Welsh accent and sandy hair that drags over his eyes. "All right, Jo?" he asks.

"This guy's alive," I say. "He's responsive. He's not even, all I did was—"

Roberts doesn't let me finish. *"Fooookin' bloody hell!"* he blurts, and shakes his head. He tears off down the hallway without saying anything else. I am again alone in the room. Well, no. I am not alone.

I have no gurney. I have no equipment. I have the cardiac monitor, which I realize I am still holding at my right side, and still have nowhere reasonable to set down. I look over at the formerly dead guy, who is now awake but dazed, and staring back at me wordlessly.

"They thought you were dead. They . . . uh . . . What's your name?"

He still looks blank. He's high, or drunk, or maybe dead after all, albeit the breathing, groaning, sitting-up sort of dead. I get on my radio and ask my partner to bring the gurney back upstairs. I drop the monitor onto a slightly less wet corner of bedsheet and place the blood pressure cuff and stickers on the guy. I try to ask him a few more questions, but he just blinks at the ground and mumbles. I get a first name out of him, and the rest is low-pitched zombie noises. His blood pressure, heart rate, and oxygen saturation come back stable. He's still breathing fine. I fold my arms and lean back. Well, here we are. We wait.

Eventually my partner walks in and we pour the patient onto the gurney. In the elevator, I tell him what happened. "They didn't even do a shake and shout! They didn't even look at him! You could fucking see chest rise, dude. He was breathing the whole time!" Andrew looks down at me, expressionless.

When we get downstairs, Roberts has herded the entire engine crew into the lobby of the SRO. The elevator door opens into a gauntlet of sheepish firefighters with their hands folded like school-children. They peer up at me with pinched looks that I'm not sure are entirely remorse. They seem to question whether I'm going to *make a thing* out of this or not. I nod slowly as I pass them, trying to make my face indicate that no, I'm not going to write them up, but maybe they should suck less next time. We get the guy in the ambulance and do a workup; nothing really comes up interesting. He just seems wasted, maybe septic, maybe just confused. We take him over to St. Matthias. I tell the nurse his chief complaint is *not dead*.

THIS IS LOVE

It's hard, in a series of essays, to describe the day in and day out grind of the work. Once you get used to the bright blinking lights and screaming sirens, the calls mush together, water drips down the page and blurs the ink. One day I take notes about some of the calls I ran that day, just to do *something* with them, to make some record of the endless parade of humanity that I carry on my shoulders. I am not allowed to take protected medical information home from work, like the patient's name or exact appearance, but I write down images, emotions, and scattered dialogue. It becomes a way of feeling as though I exist in the world, as though these people and their stories are real, rather than just one long strange fever dream. The notes become an anchor for me, a way to keep from floating away.

Most calls, despite all of the drama and emotion, are ultimately forgettable. Your brain runs on five or ten or fifteen per day and it is simply not possible to remember them all. The eighty-two-year-old with diarrhea, the drunk thirty-four-year-old at the club, the fifty-eight-year-old with a migraine. Maybe I start an IV, run fluids, or just give them a ride. I probably do my assessment, check them out physically, and recommend transport to the closest facility. I call the patient sir or ma'am as I tuck the blanket into the gurney around their hips. As we start driving I hook them up to the monitor, and then change my gloves so that I can start charting on the way over. I might ask about family or how long they have lived in the city as I punch numbers into my laptop. Probably recheck vital signs as the ambulance bumps along through traffic. Maybe glance at my phone once I run out of things to say. When we get close to the hospital I call in a report on the radio, grab one more blood pressure, and pull the cardiac monitor stickers off of the chest. Wipe down the lead cables and roll them up as my partner backs the rig into a tight parking lot. By the end of the day I will forget their face, and after a week the whole call is erased but for the one-word description in my notebook. *Diarrhea.* Who knows what that means, who that man was, what he was feeling that day. Maybe he remembers the ride just as dimly, as a slow taxi to a hospital stay. Hopefully he thinks the paramedic was kind.

Tucked in between dozens of nice people with minor complaints and mean people with minor complaints are the occasional heavy hitters, the ones that leave a mark. After several days of stomach aches and drunk folks, one day we drive slowly to a code two call to put someone back to bed. We arrive to find she has been on the floor for several days and is confused, hypotensive, and covered in infected sores. We rush her to the hospital code three, clean up the ambulance, and on our way to our very next call are T-boned in an intersection by a tiny red car that shoots out from behind a stalled Muni bus. The driver of the red car is transported by another unit for rib pain. My partner and I are fine but the ambulance is busted and the paperwork takes a few hours. We get back out on the street in time to run our last call of the day: a twenty-two-year-old who killed himself with a zip tie around the neck. My journal that day offers this: "Nice roommates, fucked up call."

The next day I am back for more routine complaints: Dizziness. Shortness of breath. Alcohol. Heroin. Abdominal pain. Fell out of bed. Another dizziness.

A few weeks later, another call cuts through the noise.

Syncope. AMA. Old gay couple.

This one I remember. An elderly married couple. Any gay men in San Francisco past a certain age; it means they lived through the AIDS epidemic. They watched most of their loved ones die. They survived. I remember these particular men so vividly: the dark room, the art on the walls. A series of watercolor portraits, arranged carefully above a cluttered desk. A large abstract in deep earth tones, made more muted by the dim light. Above the bed hung a ceramic sculpture of two faces intertwined, so different stylistically that I wondered briefly if it was made by a friend or purchased on vacation. "AMA" means "against medical advice": that is, the man refused to come with us. He spoke quietly, and eloquently, and told us he didn't want to die in a hospital. That if it was his time, he was ready. We sat with them for over an hour until we were confident that he understood his situation and was making his choice with a clear mind. The husband, almost twenty years younger, was terrified but full of love. He begged his husband to go to the hospital but ultimately respected his wishes. My supervisor burst in the door with concerns about rules and liability but softened as she came to know the situation. In the end I don't remember which one of them actually said the words that I wrote down in the margin of my notebook: "I am stubborn. He is patient. This is love." I don't think it matters who said it. We left them in each other's arms, perhaps for the last time. We should all be so lucky to find what it means to be family.

JOURNAL, JUNE 2015

An old memory comes to mind: sitting in the medical tent at Burning Man, talking to an older guy. An RN or PA, maybe. He says, "You're a junkie. You're always gonna need something more, a heavier hit. In the beginning, you're going to love being a medic. Driving fast, codes, traumas. You're going to love it. But that's going to wear off. The rush will wear off, and you're going to need something else, something more. It's not going to last."

After learning how to be an EMT and then medic school and two years in Reno, I get a job back home in Santa Cruz and I'm so blindingly happy to be back near an ocean that my second day here I take a stupid risk surfing and shatter my ankle. Surgery, cast, boot, benched for another three months. It's tremendously shitty.

After a month or two I start to get real, real depressed. I stop giving a shit about surfing or mountain bikes or anything and I just want to go back to work. I don't feel like myself without it. I miss the puzzles, the excitement, the heartache.

Things get difficult with Kyle because I don't feel like there's anything in me worthwhile enough to flirt with. I feel like a waste of space. We're at dinner one night and I'm picking at a bowl of soup and trying to make conversation. He catches my eye and says, "You really miss it, don't you. You . . . you get a thrill out of it?"

I put down my spoon and want to cry.

"Yeah. Yeah, I really do." Then I ramble a bit, trying to explain myself, but it comes out bullshit and I go back to my soup.

"WE ARE IN THAT FUTURE"

DAN QUINTO, RETIRED EMS SUPERVISOR;
FORTY-SEVEN YEARS IN EMS
SANTA CRUZ, CALIFORNIA

Generally speaking, 911 has gotten busier. I would like to say that it ebbs and flows, but it certainly seems to flow way more than it ebbs.

These days it's all streamlining, it's all economics. We all work under UHUs now, "unit hour utilizations." If your UHUs aren't high enough—that is, if you're not running enough calls per day—then they're going to take that unit away. I mean, no matter who you are, you're going to bitch about your job. But it's gotten really bad. Who wants to stay in a medical job where your company is happier the busier you are, but you don't have time to go to the bathroom, or do a proper patient assessment?

I would have never said this years ago, but I think ambulances need to be run by a third service. That is when the government provides the ambulance agency, but it is run separately from the fire department or the police. The Department of Public Health ambulances in San Francisco was third service, Denver was a third service. They were highly successful, career positions. And then they were all enveloped by the fire agencies, because counties looked at it and went, *Why are we paying for two separate infrastructures for the same job?* They thought it was the same job. It's not my intention to talk disparagingly about the fire service. But their involvement changed EMS dramatically.

Prior to them getting paramedics, they went to fires. They didn't go to traffic accidents unless they were requested, and they didn't go to the little lady who fell in the produce aisle. As they got into the paramedic business, they had to go to those calls. And they started realizing that those are the kinds of calls that exist in 911.

We had to change the educational standards for the fire service. It's not because they're not smart. But it's not the way they were taught to think. It is a different mindset. It was very rigid and streamlined. They can't get past sometimes that A and B don't always lead to C. The fire service has a training system for what they do. There's a reason for it. It may work when you need to learn how to tie a knot, or swing an axe. But there is a different mindset to do medicine. I mean, we have paramedics who were never firemen who have the same problem. But I saw it especially when I was teaching. We finally adopted some of their methods, because that was the only way they would be successful.

It was shown that way in the media, on television. In *Adam-12*, for example, there's an episode where police officers rotate onto the ambulance. Because it's not an important job, anybody can do it. You just rotate somebody through it. That's what it's like with the fire agencies. They are very good at what they do, but EMS is not their job. And it shouldn't be. The thought process of medicine is very different than fighting a fire. There are some that can change their way of thinking to run medical calls, but very few.

Another big change is that until what I consider modern times, everywhere I worked had a base station that you actually talked to and consulted with. It was a huge deal in how people cared for their patient, and how they were able to follow up and get feedback about their patient. As you gained your relationship with the base providers, they would really get to know you as a practitioner. As they grew to trust you, your orders would become bigger and bigger. You would go to base station meetings every month. You were required to go. They would review tapes, and it would be a frank review. Sometimes too frank! But then we had a forum to discuss it with your peers and with the doctors. That feedback loop doesn't exist anymore.

A lot of it went away due to finances, with ERs getting busier. They cast away the idea of base doctors and wrote standing orders instead. We still have base hospitals, but we have a nebulous relationship with them. And when we do call, nine times out of ten the attitude is "What are you calling me for? What do you want?"

It's a complicated problem, and one little thing isn't going to fix it.

Ambulances have never been profitable. We're the last to be paid, if we get paid at all. Most of the smaller companies were mom-and-pop shops, up until AMR's dominance of the industry. Your returns—that is, what you billed and what you got back—really depended on how big of an asshole you were. I knew one company owned by lawyers, and they had a collection rate that was astronomical! And nobody in the community liked them.

We do medical reimbursement so wrong in this country. We do it wrong, and we know it's wrong, the COVID-19 pandemic proved that it's wrong, and we don't want to go and change it. Because the people that would be in charge of changing it are the ones who are making money off of it.

That's my personal opinion. During the COVID-19 pandemic, everybody in Congress was talking about combat pay for first responders, and banging pots and pans. But then that was the end of it. Now we're just the guys that were taken for granted when they needed us.

We end up being the entry point for health care for a high percentage of our patients. We deal with the people that have nowhere else go, and we become their primary health care. Unfortunately, we can't do anything for them. We can take them to the hospital, where, generally speaking, they don't get the care that they need. And the hospitals often see us as bringing them these people that they don't want. Instead of listening to our report or treating us like equals, they'll cut off our report and say, "Oh, yeah, whatever. Put him over there."

What they don't see is the part where we had dragged this guy out of the bushes at the park, put up with abuse from him or his friend. But we have developed people skills, which are hard to teach, and learned how to communicate with him, and not all the time but often by the time we get him to the hospital he is in a better mood. I have a high respect for the paramedics that can complete their full assessment, every time, without skipping any steps. Nobody thinks about what you need to do to get that job, and then what you need to do to be successful in it, and then what you need to do to keep your sanity.

We've been saying for twenty years that we really need to sit back and take a critical look at how we deliver emergency medicine in this country, because it's not a sustainable model for the future. And now, we are in that future. We are here, and we ain't sustainable.

SAN FRANCISCO: SCARY NARNIA

*If the precious yellow metal hadn't been discovered in the aurif-
erous sands of the Sacramento Valley, the development of San
Francisco's underworld in all likelihood would have proceeded
according to the traditional pattern and would have been indis-
tinguishable from that of any other large American city. Instead,
owing almost entirely to the influx of gold-seekers and the
horde of gamblers, thieves, harlots, politicians and other felo-
nious parasites who battened upon them, there arose a unique
criminal district that for almost seventy years was the scene of
more viciousness and depravity, but at the same time possessed
more glamour, than any other area of vice and iniquity on the
American continent.*
HERBERT ASBURY, *The Barbary Coast: An Informal History
of the San Francisco Underworld*

*San Francisco values did not come into the world with flowers
in their hair; they were born howling, in blood and strife.*
DAVID TALBOT, *Season of the Witch: Enchantment, Terror,
and Deliverance in the City of Love*

This place is like scary Narnia.
Angel, back of the ambulance

We hop out of the rig and walk across the street to a couple of cops who look exhausted. They're both shifting their gaze around, looking at us, or up in the sky, or out at the street, or anywhere but down. On the sidewalk next to them is what looks like, from far away, an upside-down, thrusting vagina.

We both squint and walk a little slower. As I get closer, I realize that is in fact what I am looking at. I slow down even more. It's fucking Megan. She's got her shoulders and neck pressed into the ground like a circus contortionist, and her legs are spread-eagled up to the sky and thrusting up at us quickly, forcefully, desperately. A wet, open piston in a methamphetamine combustion engine. Pow, pow, pow, pow. Vagina! In! Your! Face!

It's dirty, hairy, and a little bit bloody. I find myself wondering if she's on her period or if we should transport her to our sexual assault receiving hospital. I wonder if you can even get periods when you use that much meth, and decide they should put that in medic school instead of spending so much time on the kidneys.

My partner leans over and whispers, "Don't look straight into the sun; it'll burn your eyes."

I shake my head and shout, "Hey! Megan!"

I try again, louder. "Megan!! You in there?! You got your pants upside down. Can we talk to you?"

She's busy screaming gibberish, sweating, thrusting. Her eyes are wide open and darting around the sockets like electricity. She can't hear a word we're saying. She's on fucking Mars right now. I guess I'll go get a sedative.

Everyone stands awkwardly, trying not to stare into the sun. No one wants to be the first one to put hands on her. Everyone tries talking to her or yelling at her, but it gets nowhere. Someone finally grabs an ankle and just sort of tips her back down onto the sidewalk. Now she's still thrusting but it's more of a sideways, fish-on-dry-land flopping motion instead of the bloody piston of doom. We get her restrained and give her a sedative.

At the hospital the nurse sighs. "Megan again? How was it this time?" "Oh, trust me, you don't want to know." I mention the blood and where it was located and the nurse looks like I just gave him a paper bag full of dog shit. I say, "I'm sorry, dude. I'm just trying to do the right thing."

I wash my hands for way too long and walk back out to the ambulance.

All over the streets of this city I can see brains zapping like batteries in a rainstorm, torn to shreds by meth, scattered through the avenues on an ocean breeze. Shards of personhood floating by.

Megan has a big personality and is one of the most well-known EMS clients in San Francisco. She is energetic, aggressive, and quick-witted. But she uses a lot of meth and often becomes hypersexual, thrusting or grabbing at paramedics and cops. I hear a medic complain once that she has probably sexually assaulted every single working first responder in the city, and if she were a man she would have been in jail years ago. The city has easily spent hundreds of thousands of dollars cycling her through the system—treating, transporting, hospitalizing, and releasing her again and again and again. Still, we hold a certain affection for her. We have all ducked her punches, pulled her hands out of our crotch, and yelled at her when she got on our last nerve. But we have also held her hair out of the way while she vomited, listened when she cried, and laughed with her when she landed a particularly cutting insult about our ambulance partner or a cop on scene.

I find her unconscious once, overdosed, and try to revive her but can't get a reaction. We transport her code three, breathing for her the whole way. I hear later that she spent a week intubated in the ICU following a polydrug overdose that day but eventually woke up and snuck out of the hospital to go back to using. We joke about putting one of her famous hats on the wall of the EMS office as a reminder—our all-star clients hall of fame.

A few years later, I learn that a murdered corpse found earlier that week belonged to her. Our high-volume patients often die young. I shouldn't be surprised anymore, but I still can't get past Megan's death. It feels personal somehow. It hurts like hell. I carry it around with me for years like a heavy briefcase that I don't know how to put down.

For most of my childhood, San Francisco was a blinking skyline. I'd roll a joint and walk up the hill from my parents' house in Oakland, staring across the bay at the glowing stegosaurus bridge and the tall thin pyramid of the Transamerica building. My favorite view was just after sunset, when the light began to dim and the colors took on a deep, matte hue that reminded me of a comic book. In the shadow of the evening I could handle the city, even admire its beauty. During the day it was all too harsh for me. I hated the traffic, hated the cement and buildings and cars. I would imagine grabbing a corner of the Bay Area and tearing the entire thing out from its roots like Velcro, ripping back asphalt and electrical lines and sewer pipes until the whole peninsula was raw dirt and grass.

I took the subway into the city sometimes, to see my grandparents or go to a concert. My abuelita—my great-grandmother—lived in a small apartment out by the water, with a skinny iron-gated elevator that had rusted in the ocean fog. I would use both hands to shove the gate open, trying not to catch a finger in the filigree. Even as a child I thought the mechanism seemed precarious, though at that time I never imagined trying to cram a gurney and a patient and three firefighters into it. San Francisco was a windy suburb to me, a place full of crowds but without the sense of home I always felt in Oakland.

In college I fell hard for a boy from San Francisco who worked as a builder, helping his dad create custom Victorian building-fronts for wealthy homeowners. We stayed at his parents' house in Bernal Heights for weeks at a time, where the family music collection spanned a floor-to-ceiling wall. We took buses across town and walked through our favorite neighborhoods, eating burritos and looking for bars that didn't check ID. But after the relationship ended, I didn't go back to the city for a long time.

It was the screwed-up economics of the 911 system that brought me back to San Francisco many years later. In the United States, there are three main ways to run an ambulance service: through a privately owned company, through the fire department, or through a municipal "third-service" agency. The nickname "third service" refers to the idea that the government should run police, fire, and EMS as the three branches of public safety. Third-service agencies are usually run by a public health department and are known around the water cooler as by far the best place to work. But they have become rare in modern times, and on the West Coast my options were pretty much either a privately owned company or fire.

At that point, I had spent two years in Reno and a little under a year in Santa Cruz working for two different private ambulance agencies. I loved being a paramedic, but it was hard to imagine withstanding the working conditions over the long term. In Reno, we worked four twelve-hour shifts per week and were often held over hours after our shifts were supposed to end. Even after I moved closer to the station to cut down on my commute, it was a constant battle to make sure I ate regular meals and slept more than six hours per night. In Santa Cruz, we worked twenty-four-hour shifts and often didn't sleep at all. I found myself nodding off at the steering wheel, swallowing down acid reflux during calls, and silently wishing my patients would either refuse care or die so that I could leave them at scene and go back to bed. I watched co-workers get kidney stones from pounding too many energy drinks, or end up in the same psych ward that we took our patients to. Behind all of our machismo, my friends and I always seemed injured, sick, or on the verge of an emotional breakdown.

I knew that despite how much I loved the job, the working conditions were simply not sustainable for more than a few years. There is a reason most paramedics end up training to become either firefighters or nurses. I understood that taking one of these paths would provide me with a much healthier lifestyle, but there was something about the ambulance that I didn't want to leave. I loved the street medicine, the sirens, the patient care. I found the actual work to be deeply fulfilling, and wished that there was a way to run calls that seemed like it wasn't destroying my body and mind.

I had heard that San Francisco's was one of two fire departments in the whole state of California that would hire what are called "single-function paramedics": that is, medics who staff the ambulance full-time rather than bouncing between the fire engine and "the box." The SFFD's schedule, pay, and benefits were dramatically better than at a private company, and when the chance came to take their test and apply for the job, I knew I had to give it a try. It was my first introduction to the grindingly slow processes of city politics: almost eighteen months passed between when I first tested and when I finally received a series of interviews, after which I was put back on hold.

But I did get the job, eventually, and the paramedic supervisor in Santa Cruz sighed when he crossed my name off the schedule. They were used to losing medics.

I had no time to consider a new living situation. After being in a holding pattern for almost two years, I received a formal offer letter only seventeen days before the academy was scheduled to begin. I called my parents in Oakland, and my older brother in San Francisco, and worked out a schedule of couches and spare rooms to sleep on and in during the six-week hiring academy.

A few days later, I arrived in San Francisco and put on another blue uniform. The training process was awkward: a lot of yelling and saluting and hearing how lucky we were to be there. I was issued a thin silver badge that I was expected to wear on my left chest pocket on duty.

On my weekends, I went back to Santa Cruz and shared a small two-bedroom with a local farmer, a hippie type who brought home produce and bundles of lavender from the market every Wednesday. Each week, I packed a duffel bag and drove an hour and a half up the coast for work. The commute was a bear, but I had grown attached to my life in the redwoods, and for a while I liked the separation between my two lives. Rent in San Francisco was astronomic, and I had no desire to live in the city full-time. My older brother, by then a successful tech sales type, offered up his spare room to help me make the job work. I would spend one or two nights a week with him, a couple nights in my truck, and the rest back home in Santa Cruz. I was grateful for his generosity but felt like an interloper in his space. The house was modern, with large windows and high ceilings. He kept it hermetically clean. I left my shoes outside in the garage, showered when I entered, and did my best not to let my dirty uniforms touch his cream-colored carpets. The bed was warm and soft but I sometimes felt more comfortable curled up in the back of the Tacoma at the beach.

In the locker room before my first shift, I learned that I was not the only medic who saw this as a once-in-a-lifetime opportunity. I met Flora, who came to the Bay Area from El Salvador at age seventeen. She had limped her way through academy on a torn left knee, clearly in more pain with morning workout. We sat with an ice pack after work one day, and I asked if this job was really worth potentially permanently destroying her body. She looked at me with sudden intensity and said simply, "I have a kid. I'm not giving up."

I met medics who lived two, three, and four hours away. Compared to the wages they would earn as paramedics in their own communities, this job was worth the sacrifice. The station had a couple of cots up for grabs in a small office room upstairs, but for the most part members slept in their cars. I was lucky to have part-time use of my brother's house. Our station parking lot usually had a cluster of vehicles in the back with cardboard and blankets taped up against the windows, blocking the light.

Despite the swarm of blond dudes in Oakleys at the initial hiring test, the ambulance staff was more diverse than I had been expecting, with members of many races and backgrounds. Almost a quarter of us were women, more than I had ever seen in EMS. A few weeks into my new job, a captain told us a story to welcome us to the department. Years ago, he had been called to a DOA and was met on the street by some police officers. They described a grisly suicide in an apartment, saying they could walk my instructor upstairs but he didn't need to bring his equipment or his partner. Brian nodded and took only his cardiac monitor. After confirming death, he trudged back down four flights of stairs and sat in the ambulance, staring out the windshield with his hands resting on the laptop, not quite ready to write down what he had seen. His partner asked about the patient, how Brian was feeling, then sighed and climbed out of the rig. When she returned to the ambulance a few minutes later, he asked why she had gone inside.

"If you're going to have to carry that around with you all day, I don't want you to have to do it alone."

Brian looked at all the new hires for a moment and let his message sink in. We looked at each other. At the private companies, the working conditions are so poor that most paramedics injure out or leave within a few years. But the fire department offers decent wages, benefits, and a pension. Many of the people in our hiring class did not have college degrees or backup plans. There was a good chance that we would be working together for the rest of our lives.

The city was crowded, tight, and dirty. There were no trailer parks, no dirt roads, no tumbleweeds or ATV accidents. The roads were so narrow and the traffic so thick that car crashes were usually low speed, injuries minor.

My second day in the field, my cellphone blew up with texts from friends and family. Apparently an ambulance had been stolen, driven across the Bay Bridge to Treasure Island, crashed, and set fire. "Dis you?" they asked, with screenshots from the news. I set the picture as the background on my phone. A flaming, sideways ambulance, jammed ass-first over the median, on an island in the middle of the San Francisco Bay was about as perfect a welcome postcard as I was ever going to get.

We spent most of our time downtown, doing laps in a ten-block circle nicknamed the "poop loop." Many of the city's poorest residents lived a crowded downtown neighborhood called the Tenderloin, either in tall SRO buildings or on the sidewalk just outside of them.

The closest hospital was only a few blocks away, so we might pick up a patient from this area and drive them up the hill, and then, as soon as we cleared, another call would pop right back where we'd just come from. A co-worker would sigh at the end of shift, "Yeah, we started off out by the beach but then got one downtown and got stuck in the poop loop for the rest of the goddamn night."

I learned later that this gravitational hole is actually an echo of the city as it existed before World War I. During the turn of the century, the industrialization of San Francisco brought workers from all over the country to hotels and rooming houses along the ports and downtown corridor. The proliferation of residential hotels in the core of the city allowed job seekers to flock to San Francisco, but inspired a decades-long debate about whether young men and women living alone in the big city were destroying the moral fabric of the humble family unit. Politicians also needed a tasteful way to racially and religiously cleanse their communities. Eventually in the 1920s, a group of "reformers" succeeded in writing zoning law that drew a strict line around the existing hotels and prevented the building of most types of group housing in other parts of the city. As a result, San Francisco still contains a concentrated group of ancient tenement buildings in just one area. I wondered if the people on the planning commissions that created these districts knew that one hundred years in the future, ambulances would still trace haunted circles around their borders.

Running 911 calls in San Francisco had a strange rhythm. The pace of work felt very different from Reno; each call took far longer to run. We sat in traffic on the way to the hospital, then waited at the hospital for hours to be seen by a nurse. I hated the inevitable conversation with my patient: having to explain that although we have arrived at the emergency room in an ambulance, we will be camping out in this doorway for a few hours before going inside. We joked with each other about bringing lawn chairs or cornhole games with us to pass the time.

According to a 2023 count, roughly a quarter of San Francisco's 911 calls were for homeless people. In both Reno and Santa Cruz we worked with the homeless a lot, but somehow in San Francisco the culture shock felt more extreme. In the other counties I had worked in, calls always seemed to run along a spectrum: minor to critical, urban to rural, poor to rich. In San Francisco everything seemed to be either zero or a hundred. No in-between. Our patients were either wealthy or destitute, our calls either easy or *holy-what-the-shit-fuck*. I could run simple calls for three weeks straight and then get two days of back-to-back lunacy. One night after a boring stretch I was eating lunch with a partner, waxing a little nostalgic for the constant medical excitement of Reno, and got interrupted by a call for a "confused" patient in a hotel lobby. Ten minutes later, four of us struggled to restrain and oxygenate a three-hundred-pound man who, naked and high on meth, had run screaming downstairs to try to fight the front desk crew while actively dying of severe airway burns. It took all four of us to hold him down, sedate him, and breathe for him while a nearby police officer hopped in the front cab and drove us up the hill to the burn center. Never tempt the EMS gods.

The fire department was organized into two divisions: fire suppression and EMS. The suppression side managed the traditional business of firefighting: engines, ladder trucks, hazmat, rescue units. Axes and hoses and ropes. The EMS division was newer. Until the late 1990s, emergency medical transport in San Francisco had been handled by a combination of private companies and a government ambulance service run out of the Department of Public Health. It was a true third-service 911 system. But due to budgeting and political challenges, the city eventually decided that the fire department would take over the ambulance service instead. The old vans had been boxy and white, with blue lettering on the sides. The new ones would be painted red.

The EMS division of the SFFD was housed at Station 49, which is less of a fire station and more a giant garage, tucked down on the southwest corner of the city between some warehouses and a sewage treatment facility. An old-timer told me the building used to be a slaughterhouse and said not to drink the water. The "49ers," as we were called, made up roughly 250 of the department's 1,700 full-time members. We wore the same uniforms as the suppression guys, and carried the same badges, but were totally segregated from them in our daily work and culture.

I had thought that in San Francisco I might be able to make a true lifelong commitment to ambulance work. But despite all the hiring academy chatter about the golden handcuffs, I found out quickly that the EMS division was not viewed as good a place to spend a career. Firefighting was still seen as the reason that we were here: the most important and glamorous work, and the obvious long-term goal. Each year the brass pulled five or ten of the most qualified 49ers out of the EMS division and helped them over to suppression. It quickly became obvious that the suppression members were valued in a way that the EMS division was not, and that the ultimate hope of working at 49 was to eventually learn how to be firefighters. Then our real lives would begin.

The relationship between EMS and fire is a complicated one, full of entangled history and deep resentment. It's an emotionally charged topic with a lot of built-in tension and self-serving answers. Some of the first successful rescue breathing techniques were pioneered by fire departments during the early 1900s, mostly in an effort to save their own guys from dying on the job. And when breakthroughs in resuscitation techniques supercharged the ambulance world in the 1960s, a handful of fire departments embraced these changes and began to educate their own members and develop rescue squads. But most pushed back against additional training, believing that they should keep their efforts focused on putting out fires. By the 1970s, some ambulance companies were run by fire departments, but most remained private, city-run, police-run, or volunteer. It wasn't until the end of that decade that things got really weird.

The biggest factor, oddly, was a development in materials science and sprinkler systems. In the late seventies and early eighties, improvements in building technology totally changed the landscape of urban firefighting. The population-based rate of home fires and home-fire-related deaths fell by two-thirds between 1980 and 2018. In the 1980s, big-city fire departments had a lot of staff, a lot of equipment, and not a lot to do. Meanwhile, ambulances were just as ragged and overwhelmed as they had always been. Many fire departments finally started to require medical training for their members, and even began sending fire apparatus out to medical calls to initiate care while they waited for the ambulance. This system, in which a ladder truck pulls up to a medical call and gets things started while the ambulance ricochets back and forth across the city, quickly became the standard in most American cities. It is sometimes referred to as the "cost-shifting" model. The ambulance is allowed to remain understaffed and underfunded, and fire stations are given some more work to do in between fires. A lot more work, actually: nationally, medical calls represent 71.8 percent of fire department calls for service. But it's a strange idea.

The utility of having a fire engine on every medical call is dubious. Firefighters are able to start CPR right away, which in a cardiac arrest is lifesaving and invaluable. They can provide extra support if a patient is trapped in a vehicle or too large to move with only two people. But they are not able to transport, which means that in calls where speedy movement is of the essence, like strokes, heart attacks, or traumatic injuries, this model wastes resources and time. And the logic is deeply circular: cities shuffle money away from EMS services into fire so that fire can help out with the perpetually underfunded EMS system. If the call is low-priority or located at a medical facility, the ambulance will occasionally respond "sole responder;" that is, by ourselves. But the standard for almost all of our runs is to send both an engine and an ambulance.

Ignoring, for a moment, the disturbing economic implications of this model, there are times when it is downright silly. Picture four guys climbing out of a forty-foot ladder truck and piling into Grandma's one-room apartment as she sits on the toilet, having requested an ambulance for constipation. Now she's looking up at half a baseball team's worth of muscle-bound firefighters politely standing around for twenty minutes until we can clear the hospital and get over there. More than once a bewildered patient has asked me if there was a fire in a building nearby.

It's hard to say how much this concept—a half-a-million-dollar fire apparatus pulling up to every medical call while the ambulance is still stuck at the hospital—has truly changed American EMS. It has undoubtably saved the lives of some patients who went into dangerous heart rhythms while the nearest ambulance was halfway across town. But it has also prompted cities to promise their citizens that a paramedic would arrive within eight minutes, for example, knowing full well that the engine paramedic would not have a way to get them to a hospital. This white lie has allowed private ambulance companies to keep their staffing levels homicidally low while still turning a profit.

The awkward crossover between fire departments and medical calls has also dramatically changed the career trajectory of an EMS worker. Working for a big-city fire department is an extremely coveted job. It never appealed to me; I like the medicine too much, and I find humans more interesting than buildings. But it's a well-paid, fully pensioned, city-funded career that doesn't require a college degree, and for a lot of men and women, it's the dream. And rightly so. It's an important job, and we need good people to do it. But because most fire departments now require an EMT or paramedic license, the best way to get hired is to put in a few years on the ambulance first. This means that every year, private companies like AMR and Falck are guaranteed a fresh crop of bright-faced twenty-year-olds whose life goal is to put out fires. The result of this practice is that no matter how crappy the pay or abusive the hours, there will always be a pool of eager young (mostly) men to fill these jobs. The fire department plucks a few guys out every year, so if young firefighters-to-be can endure a few years of a private company's brutal working conditions they will eventually be, as my friend Tom put it when he finally got picked up, "set for life." This has created a culture in which EMS has a much tougher time unifying or advocating for ourselves as a profession because almost all of our medics move on after a few years. Instead of a career worth fighting for, ambulance work has become an unpleasant stepping stone on the way to a life at a firehouse.

I had hoped that at the San Francisco Fire Department my experience would be different. Unlike the New York City Fire Department (FDNY), which famously pays its EMS division a fraction of what their firefighters make (despite running three times as many calls), the SFFD advertised similar starting wages for their EMS and suppression divisions. However, the equitability seemed to end there.

Suppression members were given better staffing, more opportunities for training and promotion, and more control over their schedules. They worked in twenty-four-hour rotations out of firehouses with dedicated zones. Although the downtown houses were quite busy, many of the crews in quieter areas could go days with only one or two calls. They got to live in stations where they could eat, work out, rest, and train on the job. Ambulances were originally also placed on twenty-four-hour shifts, but the EMS division was staffed so poorly against such a high call volume that the around-the-clock model proved unsafe. By the time I arrived, ambulance crews worked twelve-hour shifts, with no stations or rest areas. Instead, we arrived at the garage in the morning, picked up our rig, and then spent the day driving around the city from call to call. If we did have any downtime on a slow day, we parked on street corners or in hospital parking lots. But in San Francisco, like everywhere that I have worked, it was common to run so low on ambulances that calls were stacked in a waiting list until one of us could clear a hospital and take a new one. And although the turnover at Station 49 wasn't as high as I had seen at the private companies, within five years most of my friends were gone. One or two promoted through the EMS division or got jobs teaching at our training facility. Some left for nursing school or other work entirely. Most completed the firefighting academy and crossed over to suppression.

One of my bitterest memories took place during our continuing education classes. Like many licensed professionals, EMTs and paramedics are required to complete a certain amount of classroom instruction each year. The classes usually contain pre-recorded videos that don't change much year to year, so they provided the perfect opportunity for me to chug coffee, stare around the room, and feel my rage build. I would see three or four ambulance crews giving up a day of their weekend, often fighting to stay awake after running calls all night. This in itself didn't bother me; in fact, most medical professionals can probably relate. The part that drove me nuts was incredibly petty: while EMS members were required to come in on their days off for these classes, firefighters had the time built into their schedule. I saw their radios on their desks, turned off for the day. I tried not to let it get to me, but we all knew that in a thousand years, the department would never budget the EMS side with enough staffing to let us do something like that.

Despite all my frustrations, I never found a specific person or policy to blame for my anger. I began to read history, trying to figure out why the work that I wanted to give my life to was treated by city governments as such an afterthought. But the more I read the blurrier the picture became. I learned that historically, the ambulance has always been seen as a brutal job, and not one that was considered by the medical establishment or the public safety sector as a respectable career. From its inception back in the horse-and-buggy days, hospitals quickly realized that their senior physicians would not submit themselves to the low pay and physically demanding work required on an emergency vehicle. And ambulance shortages are common around the world—to a certain extent it is simply the nature of the beast.

I didn't want the firefighters working conditions to worsen—ask a firefighter how "easy" their job is after they've been shoveling debris for a few hours or been woken up five times after midnight. I just grew sick of seeing my friends burn out and get injured and leave the EMS side. The merger with the Department of Public Health took place in 1997. Although twenty-five years seemed to me like a long time to figure out how to run a new program, I had to remind myself that the department was founded in 1846. The city was a smattering of canvas tents on a windy peninsula back then, famously burned to the ground six times in eighteen months. For 151 years the SFFD focused on fires, and for just twenty-five they had taken on this new responsibility. The merger wasn't exactly peaceful; we heard stories of fistfights at firehouses and paramedics banned from coming inside the buildings, sleeping outside in their ambulances and ignored at mealtimes. Things were undeniably better now than they used to be, but it was hard to imagine we would ever be seen as equals.

In many ways, this treatment led those of us at Station 49 to bond even more tightly. We were the underdogs, the mistreated stepchildren of the department. We made ourselves station T-shirts with logos of black sheep and flaming ambulances. We rolled our eyes when suppression captains gave us grief for taking too long to arrive at their call, knowing that we had come straight from a hospital halfway across town while they were cooking breakfast two blocks away.

And at night, the streets were ours. For the most part, our assigned posting zones were spread throughout the city, so we sat alone in idling trucks. But on a busy night we would often find ourselves gathered at the hospitals between calls, not bothering to drive out through the neighborhood when we knew another run would come in before we made it through the first stoplight.

One night there are a few of us in front of the hospital. I'm writing a chart against the hood of a running ambulance while a few other medics smoke cigarettes or drink coffee and tell war stories. They stand in a loose ring: an unholy coven, the most sacred prayer circle of the night shift. There are unspoken rules to the bullshit circle: No supervisors allowed. Anyone else in uniform is welcome, regardless of friend groups or social standing. Anyone can tell a story. Anyone can interrupt. Cigarettes are allowed. Coffee is encouraged. If the radio begins to speak, all conversation stops for a few seconds until the unit number is announced.

"He dropped a tube for me the other day! I'm trying to get an airway, but the vomit, I mean, this guy was Mount Vesuvius. I literally suctioned for five minutes, and Bill's like, you have to do something with that, I'm like, I am! I'm fucking fixing the airway!"

"—and I was like, 'Do we *have* to go code three? He's eating chips!' And then you hear the guy go, 'Hey, man, you guys got any water, I'm thirsty!' His friend's still all stressed, telling us to turn the sirens on, and our patient's sitting there shoveling Funyuns into his fucking mouth hole."

"Right? And then Bill's like, 'Oh, you gotta go, dude, that's like, the first sign of shock, dude!' He's thirsty!' I laughed so hard in his face."

Raul pauses to take a drag of his vape. Sascha puts on a pair of gloves and opens a plastic tub of Thai noodles. We run calls, we clean gurneys, we swap stories. The night melts down to its wick.

Then I hear a shout across the street, followed by a smack, and a sickening crunch.

"Mother-fucking-FUCK! Fucking *kidding* me with this shit?"

The cussing belongs to my buddy Tom, the smack and crunch to a homeless man we all just watched get hit and thrown by a large work truck barreling up the street. Tom is particularly annoyed by the accident as he's the one who dropped off this homeless man at the hospital about fifteen minutes ago for alcohol intoxication. One of the main reasons we will transport a drunk patient is if we conclude that they are too incapacitated to walk unassisted without, say, getting hit by a truck. The emergency room took the guy in, chatted with him, and kicked him back out before Tom was even done wiping down the gurney, which is now conveniently located about eight feet from the man's crumpled body.

There's a lot more profanity as Tom scoops the guy up, throws him back on the same gurney, and takes off for the trauma center. We get on the radio to tell dispatch to drop a call on him. People drive fast in this neighborhood, especially this time of night. It's not the first or the last time an intoxicated patient will stumble out of the doors of the hospital into oncoming traffic.

It is while working in San Francisco that I first read Matthew Desmond's *Evicted: Poverty and Profit in the American City.* The book is ostensibly about housing and economics. Desmond follows eight families through the eviction process in Milwaukee, Wisconsin. It is a gut-wrenching read, compassionate and complicated, and about three pages in I realize, *Oh. This book is about my job.* Desmond writes about Arlene, a single mother of five or six kids. She lives off welfare because the money seems steadier than any job. Her youngest son has asthma and she keeps falling behind with his medications. I know before Desmond tells me that she often calls 911 for his asthma attacks. He gets sick a lot and, with no primary care doctor, they take him in to the ER. I know. I've run that call.

The night after I finish reading *Evicted* I write down some of my calls for the shift. I work downtown, from 4:30 p.m. to 4:30 a.m. That night's calls include Tag, a forty-one-year-old at a free clinic who's had pain in his ribs for about a month. After Tag is Ronnie, a fifty-eight-year-old male from a veterans housing assistance shelter. He's having a psych episode and a runny nose, in that order. He talks quickly, mostly makes sense, but veers into paranoia if you let him steer the conversation too long. His nose has been running for a week and his neighbor stole his pants and painted them a different color. These pants? I point to the jeans he's wearing. He's not sure. He says the guy crawls under his door every night and does it and then crawls back out. We give him some Kleenex and take him to the veterans hospital.

There's a drunk homeless man with a cut on his head, called in by a tourist who didn't even stop her car, just reached for a cellphone and drove on by. Then an elderly man with neck pain that has been bothering him all month. Then a ninety-one-year-old Russian woman having a breathing episode, which is more or less resolved when we show up. Her son is worried, though: she lives alone, he can't stay the night, and they can't afford a home care nurse to stay with her.

All of these patients face serious issues with housing, food, basic life skills. The 911 call is less about an emergency and more about an inability to provide for themselves. Lack of access to basic human needs like food, water, and hygiene will eventually become medical if ignored for long enough. Bare fridges lead to malnutrition, broken plumbing creates infection. Addiction becomes overdose. Some folks call us hoping for a trip to the ER when they just don't want to spend another night alone.

I tell a friend of mine some of my thoughts about the book as I'm reading it, and how it highlights the ways that my job differs from the classic Hollywood image. She says, "Wait, that's really interesting." Haley is a senior editor at a literary magazine. I met her the first week of college, when I found her to be the only other woman in my dorm plaza awake at 3:00 a.m. on a weekday. Since I began work in EMS, Haley has often provided an outsider's perspective for me. When I won't shut up about *Evicted*, she helps me work my thoughts into an essay discussing the relationship between EMS and poverty, and prints the piece in her magazine. The SFFD controls media very tightly, like most EMS agencies, so instead of asking for permission I write the essay under a pseudonym and scrub all mentions of my location. The response is positive. I feel like I have told Haley's readers a little piece of our story.

———

I often debate moving closer to the city, but Santa Cruz provides a counterbalance for me throughout my time in San Francisco. If my work week is sweat and diesel and urine and blood and tar, then my weekend is salt and sand. I live with the farmer housemate for a few years and then move into a one-bedroom on the southern end of town. I grow closer to Kyle, who is the opposite of everyone I know in EMS. He is quiet, patient, and observant. He keeps his thoughts to himself. He works as a machinist during the day and comes home smelling of chemical solvents and sweat. He surfs almost every evening, staying out so long after dark that I wonder every night if he is lost at sea.

Kyle lives in a crumbling surf palace about two blocks from the ocean. The Anchorage House, as the neighborhood calls it, is legally a two-bedroom but holds anywhere from three to six roommates at a time. A teenager lives on an air mattress behind the TV. Any time the waves are good, a parade of surfers wanders through and crashes on the couch or in vans parked on the lawn. The backyard feels tropical, with overgrown banana plants and piles of surfboards under blue tarps. A decrepit hot tub sits in one corner.

It is at the Anchorage House that I first meet Leelu, a tricolor English bull terrier who technically belongs to one of the roommates but seems familiar to everyone in the neighborhood. When I walk her down to the water, sunburned beach bros stop to greet the dog by name before they look up at me and ask how I know her. When I arrive at the house she head-butts me in the stomach to say hello, and the warm weight of her makes me feel whole.

When I feel my job start to choke the air out of my throat, I walk to the ocean, ride my bike around the neighborhood, or lay out on a towel in the grass with Lee. I stay at Kyle's house for days at a time, only swinging by my own room for clean underwear and snacks.

Between his house, my brother's place, my truck, Station 49, and my ambulance, I often feel like my life is a never-ending road trip. I weave endless circles around the Bay Area in various vehicles, feeling like the only time I stop moving is in the ocean or in the Anchorage House backyard.

I work with a jumble of partners in San Francisco. There's Jill, the impossibly cool road-biker chick with half her head shaved. Auggie, the soft-spoken basketball coach who gives me thoughtful advice on how to keep my head down and stay out of trouble. My longest run is with Andrew: a stern, broad-shouldered SF native, born and raised between downtown and Chinatown, who speaks Cantonese and knows every nurse in the city by name. I learn a lot from Andrew, even though his blunt way of telling me I'm wrong usually makes me want to curl up and run away. After Andrew I work nights with Jack, a hilarious Australian transplant who yells, "Put your dilly away, mate!" at a drunk guy with his pants down. I decide in that moment I will never again refer to the male genitalia as anything but a "dilly."

One night Jack and I are waiting for a bed at the hospital when we see a familiar patient arguing with the charge nurse as he leads her out the front door of the emergency room. She is begging him for clean clothing, saying her pants are soiled and she just wants an extra pair before she leaves. Seth, the nurse, puts his hands on his hips.

"What about the last time we gave you pants, when you walked a block away and sold them to some homeless guys for crack?"

She looks indignant. "Bitch, I'm an entrepreneur!"

I enjoy some aspects of night shift: the quiet streets, the calls, the camaraderie. The hospital staff seems more relaxed and the dispatchers don't watch our locations as closely. When we are called to a nicer house in the middle of the night, the complaint tends to be serious.

But although I am resting more than I'd been able to at my previous jobs, I still feel like I am never truly awake. Kyle is easygoing when I fall asleep in the middle of a meal or ask him three times what day of the week it is. His friends like to gather at a local late-night diner, ordering breakfast and beer and coffee for hours after a surf session. Two of the waitresses know our group so well that on slow nights they sit with us and steal our fries. One warm summer evening I get so sleepy that I ask a friend of Kyle's where he parked and walk out of the diner to take a nap in the bed of his truck. I wake up forty minutes later to the sound of the guys calling around for me and stick my head over the tailgate of a total stranger's car. I had been so tired that I'd hopped in the back of the first red Dodge pickup I'd seen, and it was dumb luck that its owners had been slower than us to finish their meal.

Leelu keeps me going. After a long week on the ambulance, I bury my face in her stomach before bed, feeling her musty smell push the stress out of my pores. She wakes me up with a grunt in the morning and we stumble down to the beach together to check the surf conditions and find out whether I should put on a wetsuit or go back to sleep.

Journal, August 2017

There's a record-setting heat wave in San Francisco and the whole city explodes. Dispatch is panicked. Calls are popping, the ambulances overheat, and the engine fans whine and screech alongside the sirens. We don't have enough crews and people are dropping in the streets. Thirty calls are pending. Engine crews are waiting at scenes and begging for ambulances on the radio. Units are crisscrossing. It's so hot in the rig that the sweat is dripping down the inside of the windows. The inside of my uniform is sticky and heavy with every step. Heat radiates off the sidewalk and penetrates every smog-covered pore of exposed skin. Many buildings in San Francisco do not have air conditioning, and in some of the cheaper SROs the windows are sealed shut.

Downtown the sidewalk folks burn and faint and overdose onto the steaming tar of the street. High above, atop thin staircases, in thick-walled single rooms, elderly people boil in their beds until they stumble into even hotter hallways and collapse. Everybody's dying, everywhere.

When I worked in Nevada I felt like I was helping these hard-working desert folk who were clinging to the edges of their lives. Here in San Francisco I feel surrounded by crowds, money, big-city corruption and big-city noise. . . . in this city there is too much life; there is a teeming, thriving, rotten pile of devils upon angels upon rats upon bruises, screaming, laughing, sparkling, tangled high-fiving neon lights; crumpled paper bags, stinking newspapers, shithole, refuse, taxi horns blaring, tripping over bodies in the street, bodies that could be dead or alive, dead bodies feeding off of the live ones, decomposing into each other, jungle layers of life and death and noise and a huge billowing cloud of meth fentanyl smoke drifting up white and chemical cross your eyes. The city is corruption, it's density, it's filth. If the desert is a long silent exhalation then the city is a scream.

After a couple of years on night shift, I eventually gained enough seniority to switch to days. With the switch came a new side of the city: blue skies, more traffic, fewer assaults. I learned a new rhythm and saw more of my brother now that I was awake during daylight hours. We chatted over the kitchen counter as he dropped frozen dumplings into a pot of water.

AJ lived in a completely different San Francisco than the one in which I worked. While I was pulling dead bodies off of sewer grates, he was on a bike ride in Golden Gate Park. While I held a meth user's sweating knees against a backboard, AJ ordered drinks. He barely ever had reason to pass through most of the neighborhoods I knew best. His favorite restaurants are an eclectic mix of Vietnamese, Chinese, and Middle Eastern, while mine were all takeout spots located within four blocks of a hospital. Even our landmarks were different: he might describe a location by a music venue or dog park, while I found my way by nursing homes and halfway houses. He found my stories entertaining, scandalizing even, but our conversations felt like they were in two different languages.

I went through phases with San Francisco. When the pain and addiction I saw in homeless encampments was too much for me, I blamed it all on the city, as though the skyscrapers themselves represented the hulking supervillains who had caused this tragedy. I said it was all the fault of rich people, and politicians, and the tech industry. I read gold rush history, telling myself that this city was founded in drunken greed and only got worse from there. Some days I made it the patient's fault, for coming to this godforsaken town in the first place. But other times my heart would soften. I'd see SF as a gathering of humans who came out west in search of a better life, whatever that meant for them. I'd smile at the languages spoken on the bus, or the huge families stepping over each other in tiny apartments. I realized San Francisco was made of a thousand human stories, no better or worse than anywhere else.

Eventually I even learned to love the city. It was gross, and crowded, and overpriced, but the pulse of it pulled me in. I carried an unconscious man out of a clearly illegal upstairs gambling den in Chinatown that looked like a racist movie set. I grew to know every hotel in the Tenderloin, hundred-year-old wallpaper hiding roaches and ghosts. I learned how to say "chest pain" in Russian and Cantonese. I knew which station bathrooms might have an EMT sleeping on an air mattress on the floor, and which of my partners were due for knee surgery or putting their kids through school. I worked with a girl who grew up in the Sunnydale projects, on the Samoan block. She took me to the Samoan community center and introduced me around, then showed me where to get all the best food in the neighborhood. I stared out at fog and hills and candy-colored houses and bricks and liquor stores and Muni buses and more fog. I ate delicious pho in the rain, broth sloshing over the sides of the Styrofoam. I teared up laughing at the punch-drunk gallows humor that we shouted out rolled-down windows to each other at two in the morning. I paid three times as much as I ever though I would for the "best croissant in America" and then cursed when I realized it was worth every penny.

I ultimately spent seven years at the San Francisco Fire Department. I earned two promotions and damaged my shoulder, wrists, and lower back. I built a complex web of love for the people I worked with and anger at the broken insanity that we worked inside of every day. On particularly hard days I curled up with my notebook and poured tears and ink onto the pages. I spent a lot of time frustrated with our management, our city politics, our hospitals, and our patient population. But in the long run it turned out Captain Brian was right— no matter how much the job could suck, I was never in it alone. The field crews on the EMS side fought and joked and shared meals together. I broke up screaming matches between co-workers, learned how to make fresh ahi poke, and closed my eyes while another medic gave me some meds and a hug during a late-night panic attack. When my injuries grew too serious and I knew it was time to leave the department, it wasn't my job or my badge or my identity as a paramedic that hurt the most to lose. It was the crew.

My last year on the job, I read Anthony Almojera's memoir of the New York Fire EMS Division. The book ends with a description of his own suicide attempt and the way that his chosen family at the department pulled him out of his darkest moments. When I closed the book, I wanted nothing more than to call Lieutenant Almojera and see if he was free for lunch. I felt sure, somehow, that we would talk about EMS and fire and trauma and food and life and family and that from one coast to another he would feel like my kind of people.

My last long-term partner on the ambulance in San Francisco was a new hire named Maggie. When I called the training facility to hear the scoop about her, I was told she was green but very competent. "You'll get along," said the training officer. "She's great."

The first day we met, I found her in the back of my ambulance organizing gear. She was skinny, with a short pixie cut and a friendly smile. She spoke with a British accent, which was a surprise. Trying to find common ground, I told her that Kyle and I had traveled to Ireland earlier that year. I said that it was beautiful but the weather was pretty shit. Maggie gave me a look filled with amused compassion, like I was a child who'd dropped an ice cream cone, and said, "Oh, did . . . did no one tell you? About the weather in the UK . . . ?"

I laughed and liked her immediately.

As a partner, Maggie was quick on the draw but nervous. She seemed afraid to make mistakes, frantically apologizing if she couldn't find a piece of equipment or took a wrong turn while driving. I could tell she was savvy enough to understand the layers of confusion and frustration and hypocrisy built into our job, but whenever I ranted or complained or asked her for her opinion she remained polite and neutral.

I understood the source of her formal demeanor. New hires at the fire department are given a classic piece of advice: for the length of your probationary year, repeat the following phrase: "I'm just happy to be here." While you are new, you do not have an opinion. You do not complain. You do not provide insight. You are a silent, happy worker bee, grateful to be given this opportunity. You must earn the right to use your voice. Maggie seemed as though she had taken the suggestion to heart, and for several weeks did not break character.

I learned a little more about her: she held dual bachelor's degrees and used to work in a high-level position in data science. I asked how exactly she ended up getting from a South London office building to an ambulance in San Francisco, as it seemed like an especially bizarre life path. Maybe she fell in love with a dashing young firefighter. Maybe she had to escape a secret life of crime. Was it drugs?

She told me she was working in finance during the 2008 crash. "I looked at what was happening all around me and I just couldn't . . . I couldn't stay. I saw a comedy skit with these men on a ship saying, 'Are we the baddies?' Do you watch any British TV? Have you seen the one I mean?"

I hadn't seen it, but I watched as soon as I could—it's a sketch in which two soldiers come to realize that their uniforms are covered in skulls and crossbones and do some amusing self-reflection. When Maggie's husband received a job offer in the United States, she followed him here and enrolled in an EMT class. In five years she had become a full member of the fire department, a journey that usually takes more than twice that. I loved Maggie's story, her intelligence, and her compassion, but was sometimes worried by her motives.

Many of those who got into this job to help save the world are the ones who burn out the fastest, when they see what we really do.

There is a moment in every new EMS partnership where you find out whether you will get along or not. Usually it comes in the form of a critical call: a real mess of a patient with split-second decision-making and unexpected complications. If you are in sync in those life-or-death moments, the next day's coffee run feels infinitely more relaxed. But Maggie and I had been running on moderately sick patients for about a month, with no real drama. She was professional and knowledgeable with patients, courteous and deferential with me.

It turned out to be a flat tire, of all things, that finally broke the ice.

We walked out of the hospital to find our left back tire flatted out one morning. We called our supervisor and entered a bizarre, day-long game of bureaucratic tail-chasing trying to get it fixed. For some reason we had just switched tire vendors and were advised to head to a new auto shop for a spare. We informed dispatch of our delay, then drove across town to find their storefront closed. There was a debate about whether our own in-house mechanics were able to do the swap, something to do with qualifications and union hours and inter-station politics. We drove to two or three more locations and made what felt like dozens of phone calls, all the while fielding questions from our dispatchers about what was taking so long. We finally made it back to our station, watched another argument, and eventually waited forty-five minutes for the fire department mechanics to drive over and do the job after all. They used a pneumatic impact wrench, a large, fast tool that Kyle and his friends call the "ugga dugga" for the sound it makes. When Maggie saw that the repair we had been chasing down all day took less than five minutes to complete, she threw up her hands in exasperation.

"That's it?! That's all they had to do? It was just . . . ?" She looked at me with her mouth open.

"Yeah. I tried to tell you, we could have had this done before we cleared the hospital."

"I can't . . ." I watched Maggie pull her hands to her face, smoothing her hair back. She had been so poised until this moment, and I couldn't help but smile as her smooth exterior finally cracked. She leaned back against the rig, crossed her arms under her chest, and sighed.

"What a fucking faff."

I put my hand on her shoulder and began to laugh. It was her body language, her exasperation, her British slang. She looked back at me and we started to imitate the arguments we had heard on the phones all day. We mimicked the voices, the radio sounds, the confusion, and giggled until we had to lean against the side of the ambulance for support. I told her I would buy her an ice cream next shift to make up for the hassle and she asked me how many different vendor-approved ice cream shops we would need to drive to before finding one that was officially mandated to allow for department scooping needs. I grinned, realizing that I finally had a partner instead of a co-worker. Which was good, because we blew that tire in January of 2020. We were going to need each other more than either of us knew.

"IT'S ALL CUMULATIVE"

A.K., PARAMEDIC/EMS CAPTAIN, DISPATCH SUPERVISOR;
TWENTY-THREE YEARS IN EMS
CALIFORNIA

I wish the public knew that we don't have a million ambulances. Not just in this city, but as a whole. Often times people will call 911 for somebody without actually checking in on them. They'll be calling out of their second-floor window, you know? I don't want to say that the public should call us less, I just want them to really take into consideration what they're calling for. The amount of times that I show up on scene, and I'm trying to figure out, *Why am I here again? What's going on?* I feel like that happens a lot. If I think about all the calls that I've been on which ended with the patient refusing or walking away from us or cursing us out, it's countless times. Countless.

The triage delays have gotten really bad. There's been crews at hospitals for two hours past their off-duty time. One was there for four hours last week. I call the charge nurse and ask, "Is there an ETA to get beds for these patients? We're running low on medics in the city."

They always give the same answer. They say, "We have a lot of sick people. We have too many patients." They will say that the ICUs upstairs are full, and that they're actually boarding their patients in the ER. Part of it is the volume of low-acuity patients. This is nothing new, but I do feel like it has gotten worse with the new generation.

Maybe I have just observed it more recently because I'm up in dispatch now. I see a lot of people in their twenties calling us for headaches or because their knee hurts. Do we still respond? The answer is yes. I wouldn't refuse to take people to the hospital, but it was one of the most frustrating things for me while I was on scene.

I'm understanding more of what goes on behind the scenes. I didn't have the best perception of dispatchers when I was in the field full-time, because I always thought of them as the whip crackers. But now that I am working side by side with them, I have a lot more respect for them. There's a lot going on up at dispatch. They have a hard job to do.

Sometimes crews will call and ask me questions. I'm happy to answer. That's one of the reasons why I'm up there, especially at three in the morning. I enjoy that, I like helping crews out. Even though I don't help the public directly right now, I enjoy checking in on crews.

PTSD is a real thing, and I certainly have it. It's all cumulative. I want everybody to go home safe at night, but it's a dangerous job. Sometimes my lieutenant will point out, "Hey, Medic 568 just got dispatched to that shooting, maybe check in with them after that call."

I grew up in this city. I have family that live here. I always try to work with a sense of urgency because I feel like that's the right thing to do. Everybody needs a break sometimes, for sure, but there's a fine line between taking too long of a break and knowing when it's time to step it up.

I just think it would be good if the public was more grateful, you know? It's a tough job.

EMS BINGO

⭐ FREQUENT FLYER Jamie Donovan!	Sedatives and restraints before noon	Uninterrupted poop 🙂	CRITICAL RESTOCK: Run out of narcan
Vehicle accident turns into an assault when the victims start fighting with each other	"It just went off!" Questionably accidental gunshot wound	THE DOUBLE PLAY: Healthy person demanding a ride for toe pain followed immediately by eighty-year-old refusing transport while having massive heart attack	⭐ FREQUENT FLYER One-eye Glen!
Drunk patient pees on your gurney	⭐ FREQUENT FLYER Susan Mitchell!	Engine captain who has run one call in 48 hours chews you out for something petty	Pay for your food and get a call before it's ready
Get yelled at by Supervisor Jones for something done by a different crew	Get sexually groped by an elderly dementia patient	Piss Test!! ☹ You wrecked an ambulance	Otherwise nice patient says something jaw-droppingly racist

EXPERIENCE IN AMBULANCE
WAS SCARCELY JOY RIDE

Four Nurses Suspended for Skylarking Claim They Were Acting as Good Samaritans

NEW YORK, Aug. 3.—For their failure to return to the dormitory at 10 o'clock Thursday night—the specified time for retiring—four student nurses attached to the Long Island College hospital, Brooklyn, were suspended temporarily yesterday morning by Miss Eugenie Speiser, acting superintendent of nurses.

The four girls had leave of absence Thursday evening. They went for a walk and were returning to the hospital when the clang of the ambulance bell attracted their attention. They decided to follow the swiftly moving vehicle, which turned down Degraw street, and came to a halt in front of No. 472. There they found that Mrs. Clara Mayer, 30 years old, had become suddenly insane and was battling with the ambulance surgeon.

Having their mission at heart, the girls thought they could pacify the raving woman. Two of them, Julia O'Connell and Irene Noble, rendered aid to the surgeon, Dr. William Donahue, who commended them.

The two girls comforted the afflicted woman, and, to please her, took seats in the ambulance and accompanied her to the hospital. The other two girls, whose names could not be learned, also rode in the ambulance.

While administering to Mrs. Mayer the nurses forgot all about the time, and it was nearly 11 o'clock when they reached the dormitory. Yesterday morning they were called before the acting superintendent for being delinquent.

Miss Noble told of the ambulance ride. Miss Speiser became indignant and suspended the four immediately. The nurses will have a final hearing next week when Miss Mary Bodine, superintendent of nurses, returns from her vacation. They are confident of reinstatement.

One of the girls, when asked about her dismissal, said:

"Miss Speiser has not heard the true story. She listened while Miss Noble told of the ride in the ambulance, and believes we were joy-riding. We were not skylarking. I'm sure we acted properly.

"Have you seen our ambulance? Well, it's terrible. No one would ride in it unless compelled to."

◆◆◆

Don't simply allow it to die—that plan of yours. Find a little capital through advertising.

Los Angeles Herald, August 6, 1909

JOURNAL: DECEMBER 18, 2015

Lounging in San Francisco on a foggy day, thinking of the past.

I remember Mikey and me staring at each other over burritos once, trying to figure out what it was that tasted so good, so filling, and suddenly realizing that it was the first hot food either of us had eaten in over a week. We busted up laughing.

I found a huge beetle at the hospital in Reno once. The little one at the eastern edge of town. You drive up one of the main roads all the way out until it dead-ends into a dirt hill. The ambulance parking sits against a huge boulder pile tucked into the side of a tall brown slope. It's situated east/west, so when you pull open the rear doors of the ambulance your patient is staring straight into the sunset.

I was working with Boon; they split us up for a few days so Mikey could take a trainee. We were unloading an empty gurney to pick up a transfer and I shouted at Boon to stop. There was the most massive beetle I had ever seen on the cement right under our feet. I told him to take the gurney so I could get a picture. It was giant and the body looked painted in desert camouflage. Tan and gold pinchers reaching up towards me, articulated claws clipping at the air. I could see dust particles clinging to his exoskeleton and I lay flat on my stomach to investigate. It was almost midnight but the air was still hot and dry, warm Nevada summer folded all around me. My new friend was illuminated only by the ambulance

*lights and he glowed reddish against the cement. I kept thinking
about how perfectly adjusted to the desert he was compared to me,
my fat soft human body full of water. Is the shell called a carapace?
Eventually Boon yelled at me and we went inside to get our patient.
When we got back out he was gone.*

   *That desert feels so far away now. I first got there as a child, you
know? This tiny, klutzy, brand-new Californian medic who didn't
know a goddamn thing about work—they took me in, they trained
me, they bled me, they beat me up and sweated with me and
brought me in and loved me. I did my best to earn their respect,
but I left in the end. Now I'm back in the Bay Area, home again
but feeling as lost as ever.*

"WHAT WE DO"

DAN QUINTO, RETIRED EMS SUPERVISOR;
FORTY-SEVEN YEARS IN EMS
SANTA CRUZ, CALIFORNIA

I just don't think that people have any kind of an understanding of what we do, or how important we are. I really don't think that EMTs and paramedics get their due for their job and for what position they hold in society. EMTs in particular.

I took an EMT class when I was in high school, at a local community college. They had one of the first EMT programs in the state. As part of the program, we had to spend one day per week at the hospital, for clinical practice. I remember very distinctly one of the first days that I was there. This woman had her daughter with her. The girl was probably six or seven, and she had broken her forearm, and she didn't have insurance. So they were sending her to the big county general hospital, but all they did was give her some piece of paper saying where to go. She asked, "Well, how do I get there?"

And they said, "I don't know. Take the bus."

And I thought, *That's nuts.* This is a seven-year-old with a broken arm. "I don't get it," I told the nurse.

She said, "Well, it's not our problem."

I thought, *It is our problem.* It's society's problem.

I was eighteen. I didn't know anything about society yet. But I remember that moment. And I've always thought back to that.

THE PAST IS THE PRESENT,
THE OLD IS THE NEW, AND
OUR PAIN IS NOT OURS ALONE

I don't remember the exact moment that I began looking into ambulance history. It may have been a slow day, the kind with enough time between calls to stare out the windshield and wonder how this all came to be. It could have been on one of those nights when every single patient seems out to get you: screaming, spitting, grabbing at cables and calling you names. Or maybe it was a totally normal week: the elderly, the homeless, the addicted; and one or two real live, light-'em-up, no shit emergencies thrown in just to keep you on your toes. But one day I looked up and wanted some answers. When exactly did ambulances shift their focus from true emergencies to social welfare issues? Why are we always stretched so thin? How did this all come to pass? I had always assumed that our role as a societal safety net was a modern development. I thought that in early history, ambulances had been a carefully conserved resource, used only in the most dire situations. I wondered at what point exactly our system began to fall apart.

I suspected I would blame the shift on the loss of mental institutions in the 1980s, or a recent financial crash. Or, if my parents were to be believed, it was one more trickle-down consequence of Reaganomics. Instead, I was shocked to find story after story of similar issues tracing all the way back to the gold rush days: lack of staffing, low budgets, and frustration with low-acuity calls taking the place of "real" emergencies. The shape of the van and its tires had changed, as had the titles and educational background of its staff. But the underlying character of an ambulance—as a struggling, barely functional system that catered mostly to the poor—that seemed to have been with us all along.

Humans have always found ways to carry their injured to the doctor. Cloth stretchers, sedan chairs, a wooden cot buckled onto the back of a camel. The word *ambulancia* first appeared in a military context, to describe the temporary medical tents built by Queen Isabella of Spain for soldiers wounded in battle against the Moors. The term soon came to refer to not just the tents themselves but to the fleet of bedded carriages designed to ferry soldiers back and forth between them. During modern times, the word *ambulance* has come to signify a specialized vehicle intended for rapid transport of those in need of medical assistance. At different points in history, these vehicles have been staffed by attendants with varying levels of expertise: sometimes with surgeons and doctors, sometimes with anyone the army could find that could ride a horse. But no matter what level of medical care is provided, almost every historical incarnation of these vehicles has faced issues getting people to show up to work.

During the Civil War the army was so low on manpower that the ambulances were driven by musicians from the regimental band. When they finally recruited a couple of teamsters, the commanding doctors complained that these men were "vulgar, ignorant, and profane," and so drunk that they occasionally had to be thrown in the back with the patients. Then a cholera epidemic pushed New York City's Bellevue Hospital to build the nation's first municipal ambulance service. The original idea was to place experienced doctors on the buggies, but the low pay, terrible hours, and dangerous conditions forced hospitals to use interns instead. That worked for a couple of decades.

Eventually even the easily abused trainees had enough. More and more medical interns chose residency programs that did not require ambulance time. As hospital-based ambulance programs began to disappear, many towns relied on police or fire department emergency services, volunteer rescue squads, or private companies. Police departments took the lead until the 1920s or so, hiring doctors to ride to emergencies with them. But by the 1930s the administrative costs were too high. Privately owned funeral home transportation became more common, mostly because a hearse was already the right shape to transport a body. Their drivers had little or no medical training, and if the patient died they would simply turn around and head for the mortuary instead.

Then there was the money.

Imagine a shoe store where a customer walks in, is given a pair of shoes, and then leaves and receives a bill in the mail. Now imagine that they are not required to provide their mailing address, or even their full name, in order to receive the shoes. Now imagine that without the shoes they will die. How many of those shoes do you think are getting paid for?

Ambulances were never profitable. Most patients were poor, and few paid their bill. From their earliest conception, civilian ambulances lost money for hospitals, lost money for police, and lost money for cities. Funeral homes scraped out a profit, barely, by paying their drivers terribly and refusing calls in poor areas.

And there were the calls.

The bell rang at all hours of the night for a sore throat, a bruise, a ride home in a snowstorm. The interns grew frustrated. The police kept calling for drunks. In a 1939 interview, a New York city ambulance driver complained about night shift: "when you get the pie-eyes and psychos by the dozens." Mayor Fiorello La Guardia gave a city-wide radio address in 1942 begging his citizens to stop calling ambulances for stomach aches so that they might be available "in the event of a real emergency."

But mostly, it was the staff.

With long nights full of non-emergencies, and without money to offer competitive pay, ambulance services could never hold on to employees. Although "rescue squads" were popular with police and fire departments, these institutions usually found medical training too onerous on top of their regular duties. Some departments embraced rescue breathing or basic first aid, but most resisted any formal educational requirements. By the 1950s, American ambulances were run by a hodgepodge of private companies, government agencies, and volunteers. Only a few hospital-based services were left. Mortuary ambulance companies collapsed left and right due to new federal minimum wage laws requiring them to (gasp!) pay their drivers a decent living. But the population in the United States continued to grow, and medical advancements in CPR and surgical techniques were pointing to an even greater need for the ability to intervene quickly in an emergency.

Mikey and I are driving through Reno one afternoon, underneath a heavy summer sky. The dark clouds along the ridgeline are threatening thunder. I'm working in San Francisco now, but I still visit regularly and like to talk with Mikey about how things are going on the ambulance.

He says they've been busy lately, like always. He's been working a lot of overtime. He shows me his phone, filled with pages from supervisors asking for medics to come in and fill empty shifts. I chuckle and pull out mine to compare.

We both stare at the screens for a minute. Every time slot in the stack of texts represents twelve or twenty-four hours that our communities will be without the resources that they need in an emergency. Our co-workers will be stretched thin, our own family members' lives at risk. But these pages come in all day, every day. There is always an empty shift or two (or five) to be filled. Things have been this way since both of our careers began. Over time you learn to take the days off that you need, put the phone away, and try not to think about it.

We drive out to the western edge of Reno, past housing developments and dogwood trees, to the end of Fourth Street.

"I want you to see the progression," he says. "The hills up the river, through the new nice houses, then the industrial, the weekly motels, downtown, to where it all peaks at the new campus." He's talking about a huge new homeless shelter built after I left. A dozen yards off the street there is a large white building shaped like an agricultural or military outpost. He describes the facility: brand new, nine hundred beds.

Mikey and I talk about how complicated our feelings can get about places like this. He mentions a day when the campus had just opened, and had called 911 so many times that he felt like the EMS system for the entire county was hijacked. At the time he was furious. But lately, he wants me to know, the place has matured. "It's better now. They have grass courtyards, and laundry, and showers," he says. "They build an on-site medical clinic. I mean, we still go there a lot when they need our help, but there are good people doing good work."

When I got in the car that morning, I had asked Mike how work was going. I didn't ask him about understaffing, or the homeless population, or the economics of the influx of new housing, or the social impacts of recent population changes, but of course that's where our conversation drifted. It had to. These issues *are* EMS.

———

In the 1960s everything happened all at once.

The Korean and Vietnam Wars proved that speed was the ultimate medical intervention in traumatic injuries—the sooner the surgery, the more likely the save. And this knowledge was more relevant than ever: car accidents were more common, and more deadly. The United States had just completed the transnational highway system, a technological and logistical Cold War triumph that created thousands and thousands of miles of pristine asphalt for Americans to splatter themselves over. In the late 1960s, more Americans were losing more blood, farther from the hospital, than ever before. The federal government noticed: in 1966, the National Research Council published a paper highlighting a major national problem: the new freeway system, increases in industrial accidents, overcrowded ERs, and no national system of emergency response. They equated the resulting suffering and death to "a public health problem second only to the ravages of ancient plagues or world wars."

Traumatic accidents and heart attacks. Both not just causes of death, but causes of young death. Unexpected death. Over the next decade, dozens of counties came up with ways to train a generation of emergency responders in the basics of cardiology and trauma care. Haywood, North Carolina. Pittsburgh. Miami. Seattle. The feds got on board. Several government acts set aside funding for ambulances, dispatching, and a nationwide regional EMS system. But all of the money came with an expiration date: local emergency systems were supposed to become self-sufficient within a matter of years . . . somehow. There was no clear strategy. Once again, everyone agreed that ambulances were vital, but no one wanted to pay for them.

Then, on top of all of these changes: Hollywood.

A dramatic soundtrack plays, sirens wail. A fire station in the foothills of Los Angeles, the roll-up door slowly lifting to reveal two hunky men in uniform hurrying through the garage. They climb into . . . a fire engine? A ladder truck? No! A little red pickup truck, stocked full of tools and heavy gear boxes. The driver, a stoic blond, gives us a knowing side-eye while his younger partner fumbles with a helmet. These two men aren't just any firefighters. They have medical skills also! After pulling a young boy out of a condemned building, or coaching a teen into landing a plane while his father lies slumped in the front seat, they pull out brown leather bags and call their base hospital on the radio. Following direction from Dr. Brackett or the sultry Nurse McCall, they provide lifesaving interventions right there on the ground. They start IVs, give fluids and medication, or deliver a baby in the middle of a wildfire. Who are these humble heroes? And what did their characters do for American emergency care?

When the show debuted, the "paramedic" was a brand-new idea. Rather than staffing ambulances with doctors, nurses, or laypeople, several counties across the country were experimenting with an entirely new type of medical caregiver: a specialist, trained in CPR and emergency techniques, who was specifically trained to work on an ambulance or rescue team (the delineation between EMT and paramedic would come later). One of the first cities to adopt these new professionals was Los Angeles, where the program caught the attention of the producers of *Dragnet*. Rob Cinader and Jack Webb worked closely with the LA Fire Department to create a wildly popular television series called *Emergency!* The show ran for seven seasons and is often credited with introducing most of rural America to the concept of paramedics. Suddenly every small town in the country wanted a team of brawny dudes to rush into their emergencies and save the day. The medicine and rescue techniques used in the script are surprisingly accurate for the time period. But the show is told from a fire department's perspective: medical interventions are seen as a cool addition to firefighting and extrication, rather than the main event. The emergencies are dramatic. The saves and losses are final.

When I first became a paramedic, my teachers and chiefs had all come of age watching Johnny and Roy, the show's lead characters, and joked about them all the time. But a lot of those same guys had a real bitterness about the job, and I always wondered how much of that came from subconsciously comparing their actual lives to the heroic-yet-adorable antics of the two guys they had grown up watching on TV.

I spent years wondering why paramedic school spent twenty minutes on abdominal pain and two weeks on cardiac arrests, when my abdominal-pain patients outnumbered my codes forty to one. And why did we spend so much time on burns and amputations when these patients were so rare? Why didn't we spend a month learning about alcohol withdrawal and liver failure and methamphetamine psychosis?

I don't usually stop to appreciate just how earth-shatteringly revolutionary it must have been the first time a heart was successfully defibrillated. The techniques developed by Peter Safar, Claude Beck, Frank Pantridge, and the rest of their cohort fundamentally changed the capabilities of an ambulance. The EMS of the 1960s imagined a future in which cardiac arrests, strokes, and traumatic accidents would no longer spell death for the American people. It must have been such an exciting time to be on the front lines, pushing the definitions of medical care, experimenting with brand-new technology, changing the laws of life and death. But nowhere in that vision was anything about the poor, the drunk, or the alone—what the author of the first federal paramedic curriculum called "squalor and misery . . . the decay, the violence, the depravity." The original charge of the ambulance, our origin and our inevitable future. Or, as a partner once said after a particularly weird day, "I tell you, man, this job is like riding through the sewers on a glass-bottomed boat."

The 1970s and '80s were full of governments revving the engine and then stalling out; in the words of historian Ryan Bell, "an incomplete revolution." Congress passed the Emergency Medical Services Systems Act in 1973, which provided grant funding to local governments to set up their own regional EMS systems. But when the federal money ran out, the local governments wanted nothing to do with them. The program was eventually dismantled by President Ronald Reagan in 1981.

So the ambulance programs continued to struggle. With money, with staff, with call volume. As they always had. And the minor emergencies, the sore throats and drunks that frustrated the first paramedics in the 1880s? The poverty, the addiction, and the mental illness that a New York ambulance surgeon described in 1902? The tummy aches and flus that plagued La Guardia's New York in the forties? Those calls didn't just go away.

Mikey gears up Sun Valley Boulevard, left on Seventh, then down Chocolate Drive, a deeply rutted dirt road that borders trailers and the open desert. I can't decide if the whole scene is tamer than it was a decade ago or if I'm just more used to the desert now. When I was twenty-five, this street was just about the wildest moonscape I'd ever seen in my life. Dust clouds, porch swings, half-dressed little kids leaned up against a shotgun rack, blowing gum bubbles at the sky. Teenagers riding dirt bikes up to Dollar General to pick up groceries. I was a city kid back then, as blown away by Nevada itself as I was by the medicine.

I make Mike double back up the main road to see if my favorite panaderia is still open and we buy flan and fresh churros wrapped in greasy paper and stand outside for a minute, licking the sugar off our fingers.

"Look, if we were only used for true emergencies, you could run the city on like four, maybe five ambulances. We'd all be out of a job."

"Yeah, tell me about it." I know the same thing is true in each of the three counties I have worked in. It's not even an American problem. I had just finished a memoir by an Australian paramedic titled *You Called the Ambulance for What?* He tells story after story of citizens with stuffed noses and sunburns calling 000, the Australian version of 911, then pointing to the pension card on their night table indicating that the call will be paid for by the government. His writing style is entertaining, but underneath the humor he is furious. He feels that the system is being abused and his emergency skills are being diluted. New York Fire Department lieutenant Anthony Almojera describes a functionally similar experience but comes at it with a different perspective. He grew up in a rough neighborhood and lost friends to diseases that he says could have been prevented by better insurance or more mental health resources. He sees his role as caretaker for the folks who can't or don't know how to take care of themselves, even if it means arguing with hospital security about storing a frequent caller's shopping cart full of her belongings for the thousandth time. Almojera's writing reminds me of a favorite captain of mine. No matter how angry and frustrated I became with my work, Miguel would answer the phone as though he was thrilled to hear from me. "Joanna!" he'd say. "Talk to me. How can I support you?"

Mikey takes his last bite of flan, says that's gonna ruin his diet, and continues. "A doctor at an urgent care that doesn't want to make a decision. Security at a casino, with a drunk guy being problematic. A care home killed someone and is panicked and doesn't want to deal with it. A homeless guy is shouting on a street corner. Call 911." He looks down at the city. "Call us whatever you want. We are the make-the-problem-go-away button."

I learned quickly as a paramedic that most of our calls would not be life-or-death emergencies. That our patient load would be mostly low-acuity, mostly primary care. Modern paramedics usually think this is a new phenomenon, caused by cellphones, or lack of education, or lack of primary care availability. Many of us blame the opposing political party. I think we all agree that the situation is currently the worst it's ever been—we know for a fact that things weren't this bad in the past, because they *couldn't have been.* Our hearts will not let us accept any other truth. But the more ambulance history I read, the more reflections I found of the current job. I kept finding examples of non-emergencies, financial hardship, and understaffing. It was a house of mirrors.

I still get frustrated that the job is not a well-paced day full of nice people with interesting medical complaints. That we are treated as disposable by our management, held late, denied breaks, and used up until we injure out and get traded in for a newer model. Looking back at history and seeing that we have been plagued by these same issues for hundreds of years could be depressing, but personally I find it soothing. I find comfort in knowing that our pain is not ours alone. I can tell myself that I am part of something bigger.

I once got to spend a few months as a desk captain at the ambulance station while a supervisor took his paternity leave. One of my duties was giving a short morning meeting to oncoming crews to tell them about any road closures or important news of the day. The announcements were boring, and one of my morning teams started requesting a funny quote or a joke. I started with dumb one-liners, but one day I didn't have anything on hand and instead read aloud from the history book I had stashed in my backpack. I chose a section from back in the 1860s about Bellevue Hospital commissioners fighting with the police department about using the ambulance too often for drunk patients instead of saving it for "a real emergency." I wasn't sure if the humor would hit first thing in the morning, but the EMTs and paramedics busted up. Encouraged by the laughs, I held up the book like a children's read-aloud, showing a black-and-white picture of two tired-looking officers in uniform and told crews to think of these brave young men; "No really, later today when you are running on a 'police evaluation' for some drunk guy for the fourth time in a row, I want you to think of these dudes being annoyed about the exact same thing a hundred and twenty years ago and know that you are connected to a beautiful American tradition."

In the opening of *Cannery Row*, John Steinbeck writes, "Its inhabitants are, as the man once said, 'whores, pimps, gamblers, and sons of bitches,' by which he meant Everybody. Had the man looked through another peephole he might have said, 'Saints and angels and martyrs and holy men,' and he would have meant the same thing." I think maybe he was talking about working on an ambulance.

COVID

What you've got to understand is that, in the beginning at least, we had done this all before. Every winter, we stood around a windy courtyard holding stapled packets titled things like "Emerging Infectious Disease (EID) RESPONSE PLAN: Policies and Procedures Manual" and cracked jokes as our radios beeped and muttered on our hips. The instructor would stop in the middle of a paragraph to listen to a page or answer a phone call. The papers would tear loose and fly around our feet in the breeze, full of caps lock and acronyms.

"PURPOSE: To ensure that our employees are protected from risk of exposure in time of pandemic.

"POLICY: The following policy will be adhered to at all times when encountering patients who are either highly suspected to have or are confirmed to have an infectious disease including but not limited to: Severe Acute Respiratory Syndrome (SARS); Middle East Respiratory Syndrome (MERS); Ebola Virus Disease (EVD); Influenza Like Illnesses; and Noro-like Viruses."

Every year we stood around for twenty minutes with our packets and our boxes of masks and Tyvek suits and practiced for the next Big Scary Pandemic. We donned and doffed our masks, we duct-taped ourselves into bunny suits and chased each other around the parking lot yelling, "You got Ebola!!!" We were told that in the event of such an emergency the dispatcher would ask screening questions about recent travel or contact with exotic animals. I always imagined a 911 caller holding a cellphone in one hand, with a plane ticket and a dead bat in the other, looking suddenly awkward and saying, "Well, er, the thing is . . ."

These trainings were crammed between our shifts, and if ambulance levels dropped too low we would stuff the packets into our pockets and head back out onto the streets. As we drove away, the supervisor might yell at us to read the rest online. During the latest Ebola scare, we spent several hours learning a complicated, thirty-step suiting-up process, while trainers emphasized that even a small mistake at any one of these steps could lead to a fatal compromise in sterile field. Put your hand in the sleeve like this; remove the gloves from the packaging like this; duct-tape the seal of your boot closed like this. If you do this side first, you could die. If you pull this flap the wrong direction, you could die. You could spread the disease to your family. You could flame an outbreak. All three layers of gloves in the right order, or everyone dies. We practiced exactly once. We then stuffed the suits into bags, shoved them down to the bottom of the gear pile under the bench seat, and never looked at them again.

When terrorism was the trendy fear, we learned nerve gas antidote administration instead. We heard how to inject ourselves with 2-PAM in case of an attack, yourself first and then your partner. "Remember: you will be vomiting, shitting, bleeding, and crying at the same time, so pull it out of the packaging like this and stab it into the meaty part of the side of your thigh." Those kits went behind the driver's seat. They collected dust, expired one by one, and eventually got thrown away. We still find some packaging stuffed in a bin from time to time and laugh. *Hey, remember when we were supposed to be scared about this?*

I've had many, many sick people breathe on me over the years. I've had drunk guys with hep C spit blood at me, I've had AIDS patients bleed all over my pants. I've had so much pneumonia coughed in my face that I should probably have it growing in my eyes. One time we transported a guy with a massive infection in his leg and the doctor recognized him and said, "Oh, shit! This is the guy with nec fasc! This dude's got nec fasc!" *Fucking seriously?* Necrotizing fasciitis is an extremely deadly flesh-eating bacterium, famous for its speed and fatality. I stared at the man's swollen, pus-filled leg, which had just been on my gurney, in my ambulance, pressed against my seatbelts. We had the wound covered with a blanket. I asked the doctor if we'd just had an exposure. He was an athletic frat-bro type. He squinted his eyes for a few seconds and said, "Nah, it was a while ago. You're probably fine."

If you receive an actual needle stick, or someone spits in your eye, there's exposure paperwork and testing. They can prescribe antivirals. You have to be careful with your romantic partner at home. You do a whole thing. The restrictions can last for a full year. But how many little droplets here or there just get wiped away, washed down, and we hope for the best? We've all wiped blood off our forearms and tried not to think about it.

I once met a war and disease photographer who told me over a bottle of bourbon that while covering the Ebola virus in West Africa, the media would meet at the bar every night, get hammered, and then pass around a thermometer. The reporter with the highest temperature had to pay for the drinks.

By winter of 2019, Maggie and I have gotten to know each other a bit better. We swing by her house for a change of pants one day and I am introduced to her husband, Charles, a tall, smiling man who is "very pleased" to meet me. Their dog, a mid-sized black-and-white shepherd, presses his wet nose into my palm to request a treat.

Maggie realizes that she and I both tend towards an energy crash about eight hours into our 6:00 a.m. shift, sometime after lunch. This begins a campaign of afternoon sugar hunts: each day around two or three we search for a bakery or coffee shop in whatever neighborhood we find ourselves in between calls. On days when we manage to find something before getting a call, we dig into muffins or cookies and spill crumbs on our laps. Later, when the whole world gets weird, we cling to this tradition.

I'm in the back of the rig flipping through my phone and find a story about the first California woman who died from COVID. The story says she was on a cruise ship which has since been quarantined and investigated by the Centers for Disease Control and Prevention (CDC). I turn to Maggie.

"Dude, was this the same boat? Maggie, I think this was the boat!"

I thumb frantically through news articles looking for the name of the boat and its docking location.

A week earlier, we'd run a call on a woman inside of one of the massive cruise ships that often dock in SF Bay. I had been joking at the time about how disgusting cruise ships always are and how we should probably wear masks and hazmat suits when we went inside. It had not yet occurred to us to be concerned about the brand-new virus wreaking havoc in China. When we arrived, we wheeled our gurney past large crowds of tourists getting on and off of the boat. Today was the San Francisco "port day," and everyone wanted to check out the city. We were led in through a side entrance, up an elevator, and into the medical center. Our patient was an older woman with a minor injury that needed to be seen by a specialist. A young doctor with a fancy accent gave us the patient's report and

X-rays on a disc. We chatted for a minute, then helped the injured woman onto our cot and rolled her down the gangway and out to the ambulance.

Maggie looks over at my phone and sees the article I'm reading.

"No," she says. "There must be a ton of cruise boats, what was it called? When was that run?"

The news gives the dates that the sick passenger was on the boat, and the name of the cruise liner. I thumb around. I check our old records, which list the name of the ship where we picked her up. It was totally the same boat.

We both shriek. Should we, like, tell someone? I don't know! We were there for, what, twenty minutes? I check the call notes. Maybe half an hour. We wore gloves . . . ? We were hanging out in the medical center of the first boat to dock in California with a COVID outbreak on board.

We eat our scones. We shouldn't laugh, but the whole thing is too ridiculous to hold it in. I can't believe we were on the stupid pandemic boat. Which has since, by the way, been quarantined out at sea. They are currently airlifting virus testing kits down to it from a helicopter with a lot of news coverage and fanfare. The day we ran that call we watched a couple thousand people from that boat line up to head out into the city, eat at restaurants, get drunk at bars, and presumably cough in public restrooms and lick silverware all day. *What the hell are they quarantining?* I wonder. *They were all already here. It's way too late.* This type of wildly obvious contradiction becomes a point of exhaustion for most health-care workers throughout the next couple of years.

We debate what to do. We haven't been given any official policy yet. Maybe there's a phone number, 1-800-Do-I-Have-Corona, that we can call and report ourselves to. I had a sore throat last week but I've been fine since then. Maggie has a pretty nasty cough. She's been doing her best to open windows and wipe down the steering wheel, which is common courtesy when you show up to work sick, which we all do. We only get so many sick days per year, and we get exposed to a ton of bugs. It's our job. Every winter we all cough and apologize and keep working.

We stare at our phones, wondering if they will soon start ringing with blocked numbers from CDC officials when they are done circling the anchored boat in their helicopters and rappelling down food kits or whatever Hollywood drama they're on about. We run a call—a woman in her twenties who fainted at work and seems particularly scared about taking the subway. She never says the word *COVID* but instead keeps dancing around it, saying, "You know, all these new . . . flu . . . the flu, and everything." We reassure her, tell her she's not crazy for being afraid, we're going to take good care of her, just make sure you wash your hands before you leave the ER. We tuck a blanket around her and double-check her IV. I lean to Maggie as we walk out of her room and whisper, "Should I tell her we were on the fucking boat?"

Maggie elbows me in the ribs.

After debating all day, Maggie and I decide that we should tell someone we were on the boat. The supervisor working is my favorite one, but he seems pretty burned out today. There's a lot going on, people shouting, ambulances coming and going. I tell the supervisor our situation and ask him if we're supposed to like . . . do something? Or report something? The captain is simultaneously checking his computer, his phone, his paper schedule, and standing up to go do something outside. He raises his eyebrows and looks at us over his glasses like a tired schoolteacher. "I think you're fine," he says, and walks away. I look to Maggie, who coughs while trying to cover her mouth. She shrugs and we head to the locker room to change.

I had planned to sleep at my brother's house that night, but I can't stop thinking about his cleanliness and his tendency to take things seriously. I picture him grilling me with questions about the pandemic, pretending to be okay with my presence and then wiping down every surface after I leave.

I stand in the locker room for a few minutes, then decide it's not worth the headache. I have a sleeping bag in my truck. It's a cold night and as I try to get some rest I wonder if I should be staying inside to keep my immune system strong. But then I picture having to either lie to my brother or tell him honestly about my day, and I don't like either option, so I rub my feet together and pull an extra sweatshirt over my eyes.

At Philz the next morning Maggie debates cream in her coffee. She always drinks it black, but for some reason this morning cream sounds good. I raise my eyebrows at her. "You know why your body's craving all that extra fat and sugar, right? All those little 'rona viruses need something to feed on!" We chuckle. I hope my parents are safe.

About three weeks into all the craziness, I get a text from an old friend. "So, what's it like being a paramedic during a global pandemic?"

I type "Haha" and hit Send.

I shake my head, and add a photo I took of Maggie and me holding vitamin C packets over tiny paper hospital cups of water. I had decided that I would boost our immune systems with vitamins, as though that would help with the coming apocalypse. I write "lotta this" and send the photo. Then I describe our last call—we had transported a woman who called us because a girl at the nail salon seemed sick, and now she felt anxious and light-headed. "We were, like, okay, so basically, you saw an Asian person cough?" I type. "Anyways me and Maggie are just out here eating tangerines and licking doorknobs how are you?"

One night on the phone, my brother and I aren't arguing, exactly. We're just tossing the ball back and forth. *It's killing a lot of people. The flu kills a lot of people! No, people are dying. Yes! People die! That is how diseases work! But they're suffering! Yes. That happens! Pneumonia kills a shitload of people every year!* I think back on how many patients I've treated who were septic, barely breathing, and actively dying of bacterial or viral pneumonia. So, so many. So many. The wet, rattling cough. The wheezing gasps for air. The hot, thin skin.

Yes, this one does seem worse. I'm sure it's going to kill more people. How many? I don't know, some? A lot?

I don't know anything. Nobody knows anything. At work, everybody is making fun of this thing while secretly feeling a little bit scared. The system that we worked in had seemed to be on the brink of collapse for so long that we all wondered how screwed we'd be if a real disease actually broke out. The only two possible emotional responses seemed to be fear or laughter and, well, we are paramedics.

So far, our coronavirus protocol is like this:

1. There's a PowerPoint presentation we're all supposed to watch online, but the security controls on our work computers won't let us access the website and the link doesn't work from home. It's written on the whiteboard, "Mandatory! Coronavirus training update online!" Several of us point out to our supervisors that the website isn't accessible. They frown and say they'll pass it up the chain. The bulletin on the whiteboard stays up. No one ever watches the presentation.

2. We are given new wipes for our gurneys and equipment. The canister looks the same but the top is orange instead of purple. We are told to use the orange wipes if we suspect coronavirus exposure, the purple for regular patients. What if we were on the coronavirus boat a week ago and this patient clearly has some sort of bacterial gut infection causing him to shit his pants for a month and his diaper touched my leg while we were moving him and the patient after him had pneumonia and the patient before him was a baby? Which wipes do we use for that?

3. Our dispatches now say that the patient has been asked coronavirus screening questions. They do not say if the patient screened positive, or even what their answers to the questions were, simply that they were asked. We are on our way to an older man with a fever and possible sepsis and I go back and forth with dispatch asking if the man had screened positive. "We ask all patients those questions now." Yes, but what did he answer? "It's for everyone now, everyone gets the same questions." Yes, I heard you, but did he screen positive or not? "We just had to ask because of the fever." Yes, but what did he say? "It's just on the list now, we have to ask." *Oh my god. I give up.* Maggie says, "I hope someone puts this on the news later," which is not out of the question as our radio channels are all publicly recorded lines.

4. We are required to wear our personal protective equipment (PPE) on any call for which we suspect a potential coronavirus exposure. Scratch that, wear them every call. Wait, no, maybe just exposures. No, definitely every call. The amount and style of PPE that we are issued changes daily and includes but is not limited to N95 masks (issued by a captain), simple surgical masks (if you

can find them), gowns (I think I saw some yesterday?), gloves (plenty of those), face shields (I heard they're going to order some soon), and boot covers (your guess is as good as mine).

I think a lot about sterile field this week. On an ambulance, everything touches everything. I change my gloves a few times per call, but we simply aren't able to keep things perfectly clean. I open the front door with my clean gloves on, then I touch the patient. Then I open the back doors with my dirty gloves. In the back, I touch shelves, I carry equipment, I touch the IV tray. We can't change gloves every time we open a cabinet or grab a box, and we don't have surgical techs to pass us the equipment or take notes for us. We wipe the gurney down after each call, but a lot gets missed.

I hear about how many of the tech companies are having people work from home and having meetings online instead of in person. I watch cultural splinters begin to develop as certain population groups are told to stay home for their safety, and others are told to buck up and go back to work. Resentment grows. I think about Victorian England during the bubonic plague, and money, and Marxism, and how the working class will keep cramming onto buses and subways like they always have to show up and punch the clock. My job, of course, is to walk straight into where all the sickest people are and do my thing. Then I think of what ICU nurses must be going through and feel like a baby.

My brother calls me asking if we have enough hospital beds to withstand an actual epidemic, and I snort. I think of the hours and hours I've spent standing in hospital hallways because the ER is backed up when there are no beds upstairs. That's how you get to five ambulances hanging out in an ER hallway while 911 calls go unanswered outside.

The unanswered calls are dubbed a "response time" issue on our end, which means we're getting forced overtime again tomorrow. So basically, AJ, of course there aren't enough ICU beds. There haven't been for years. San Francisco is overwhelmed and understaffed on a good day. So is every other major American city. Every time there's a heat wave we have to call for mutual aid.

AJ tells me that I should come back and stay at his house again. He says we will take turns in the kitchen; we will buy sanitizing wipes. He wants me to know that I have somewhere to go. But his house seems so clean and so safe, and his carpets are still white, and I feel dirtier than ever. I tell him I love him. I tell him no.

My brother hangs up and I overhear a captain lecturing some interns about corona; he rattles off a bunch of info that I was supposed to read in the online presentation that never opened. He shows them how to slice a plastic catch basin in half, cut slits in the top and bottom, and shove it in the side window to create a little air vent that will pull air into the back as you drive to ventilate the ambulance a little better. Says that's what they used to do on hot days way back when before they had air conditioning in the rigs. It looks pretty silly.

When I start to see news reports filled with shock and handwringing about potential hospital bed shortages, my initial reaction is not concern or fear. Instead it is a deep rage. I feel like I have been watching a house on fire for years and screaming and screaming and everyone keeps walking straight past me and then one day someone says, "Oh my god, did you know that house is on fire? My god, someone should do something!"

Dude.

It's been burning the whole time.

———

The government of San Francisco works out a deal with some privately owned inter-facility ambulance companies to send stripped-down transport ambulances out to COVID patients who are stable enough not to need advanced intervention. These are the units that have never run 911 calls—they are paid instead to take medically fragile folks to and from places like nursing homes or dialysis appointments. They tend to be staffed by twenty-year-old brand-new EMTs, rather than experienced paramedics. It frustrates me that we are sending our lowest-paid, least trained, least protected employees out into the thick of it to transport the most contagious cases. I know that's how it works, and that this is resource distribution in an austere environment, but I still clench my jaw. I buy the kids sodas at the hospital when we run into them and ask about their day. They actually seem happy, excited to get overtime pay and be part of something historic. Honestly, I remember that feeling. When I was twenty I would have loved to be part of something big and scary and dangerous. But the grownup in me can't help but wish I could shut the whole thing down.

Maggie and I gown up for call after call. Everybody has COVID symptoms. After every patient we are supposed to wash our hands, decontaminate the ambulance, wash our hands, remove our gowns, and wash our hands again. Only there's no running water on an ambulance, so instead we squirt sanitizer on our dirty palms and hope for the best. One Friday we are called to an upstairs apartment with a large family. The father was transported to a South County hospital several days ago and confirmed to have COVID. The mother has symptoms now. Fever, cough, weakness. At this point we've run a dozen calls for folks who thought they had the symptoms, but this is our first official confirmed case. The virus is still brand new, a terrifying unknown contagion that could end the modern world as we know it. We still have no idea if we are walking into a house filled with the common cold or with the next Ebola.

A captain meets me at the scene to help and we put on our equipment carefully. Gloves, gown, second pair of gloves. We still have N95 masks at this point, though mine is about a week old and fraying at the edges. We don't have face shields yet. Captain Watson pulls a thin papery bag out of a hairnet packet and tries to put it on his head to cover his hair, but it won't fit—the opening is the wrong size. I stare as he tries to slide his head into the narrow opening. A large pocket of material flops down cartoonishly over his eyes.

"I think," I say to him, "you're putting a boot cover on your head."

We lock eyes and he pauses. He pulls it down and stares. Both of us know on some level that this should be funny, but there's a palpable fear in the air, and instead he whispers back, "That's . . . hysterical." We both turn the corners of our mouths up but nobody actually laughs. We put on the rest of our gear and quietly push the gurney towards the building.

The daughter, who looks like she's in her thirties, has a scarf wrapped around her face and neck to cover her mouth, and her eyes look around the room and never stop moving. There are children underfoot, and we hear muffled voices in other rooms. The apartment is stuffy and full. We sweat under our gear. We help the mother onto the gurney as we learn that she is eighty-two years old and not an English speaker. We can't get to our phones without breaking every contamination rule, so we can't call a translator. There's not much to say anyway. The daughter tells us her symptoms and helps us lift her off of the couch. On the way to the hospital I have the air conditioner and the exhaust fan blasting, but our ambulance windows only open about three inches so it seems pretty futile. My plastic glasses fog every time I exhale, so I can't see much. Her oxygen levels look good. I can't start working on my chart because we've left the laptop in the front of the ambulance to keep it uncontaminated. There is no medication I can give her besides oxygen, no more testing I can run. I sit with my hands in my lap, trying not to touch anything. The patient and I stare at each other over our masks and through the fog of my glasses. She looks tired, and afraid. She's feverish and weak but not actively coughing. We're transporting her to a different hospital than her husband, not that they would allow visiting between rooms anyway. I know they may never see each other again. I put a hand on her knee and give her a squeeze. She looks up at me but her face doesn't change. We ride to the hospital this way: in silence, my hand on her knee, through double layers of gloves and plastic and fog and recirculated air.

Maggie and I listen to loud music on the ambulance all week: Etta James, Luther Allison, Tracy Chapman. We are filled with nervous energy and the rhythm helps us keep ourselves together. Then, on Wednesday, the city comes to a screeching halt.

There is no official lockdown yet. But everything is eerily quiet. The stoplights signal to empty intersections, gas stations sit dry. We keep checking to see if our radios are on because we've never gone this long without hearing calls go out. We run only four calls the whole day: a dead guy in the morning, a little girl with asthma, a toddler who fell off a play structure, and an old man who needed help up some stairs. We get home from our shift on time for the first time in months. We wait for the other shoe to drop.

A few days later the shelter-in-place order is announced. Maggie and I are sitting in a shaded parking lot out by the water. We are enjoying the quiet moment, playing word games on our phones, watching a man teach his three-year-old how to ride a small red tricycle near the entrance of the lot. When the alert comes beeping through our phones like a tornado warning, we stare at each other and start flipping through news apps like addicts. A few minutes later the man leaves his kid on the tricycle and walks slowly up to our ambulance to ask us if we know anything. Is he supposed to go home? Can he finish the bike lesson? What about work tomorrow? We throw our hands up: *Honestly, man, your guess is as good as ours.*

The morning after lockdown begins I leave for work at 4:00 a.m. It's dark and raining and the highway is empty. My heart races. The wet reflection of neon on the blacktop looks pixelated and I feel like a side character in a dystopian sci-fi movie. I decide to lean into it and play the loudest dubstep I can find, heavy bass grinding through my car speakers. I think of the sharp white of a hazmat suit against the dark of the night; I watch my car headlights cast yellow cylinders into the empty road. I pass an electric sign that, instead of warning about road construction or traffic delays, reads "AVOID TRAVEL. STAY AT HOME. BEAT COVID-19." The letters glow in the wet night.

The proper medical terminology for the putting on and taking off of PPE is "donning and doffing." The formality suggests that rather than casually tossing my sweaty gloves and mask into a parking lot trash can, I will use sterile technique to remove these items without infecting myself in the process. There is a common exercise in para-medic school in which a giggling instructor sprays shaving cream all over our gloved hands, then watches us practice removing the gloves without getting any foam on our skin. But while safe glove removal is second nature to a seasoned paramedic, my movements with the mask are clumsy. I have worn an N95 mask at work before, on a patient with a particularly contagious disease, but on completing the call

I have always grabbed the outside of the mask, pulled it from my face, and tossed it in the trash. Now I am expected to wear the same mask for days or weeks on end, so I must use it in such a way that the inside surface remains disease-free no matter what gets splashed onto the outside.

At first, every time I don and doff my gear I feel a wave of fear. Did anything touch anything? Did a particle of virus touch my sleeve and then my sleeve touched the inside of the mask and now I'm smashing it onto my face to rebreathe for the next forty-five minutes while I transport this patient? I grow angry at patients, angry at people for calling 911 and exposing me to their germs. We run out of purple-top wipes, then orange tops, then alcohol. We are instructed to mix our own bleach solution every morning, 1:9, in a spray bottle. The mist stains all our uniforms with pointillist orange tie-dye.

The masks get soggy after a few days. They are made of paper and elastic, not meant to be reused dozens of times. There is no easy way to protect the interior between uses. We experiment with storing the masks in cardboard boxes, cutting various shapes out of cheap felt ambulance blankets to hold against the infected exterior of the mask while pulling it on and off. It's not a perfect system. We make new ones every couple shifts as the tape gets worn or the cardboard starts to sag. One day I draw googly eyes on them in Sharpie while Maggie is in the bathroom and she comes back and screams. We call them our COVID Friends.

After a couple weeks Maggie sees an internet video where a guy makes a similar device out of Tupperware. We hold different containers up to our faces to see which might fit the closest, and find some Thai food takeout bowls that seem to do the trick. We use a pair of trauma shears to snip tiny bites in the sides for the straps of the mask and try it out, holding empty noodle cups up to our masked faces in the front cab. It works surprisingly well, and we find ourselves smiling behind the plastic. Way better! We clap our hands like little kids for a minute, pleased with our innovation despite our fear.

One night we are standing in line with our gurneys, waiting for our patients to be seen at the county hospital. Two of the older paramedics begin telling stories about working in San Francisco in the late eighties and early nineties. "Do you know what they used to call it?" Bob has his hands on his hips like he's a teacher and we're a bunch of preschoolers. He looks at us expectantly. "You know what 'GRID' stands for?"

He's talking about AIDS, of course—initially called "Gay-Related Immune Deficiency," because the disease was first identified in gay communities in New York, Europe, and San Francisco. During Bob's lifetime, our city was an epicenter for one of the worst disease outbreaks in the history of the world. The hospital we are standing in now housed the very first ward dedicated to caring for AIDS patients. The fire department whose badge I now wear had been heavily affected by the fear and homophobia and compassion of those early days.

Bob talks about how scared everyone was, how they didn't know what was happening. He says, "There was a lot of ugliness back then. People would wonder about certain types of people. A lot of people were scared. They were scared of certain kinds of people, no one knew what was happening, we didn't have gloves, we didn't know how it was passed . . . You saw a lot of fear, ignorance . . . A lot of ugliness . . ."

It's a natural comparison, but I'm not sure what to make of it when I weigh what I know of AIDS history against what we are going through right now. It is spring of 2020 in this hospital hallway. Are we overreacting? Are we underreacting? There's so much loud noise everywhere and it never stops. There's no signal in the noise.

———

For a few months the news reports make it sound as though many, many first responders will die. I read essays about Italian nurses and Chinese doctors dying in their scrubs. Kyle and I discuss how burned out I had been at work the last year and whether this is the time to step away. I shrug and tell him, "Well, obviously I can't quit now."

Kyle remains stoic throughout the pandemonium. He cooks meals and takes me for walks along the water. He pores through statistics with the analytical focus that got him through his math degree, then tells me he is pretty sure my friends and I will live to see next year. When more and more of our friends are sent home from their jobs to shelter in place, we both hold our breath for a moment. We wonder if he will receive a reprieve as well, as his role as a machinist seems to fall in a bit of a gray area. But his job is soon declared "essential," like mine. For the rest of the pandemic, both of us will continue to put on our boots and drive to work and punch the clock, no matter how much things change around us.

Maggie and I pull up to one of the dozen hospitals in San Francisco and they've got big white military tents set up in the ambulance parking area. Which means there's nowhere to park the ambulances. I swallow my annoyance and swing the rig sideways across the entrance. There's a card table set up outside with a sign that says "STOP! Triage outside before entering Emergency Room."

No one is there. I say something sour to Maggie, something like, *If they won't give us anywhere to park and don't even bother having anybody here we're just walking straight into the ER like we always do. Fuck these guys.*

My anger is misplaced. It's been building for a decade now and it erupts out of me at all the wrong times. The truth is that parking at this particular emergency room has always been lousy, like it is at almost every hospital in San Francisco. I'm sick of trying to wedge my ambulance into a tiny spot at a weird angle with a post in the way, and then pull the cot out on an incline that hurts my back because they built the step without thinking about us and the city *still* won't buy us electric gurneys. I'm tired of people pulling up to the ER entrance and then casually leaving their Teslas in the way of an ambulance when they walk inside. Truth be told, I'm still mad about that time four years ago when a different hospital took away three of our spots and glued an "Uber Parking" sign on top of the "Ambulance Parking" sign in their pull-through.

But the reality is it's not even about any of that, either. The reason this COVID tent is causing an acidic burn to rise up out of my gut and into my chest is that this particular hospital is crueler to their paramedics than anywhere else I have ever delivered patients. I know I shouldn't blame the nurses, who are just as frustrated with their management as we are, but they roll their eyes at our reports and throw our EKGs in the trash and avoid eye contact when we bring in a sick patient. They leave us five, six, seven in line, butt-to-butt in a small hallway next to the triage desk with two patients on hospital beds crammed in next to us. This is the hospital where, my first week in San Francisco, I saw a nurse casually using thick Velcro straps to secure a row of patients into chairs when they were too unconscious to sit up on their own. Rather than being placed into beds, the patients were left slumped in hallway chairs with their chins in their chests, drooling in their laps as the nurse wrenched the strap tight enough to hold them almost upright, one after another down the whole line.

If I'm being completely honest, underneath all of *that* is a whole other memory. The real, real reason that I'm so mad about the COVID tents is this guy I brought in with an abdominal aortic aneurysm about three years ago. A "triple A" is a rare but deadly condition in which the aortic wall thins, balloons outward, and finally bursts. We found him in the living room of a cute upstairs apartment, with his family huddled in the kitchen. They said he pulled a muscle in his back. He presented with back pain and stable vital signs, and we started the transport code two, no sirens, but something didn't feel right. A few blocks from arrival I knew something was wrong, but at the time we still had eleven hospitals all using the same radio channel to take reports from ambulances. I had already told our receiving hospital my patient was stable, and there was too much chatter for me to break in and tell them his condition had changed. I kept pressing the button to speak and getting interrupted by other units telling other hospitals about their patients. I never got the chance to say a word.

When we got into the ER, the one which had now filled their ambulance parking with a proud display of flapping white disaster tents, there was no nurse at the station. There weren't any nurses anywhere. My guy looked like shit. My partner at the time said, "Jo, he's *gray*." I said, "I know, that's why I'm trying to find a nurse." I walked around frantically, trying to get someone to make eye contact with me. It was about five hours until someone did. Or maybe two minutes. Or ten? I don't know. It felt like too long. Eventually a young doctor made the mistake of walking past the charge desk and I said, "Hey, I'm really worried about my patient, can you—" But she walked right past me. I felt like a kid trying to get my mom's attention, tugging on her sleeve while she took a phone call.

Eventually a nurse stopped by the desk to put something in the computer and I said, "Look, we brought him in code two, but he doesn't look good, I'm really worried, can we get a room," and she took a deep breath without looking at me and slowly typed in the computer, explaining that they were quite busy but she would do what she could. Then a different nurse walked by our gurney on her way to somewhere. She stopped suddenly and said, "Hey, this guy looks terrible," and gave me a look like I was an idiot. I said, "I know, that's what I've been trying to say," and she said, "What the fuck, he's got no blood pressure, he needs a room." I said, "I fucking know."

Now we had some movement. We wheeled him to room 31, way in the back of the ER. They tried to clean the room and get him situated but they couldn't get a blood pressure reading and three of the nurses started arguing about what to do and finally someone overrode someone else and said he needed to get into a code room. These are special rooms in every ER that are set aside for critical patients. They are bigger, to accommodate a larger team of caregivers, and stocked with more equipment. The nurses quarrelled about which one might be empty and finally our patient was put back onto the gurney, half gowned, and wheeled back to the front of the ER, where they stood him up and moved him over and tried to finish getting his gown on and get everything plugged back in and he leaned back into the bed and died.

I stood in the rear of the room, clenching my jaw, while they worked the cardiac arrest and declared him. A doctor waved an ultrasound over his chest, squinted at the imaging screen, and muttered something about a "massive triple A." Then he grumbled time of death and walked away.

About twenty minutes later my partner had her hand on my shoulder, saying, "Jo, he was gonna die today. Nothing you could have done would have changed that. Today was his day." I was staring into the windshield, replaying it over and over, wishing I'd looked harder for a nurse, or gone code three from the start of the transport, or screamed like a maniac in the hallway instead of trying to stammer my concerns like a shy teenager.

I crawled into the rig and opened my laptop, willing myself to get over it and start doing my paperwork for the run. My phone rang. It was my dispatch supervisor, calling to tell me that the doctor had complained, and wanted to make sure the paramedic knew that "that guy she brought in code two had died," and that I was spoken to about my poor judgment. I burned with shame and grief and frustration and I buried it for years. But this *fucking COVID tent in my fucking parking lot* pulls all those emotions back out and throws them all over my face.

I don't say any of this to Maggie. Instead, I continue complaining about the new triage process, and she gently offers to take over so I can go get some water. I'm still standing over today's patient in what's left of the ER parking lot, shoving my feelings out of the way, when a nurse finally materializes and stops us. He makes us wheel our gurney back behind the card table and asks our patient's symptoms. He pulls open a drawer filled with two different wristbands. Fever, cough, difficulty breathing? Okay, orange. Blue. I don't remember. Our patient gets the "not COVID" wristband and is led into the main ER.

As COVID proceeds, we all hear a lot about health-care workers and heroism and trauma and burnout. I think it's hard to explain sometimes, how hard it is to hear pundits and newspapers and family members talking about our courage and dedication or whatever as though all of our brave sacrifice started out of nowhere the day the lockdown began.

The EMS members at SFFD have a group Facebook page that we use to vent or locate lost stethoscopes and jackets. I rarely post, but one day Maggie and I are arguing about music and I break my social media silence and write a message to all of the ambulances:

"Hey morale is in the shitter so I'm spending the day force-feeding my immigrant new partner Bay Area music history lessons to remind both of us why we work in this foggy drug filled cartoon of a city in the first place. She is British so she's way too polite to say no. Today is early 90s hip hop day and I'm looking for suggestions. So far we've just been binging on Hieroglyphics/Souls of Mischief and some other Oakland shit. Tomorrow is punk rock day. Anybody wanna get in on this?"

The post explodes. I don't usually use Facebook—in fact, I only really keep the account to check our page for work announcements—but suddenly we are glued to our phones. As luck would have it we are in one of the few ambulances today with a working aux cable and I hook up my phone to the rig radio. The song suggestions Don't. Stop. Coming. Everyone sends us track after track, texting and posting and stopping us in hospitals to high-five or play a beat. The musical soul of the Bay bursts through all of the bullshit and we dance in our rig all day. Underground hip hop, hyphy, punk, ska, East Bay Hardcore: the mid-nineties music scene that Bay Area kids grew up with was dirty and rebellious and conscious and lyrical and stoned and for twelve hours it dumps through our crappy ambulance speakers. After "Now You Do" by A-1 and Flosstradamus, Maggie bursts into giggles. She says, "'He's got a big mouth like a pelican bird!' That's a great line! That's really pleasing!"

I teach her about hyphy and East Coast/West Coast rivalries. One medic recommends a particular Spotify playlist and I have to explain the word *slapper* to Maggie. One guy starts giving us jazz songs written in North Beach in the 1970s. Another posts a song recorded by one of our own medics at the department. We miss tons of radio traffic and almost blow out the sound in the rig. It's an amazing day.

———

We get sent to a "man down" at a bus stop, phoned in by a passerby. I hop out of the driver's side to see if I can find the patient. It takes so long to put on my mask and goggles and everything that I'm still adjusting myself as I look around the scene. It's a three-sided bus shelter with a bench seat on the inside. An older Latina woman leans against the outside with a grocery bag, ignoring us completely. A tall white man sits on the bench seat, slumped onto the inside of the wall. As I move closer, I see that his face and hands are blue, and his skin looks sweaty. From here it looks like an overdose.

Maggie is already walking towards me with the gurney, so I decide it will be faster to just get him into the rig and sort him out there than try to bring all our equipment to him. We have new procedures every day now and I'm insecure about running a call in the middle of the street—I don't want to end up on YouTube fumble-fucking around with my gown and mask as my patient dies.

Our guy clearly needs Narcan and oxygen, but we just got an email yesterday saying that high-flow oxygen has been determined "high risk" because it can blast all the viral particles right into your face. They have told us to use extreme caution and "full PPE" when applying oxygen but haven't actually defined what that means, or given any specific instruction on how to proceed if your patient isn't breathing. And the amount of PPE we have available is constantly changing. I start pulling out equipment and try to figure out what to do. "Okay," I tell Maggie, "let's bag him, but don't hook up the oxygen until we're gowned up."

I pull a bag valve mask out of the wall, which is a device used to provide rescue breaths to a patient who isn't breathing on their own. It has a face mask attached to some oxygen tubing and a big, football-shaped plastic sac. The rescuer plugs in the oxygen, then holds the mask to the patient's mouth and squeezes on the "bag" like a fireplace bellows. Without any oxygen attached, the squeezing motion will still force room air into the patient's lungs, which is better than nothing. I hand the bag mask to Maggie, inject some Narcan, and start putting him on the monitor. He looks like shit.

Someone passes me a shrink-wrapped PPE kit and I look up to see that the engine has arrived and gathered around the back doors. I put on the shitty white gown as the guys crowd towards the rig to help out. The firefighters standing outside are gowning up, but the engine paramedic has already hopped in with us. He and Maggie are using two hands to hold the patient's head in place and breathe for him, so they aren't able to put on their own gear. We hop around taking turns ventilating the guy, putting monitor leads on, stuffing one arm into a gown, or pulling goggle straps over our heads. It's a tiny space in an ambulance. People are trying to help each other— "I can tie that for you while you hold the mask onto the guy's face, okay, move one arm, okay, do the other." It's a zoo. Men and women keep jumping in and out of the back doors.

While we are doing all of this, the man's pulse is slowing. I think to myself: *This guy is about to code.* I think: *His face is blue, but we still can't turn the oxygen on because there are people who don't have their gowns on yet.* I think: *Fuck.* To be honest, I don't think these gowns do much to protect us, and we're already stuffed together like a pile of greasy sardines leaning over this guy's face. Is fifteen liters of oxygen really going to make a difference? But everything is so overwhelming and complicated and screwed-up right now that a simple protocol feels like a guide rope through the shitstorm. I feel responsible for the safety of the engine crew, Maggie, and the patient. And Kyle. He is always in the back of my mind these days: still stoic, still calm, still supportive. But the last thing I want to do is bring my germs home to him. I decide the gowns do matter, because something has to, and that we will not plug in the oxygen until we are all suited up. I cling to this arbitrary choice like it's keeping us alive. I notice Maggie and Polarzi, the engine medic, are putting on hairnets, which seems like a good idea, but it doesn't occur to me to take one for myself. We still don't have any face shields.

Eventually all of us get our gear on and I look around. I'm holding the end of the oxygen cord like it's a live wire. When I finally plug it in and watch the reservoir fill, it's too little too late. I thought the Narcan would kick in by now, but he keeps getting worse instead of better. My head is still spinning with all the PPE shit, the COVID shit, the doomsday shit, the tangle of it all, and I'm trying to remember how to treat an unusual cardiac call. Polarzi says, "Should we pace him?" I look at the heart rate on the monitor, which is dropping lower every second. Polarzi is right. I nod at him to go ahead. He presses the buttons on the monitor, trying to remember the sequence to send rhythmic electricity into the patient's heart. It's a procedure we do for the type of slow heart rate we are seeing in this patient, uncommon but not unheard of. I've done it maybe a dozen times over the years. It's simple enough, but it's not a built-in muscle memory, so we have to step out of our discombobulated COVID brains and remember how to actually think through a problem.

I'm holding the patient's wrist to make sure that his pulse rate matches what the machine is telling us. The cardiac monitor begins showing what's called "electrical capture": a green squiggle that means that the pacemaker is trying to do its work. But instead of lining up with what I see on the screen, I feel the man's pulse weaken and disappear under my fingers. We turn the pacemaker off and start CPR.

The chest compressions bring up some fluid, so now we've got to suction, which is another one of the high-risk procedures we're supposed to be afraid of right now. Suctioning is usually easy: a long plastic tube attached to a bucket is inserted into the patient's mouth, then used to vacuum up any liquids that are threatening the airway. But as with the oxygen delivery, this procedure now requires "extreme caution." And as with the oxygen delivery, we have no idea what this means. We're all wrapped in sweaty bedsheets like a COVID apocalypse fever dream and I wonder if maybe I am hallucinating this whole thing.

I grab another kit from the cupboards and drill a hole in his knee to give medication. I push the first dose of epinephrine. Maggie, hunched over his face with the suction tubing, pulls fluid out of the man's mouth. When she has cleared enough to see what she's doing, she inserts a tool used to keep his airway open. Meanwhile, the lock pops off the tubing in his knee and I can't get the hose to stay on and the pressure squirts saline all over my stupid tissue-paper plague costume. I ask if we should try a King tube in his airway, but Polarzi says the basic one that Maggie placed is working, and I say, "Good call, fuck it." We do a rhythm check: still no pulse. I try to get a second epinephrine in but we got a new brand of medication again this week and the tube is a weird shape and the top is stuck on it somehow and I swear I spend a full minute jerking around with an epinephrine dose trying to get the damn thing to work. Eventually I throw it on the ground and grab a new one, which works fine.

We debate transporting; we're a block from the closest ER. Usually we would work an entire arrest at the scene, as interrupting chest compressions to package and transport has been proven terrible for outcomes. But this man is already in the back of our ambulance, the COVID protocols are making everything ten times harder, and we could be inside of a fully staffed emergency room in less than five minutes.

We try to figure out who's going to drive. We are all theoretically covered in poison now, and the front seat of the ambulance is where Maggie and I will spend the rest of our shift, eat our meals, and use our charting computers. It's supposed to be a clean area. Anyone who's been in the rig would have to remove their now-contaminated gear, sanitize, get up front to drive, and then get out and put on a new set again at the hospital. There's a back and forth. There's still one engine guy standing at the back doors of the ambulance, who has been passing us equipment and helping out but hasn't actually stepped up into the workspace yet, so is he still clean? Sort of? The patient keeps trying to die on us, so we decide he's clean enough and tell him to get up front.

We get pulses back right as we arrive. When we pull the gurney out of the ambulance the cords are tangled up in the oxygen tubing and the bag valve mask keeps slipping off the patient's face but we make it work. His oxygen saturation and end tidal numbers are better than you'd think. This probably means that we managed to give him good chest compressions despite everything, which is nice.

We get him inside. The doctor is calm, he talks slowly, he takes us seriously, the hand-off goes well. I start gathering our shit and leave to get the laptop out of the ambulance for a signature. I stop at the trash can right outside his room to try to doff my gear and go through three pairs of gloves just trying to figure out what order to take everything off in so that I don't contaminate myself in the process.

Maggie and I debate whether to keep the masks for another day or ask a supervisor for new ones. We are supposed to keep using the same paper masks until they are "visibly soiled," whatever that means.

When I walk back in to check on things and get my signatures, I'm a little surprised to see that the patient still has a pulse. I wonder what medications they have dripping into him. They're putting in a urinary catheter and drawing labs and he has been intubated. I stare for a minute at the white plastic tubing snaking out of the patient's face towards the vent and it occurs to me that I'm looking at one of the precious few ventilators left in the country right now. Everyone on the news won't shut up about how we're running out of these lifesaving machines, and here is one hooked up to a guy from a bus stop who I didn't think would live another ten minutes. I wonder how viable the man is, and how long he will be kept in the ICU. I stare at the vent for a few minutes, thinking of the nationwide struggle for these devices, how many people might wonder right now if he needs or deserves this thing. I don't know the man. I don't know his story. Does he deserve a chance any more or less than anyone else right now? I followed my protocols as well as I could. I think I did my job. My mask is itchy.

I'm lying in the back of my truck. I have given up entirely on sleeping at my brother's house and spend all my nights between shifts on a small camping mattress in my Tacoma. I have to face the wrong direction because the ground has a bit of a slope to it and we are required to point our cars nose out in the station parking lot. It's quiet enough. The bed feels comfortable, but the streetlights are bright. The pillowcase I bought for my new set-up is slippery and it keeps sliding around under my head and my mind is just racing, racing. Spinning and racing. My stomach has been upset, which I'm pretty sure is just from stress and too much takeout food. I feel like someone injected me with stress. Everything is shaky. I can feel my heart beating a little faster; I feel like I can't slow down. I'm tired and anxious at the same time. I try baking bread in my head, a trick I learned from a PTSD therapist to keep grounded. I keep thinking about corona, and panic, and fear, so I try to close my eyes and bake a loaf of bread to get to sleep. I stir the flour . . . no, start over. I reach into the cupboard. Images of trains full of Jews in World War II, military coups in Central America, real historical precedent for widespread social collapse. No, start over. I turn the oven on and set it to 350 degrees. I pull the flour out of the cupboard, and the baking soda. I think about hazmat suits, and respirator masks, and tents set up in front of the hospitals. I turn the oven to 350. I pull the flour out of the cupboard. I smell the inside of an N95 mask. I think about running out of masks. I think about hospital hallways lined with cots of young dying men during the Great Flu of 1918, a nurse holding a pale hand weakened by an unknown disease, a speck of blood on her apron. I turn the oven to 350 and pull the flour out. I get the sifter out from the other shelf. I decide I'm making a rye loaf and I measure out three and a quarter cups of white flour, evening out the top of the cup measure each time. The flour is soft and clean. I use a butter knife against the cup measure, because my hands are infected now, my hands are a vector. I wonder if I will sicken whoever eats this bread. I think about the yellow gowns at the hospitals, the thin paper flapping against medical scrubs, the same gowns we used to wear before all this when transferring an infectious patient, how much I hated them on a hot day. I wonder how long we have, whether this is all overblown and it's just my anxiety, or whether we are really in for it. In San Francisco on a good day it feels like we're on the brink of collapse; it feels like we already have collapsed. I think of the Tenderloin, the walls of human debris, the drugs and shit and piss and homeless shelters full of sick half-humans lying on floors and cots and rich people with their flying cars zooming by the windows, how primed we are for something to spread. I picture Selma Dritz—the doctor in the STD clinic in the Castro in 1983 who saw how the men were fucking, saw how the illness would explode, tried to sound the alarm but no one would listen, thinking *holy SHIT this could get really bad.* I think about how often I've had the same conversation with my co-workers, standing in line at a hospital, waiting forty-five minutes for a bed, running out of supplies, walking through shelters full of coughing people, tired people, thousands of people with no hygiene and no immune systems and nowhere to go, thinking, *God, fuck me if something happens,* if something respiratory comes or another heat wave, or an earthquake. My hands feel like poison vectors and my ambulance feels small and the back of this car is full of hot air and my stupid slippery wrinkled pillowcase won't stay put. I breathe in for four counts and out for eight. I turn the oven to 350.

During a bubonic plague outbreak in London in 1665, the city paid for sedan chairs to transport infected patients to and from home and hospital so as to limit their exposure to the general public. Two unlucky bastards would heave a chair up onto their shoulders and then pick their way through cobblestone streets with a disease victim slumped over their heads.

Almost two hundred years later, in 1832, a cholera outbreak in Manchester inspired another innovation in medical transport. Though the United Kingdom had faced plague, smallpox, and scarlet fever, the scale and speed with which cholera could decimate a population was new. The disease can kill a new victim within a matter of hours. Manchester designed horse-drawn "fever vans" to pick up contagious patients and transport them to the hospital, and several years later London followed suit. Across the Atlantic, the United States was facing the same fear. In 1866, the city of New York appointed a celebrated Civil War doctor named Edward Dalton to be its "Sanitary Superintendent," a new position that proved relevant almost immediately. Just a few months into his tenure, Dalton learned of a cholera patient in a crowded tenement building downtown. Recognizing the need for swift action, he ordered the construction of a series of "flying wagons," which soon became famous for their rapid response. The carriages would be staffed by a sanitation inspector and a medical attendant, and would be kept at the ready at all times.

Within one hour of receiving news of a suspected cholera case, the crew would arrive at the location, confirm or discredit the report, and set about burning and sanitizing the patient's belongings. If the victim was still alive, they would be loaded into the wagon and transported to a local hospital. If not, the body was taken away to be disposed of properly. The flying cholera wagons were so successful that only three years after this outbreak, Dalton helped the city commissioners establish permanent ambulances at their hospitals modeled after their design. Although military advancements set the stage, in the end it was a disease that inspired the United States' first municipal ambulance service.

The last thirty years or so have been strangely free of infectious disease, at least in upper-class America. There is a lot of talk on the radio of these *unprecedented times*, a lot of shock and panic and *how could this happen*. But the threat of a mysterious virus lurking in the air that could get inside you and break down your lungs, cripple your body, destroy your way of life: this is a fear that most humans have lived with for most of history. Back in 1866, as cholera ravaged Northern Europe, the craftsmen of John Woodall and Son designed a brand-new style of carriage that replaced the cotton and leather seats with enameled wood to reduce infection spread. They even fashioned a mattress and pillow from early Indian rubber. Today our bench seats are upholstered with plastic for even easier wiping down.

I think it helps to try to understand how desperate things already felt on the ambulance before the pandemic. Long before we'd ever heard of COVID-19, we stood in parking lots reading our infectious disease outbreak handouts and learning how to wipe down door handles and steering wheels, all the while the radios begging ambulances to clear from hospitals, calls waiting in a queue, ER waiting rooms overflowing out onto the street, violent patients ripping themselves out of restraints and attacking crews. We were already fighting a battle out there. COVID-19 may be a new contagion, but the evolutionary arms race between humans and infectious organisms is the whole reason that ambulances exist in the first place. And that overwhelmed feeling? That feeling that nothing we are doing is working, that this battle is bigger than us, that we are very small and looking out at a very large fight? That's just a normal day at work.

For a few months our call volume vaporizes. Days usually filled with drunks, abdominal pain, traffic-filled transports, and long hospital wait times are suddenly twelve hours of tense silence punctuated by the occasional life-threatening emergency. The only calls are either for COVID symptoms or for people who thought their emergency was so important that it was worth the risk of calling us, of exposing their houses to the outside world, exposing their loved ones to the germ-filled hospital. When we arrive, families are full of fear and adrenaline. "We didn't want to call," they say, "thank you for coming, we thought she would die if we didn't call." People wear masks and wait in the other room. We whisk away their loved one, perform emergency care the best we can, arrive at the hospital and are quickly rushed into a room. A doctor even meets me outside at the back door of the ambulance one day. I do a double take as he stands in the wind and says, "Whaddya got?" like we're on an episode of *Gray's Anatomy*.

At work, we keep having the same conversations. *This is what EMS was supposed to be*, we whisper in awe. Scary and important. *People are only calling us when there's actually a real emergency.* People only call when they think they really, really need our help, and Maggie and I go from running ten calls per day to two. Transferring our patient at the hospital is efficient; instead of waiting in a line at the ER in a hallway full of gurneys for forty minutes we are brought straight inside.

We hold our breaths.

The world seems to rupture into two sides: folks who are still hiding inside, and people who are out in the world, moving on with their lives.

"What's it like?" everyone keeps asking us. People are cracking open the doors of their houses, afraid to go outside, afraid to buy groceries or talk to us. "What's it like out there, are you guys okay?"

I mean, no, we're not okay, but that's nothing new. We haven't been okay for a long time. Honestly, it was really weird and scary for about a month, but somehow that was also one of the best months of work I've had in a long time. I felt important that month. Needed. There was something invigorating about 911 getting used sparingly by grateful folks with urgency in their eyes. Now COVID is just one more thing. It's just one more big broken screwed-up thing in a big broken screwed-up city. Are we drowning? Sure, we're drowning. But we've been drowning for years.

Journal, spring 2020

Things were so exciting for a minute there. They felt so real. But one day I look up and I'm just back to the grind. I still go to work, I still get paid, now I scratch at a little ring of acne that's formed where the soggy edge of my mask grinds against my cheeks all day. Lots of people keep dying, but the media begins to move on. For a few months there was this sudden and terrifying common enemy. It reared up like a wave and bent and hollowed and crested but instead of crashing it lost all its power and broke into a million tiny pieces and instead of being drowned tragically in the fight we're all just up to our knees in dirty foam. We're back to where we were before, but with sad eyes and wet socks.

One morning we bring an old Italian man with a bunch of broken ribs to the emergency room: he's in his seventies, in a beautiful apartment on the north side of the city. The family looks like a cartoon—siblings and grandchildren and cousins underfoot, all talking over each other and waving their hands. A younger woman leads the man's wife out to say something before we pull away. The wife comes out wearing an apron and squinting like she just stepped out of a pasta sauce commercial and leans into the ambulance and shouts something in Italian. He shouts back. There is more hand waving, pointing at pockets, more Italian. The man digs his wallet out of his pocket and hands it to us, the woman gestures, and we pass it to her. She waves her hands upward and he does a hand motion with all his fingers bunched up and she shouts again and waves. We all smile at each other and we shut the back doors and drive off. No one seems scared of COVID anymore; he's just off to the hospital to get his ribs fixed up like it's no big deal. I give him some fentanyl on the way over but I can tell he's still hurting. He closes his eyes and stays very still. When we get to the emergency room, they leave us waiting an hour on the gurney in a hallway with this poor old man and his pain. When we finally get a room, we wheel over and see a "STOP! Isolation Precautions Required!" sign taped to the door. There is already another patient in the room, the two beds separated by a curtain.

The thing about broken ribs is you can't really take a full breath because of the pain. It's very easy to get respiratory infections when your ribs are broken, and if you do get sick it's difficult to heal. The thing about broken ribs on an elderly patient in the middle of a deadly respiratory pandemic is that we don't want to put the guy in a room with a COVID patient. We stop the gurney outside the room and stare at the sign while our brains record-scratch. I ask the nurse about the patient inside. She sighs. "I'm pretty sure that guy was negative." "Umm . . . can you check? How sure are you?" How quickly did we go from mass casualty incident tents and military ship hospitals and outdoor screenings to "I'm pretty sure that guy's negative." I mean shit, I know, American health care and all, but *fuck me*.

We wait in the hallway for a while until two different nurses tell us to just put him in there. I walk in first and creep around the other guy's bed, wondering if I should break some privacy laws and eyeball his paperwork real quick. The patient looks up at me and I think of asking him outright but he seems confused. He's not coughing. After a few minutes another doctor yells at us and we give up and put our guy in the room. There's nowhere else for him to go. We walk out hoping we have not just made a widow out of the nice pasta lady in the apron.

Every time our local governments try to tighten their lockdown protocols, the whole Bay Area descends onto Santa Cruz. With no bars, clubs, sports, or social gatherings allowed in their own cities, a day trip to the closest beach town seems like a good way to get out of the house. But the leadership in Santa Cruz has its own concerns about infection numbers. The county closes off a bunch of parking lots, as though this will somehow help, so cars line the sides of the freeway up and down Highway 1. The beaches, parks, and outdoor areas are packed with drunken crowds. Strangers park their cars in Kyle's driveway and on his lawn, looking for ways to get to the water. Then the city closes all of its public restrooms, so tourists pee on the ground and crap in the bushes. Neighbors gather in front yards to complain that the rules are too strict or not strict enough. I spend more time at my own house on days off, as Kyle's neighborhood, much closer to the beach, feels suddenly impossible.

Kyle remains unfrightened by my germs. He seems to accept that we will take this walk together this year. I peel off my work uniforms in the garage and shower before I hug him, but we share meals and a bed as we always have. When I occasionally panic about infecting or killing him, he smiles and brushes off my concerns. He jokes that he will probably somehow get COVID from his job before I get it from mine anyway, because the universe has such a twisted sense of humor.

Maggie and I walk in the door to an SRO room as a cloud of flies buzzes out to greet us. Everything is covered in shit and mold and rotting food. We expect the usual scene, alcohol bottles or crack pipes and a patient too loaded to notice the mess. I brace for an argument or a fight.

Instead we find a thin man in his seventies, curled on the floor between layers of feces. We try to pull him onto the bed to examine him but his legs are contracted and there is so much filth that it is hard to get a good grip or find somewhere to put him. Eventually we scoot him onto our gurney and start to wipe down his body. We check his vital signs as we talk.

He speaks quietly and beautifully, a little confused at times, but we slowly learn his story. Someone is supposed to come over to clean his apartment and bathe him and make sure he gets fed, but due to shelter-in-place the services were stopped. He doesn't seem embarrassed about the state of his room, only sad. He says, "It used to be better."

We ask him about his life as we get him cleaned up. He is a veteran with a master's degree in education and social work. He had wanted to be a military professor, but back then the job was reserved for white men only, and he is Black. So he volunteered in jails and at youth programs. He still helps out at a nearby school, or did when he could still get around outside on his own. When he got cancer the hospital treated him but let his legs became so severely infected during his hospital stay that he is now unable to walk without assistance.

He pees into a urinal and then empties it into a bucket because he can't get to the bathroom. The home health aides are supposed to empty the bucket, but they haven't been to his room since lockdown. He says he is supposed to get physical therapy soon, or was before the lockdown, and he wants to get back to walking so he can return to work and to helping people. He tells us he spent his stimulus check on sugar cereal, and lets out a chuckle as we pull a box of cookies-and-cream chocolate squares down from on top of the fridge. He tells Maggie and me to please to help ourselves but our gloved hands are covered in feces.

I check inside the fridge. Milk cartons, a package of fake cheese, and a couple frozen dinners. Everything else is rotting and blanketed in mold. His food delivery has also been cut off. "Non-essential," my ass.

We clean the place up a little, filling two large garbage bags with poop and trash and rotted food. I fold some towels and stack them on his bed. Maggie takes the trash downstairs to try to find a bin while I stay and organize what is left of his food and belongings. We slowly wipe off his legs and back. We get him some water. We drive him in to the hospital to get looked at and I fill out an Adult Protective Services report on the phone. The APS guy has a thick West African accent and he spells his name slowly for me to put in my paperwork, *H* like house, *E* like elephant, *T* like Tom, *H* like house, *E* like elephant. He thanks me for calling and says he will open a case for our patient.

As I get off the phone I run into my friend Nora, who says she just got into it with a nurse because they wouldn't let her back into a patient's room to give him the jacket he had left in the ambulance. The nurse had explained that no one was allowed in right now because the patient was COVID positive. Nora pointed out that she was the transporting paramedic who had just dropped him off. The woman wouldn't budge. It's policy, she said. You could get exposed, she said. Nora asked: Have you ever seen an ambulance? Do you know how air works? Nora tells me they went in circles for a minute until she finally just hung the jacket on the doorknob and walked away.

I know the nurses are even more frustrated and exhausted and bullied than we are. I know I'm wrong to be angry at them. These are the same men and women who I have worked alongside for years, who have helped me understand my most difficult patients and fixed my mistakes and left out cookies for us in the break room. And I know that their management has changed policies on them just as often as ours has, and they know far better than I do what will happen to all of my patients once they're no longer mine. But it is hard not to explode at someone. I just keep thinking of all the layers of hypocrisy in this job, all the things people don't see, how everybody fears the wrong things, and how this whole situation is just going to fold itself into one more sheet of laminated bullshit.

By late summer of 2020, the adrenaline rush has melted away. I'm not sure what the last four months were. A social experiment? A bizarre fear exercise? The overflow tents at hospitals sit unused, gathering dust. The talking heads have used their political capital and the counties have spent their money. The war metaphors and calls for unity are fainter and more easily ignored. There are some improvements, of course. We have more masks now, more gowns, and more test kits. We have a better idea of what we're dealing with. But the rally cries, the brave stomp of boots in lockstep, the cheering of distant crowds and uneasy hope in strangers' eyes; that stuff is all gone.

Maggie and I keep looking for cookies. Every afternoon, we trawl the city for baked goods, trying out Chinese bakeries, gluten-free cafés, and Persian tea houses. One morning we stumble on a free pile of treats at a hospital and Maggie takes a bag, then writes NOT UNTIL AFTER 1400 in Sharpie and throws it on the dashboard. She has decided that we will wait until afternoon for our tea-and-cookies time, like proper adults.

Then, during the hottest stretch of summer: wildfires. California always burns for a few weeks, but this year our fire season is particularly dramatic. The sky is choked with smoke for months. I am still sleeping in my truck at work, and I wake up coughing every night. Finally I clean out a shed in my parents' Oakland backyard and start spending nights there, using a gallon jug of water to wash my hands after I pee against the fence. If the neighbors see me I figure I will flash my paramedic badge and ask if they have a better idea.

One morning we pull the ambulance onto the sidewalk at an "encampment resolvement," which is my new favorite San Francisco euphemism for the city kicking homeless people off the sidewalk. One of the encampers in need of resolving is a man in his forties wrapped up in a sleeping bag refusing to move. He looks sick.

I sit down next to him on the sidewalk and we talk for a while. He's sweating and agitated, and his breaths are shallow. Clear lung sounds. I wonder how close I should sit to him, but it's hard for us to hear each other through the masks, and I've simply lost the ability to be hyper-vigilant every second of every day. He doesn't want to go to the hospital; he's too tired and feels too shitty. He just wants to stay under his sleeping bag and rest.

At one point he rips off his mask to go into a coughing fit that shoots a glob of spit onto my forearm. Oops. I bring my arm towards my masked face and stare at it closely, wondering if I will be able to see tiny viruses, crawling around invisibly like a flea circus. Eventually I snap out of it and walk over to the ambulance to clean it with something. We've run out of sanitizing wipes again and all we have is straight bleach, which is terrible for your skin. Bleach burns or COVID, COVID or bleach. I rock my head back and forth a little, grab the bottle and rag, and scrub my arm for a minute. Sure. Whatever.

When I walk back out to the sidewalk another man is shouting about his belongings while waving some sort of string instrument. He's built a structure out of pallets and trash and parts of a tent, with separate rooms and everything. Some cops and public health department workers stand around trying to negotiate. Everyone looks tired.

The public health workers are in white full-body bunny suits with boot covers and goggles. The cops wear regular uniforms. Nobody seems to have issued them protective gear; they have even been wearing homemade masks this whole time. We are somewhere in the middle, with our gowns and sodden paper N95s. An officer looks at my blue plastic gown and says, "Those look cheap." I say, "Yeah, they are."

We call our guy's doctor and she says he probably doesn't have COVID because he's been sick for too long, but he hasn't had a test yet. I cradle the phone and mouth to my partner, "What the fuck?" We end up forcing our patient to get in the ambulance with us. The captain says we're allowed to compel him because something about quarantine. I have no idea what he's talking about, but everyone seems to go with it. On the way there the guy stays agitated and keeps pulling the blanket over his head. When we get to the hospital, they give us a white sheet to lay over him. Apparently this is the newest COVID thing this month, because of the "fomites." Whatever those are. The nurse says, "Yeah, we're doing this now, in case they're shitting on the gurney or whatever . . . So it doesn't float around, I guess? It's supposed to go over their head and everything. I don't know, you guys cool with it?" We say sure and we drape the sheet overtop so he looks like a kid's ghost COVID corpse on the way down the hallway.

The COVID death count on the hallway whiteboard says "74" today. When we get to a room there is an IT lady in there with a drill screwing the phone to the table because she says they keep disappearing. We ask if people are really stealing phones and she says, "Well, they break all the time. People bring them to the front to fix them, and then I can't find them and they get lost, so I'm drilling them down." The broken phones. So they don't get lost. We wait outside the room with our Halloween plague ghost until she's done.

When we get back outside to the ambulance the air is still thick with wildfire smoke. I'm supposed to decontaminate my safety glasses but we only have bleach, which isn't supposed to go anywhere near your eyes. My eyes burn anyway from the smoke; I'm sure today I won't know the difference. It's already on my arms anyway. I spray some more bleach onto a towel and start wiping. Wax on, wax off.

Eventually, everybody gets COVID. *Everybody.* The last of my coworkers gets it, my dad gets it, Kyle gets it. By now most people are vaccinated, the Omicron variant appears to be less deadly, and the *New York Times* has finally stopped using the word *harrowing* in every other headline. And in the silliest plot twist of all, Kyle's joke about his workplace being more infectious than mine proves true: in the end, he gets sick a few months before I do.

When I finally get infected with COVID, the department is still requiring a ten-day quarantine before returning to work. I have a hard time tracking down a test, but when I eventually see the double line pop up I'm not surprised. I enjoy my two weeks off. If I'm being honest, I absolutely love it. I spend the first four days bumming around in my bathrobe, achy, sleepy, enjoying the excuse to watch TV and drink tea all day. I text Maggie photos of soup and couch pillows; she replies with encouraging quips. I relish having the extra time to recover, wishing that every time I got sick on the ambulance I had two weeks to convalesce instead of having to come back as soon as I could physically withstand the work. When I finally do return everyone says, "Oh, hi, how was it?" like when you take a school exam in the morning and the afternoon class wants to know what to expect. "Not that bad," I answer. "Two weeks off was nice." Everyone laughs and nods, says, "I know, right?" and moves on with their day.

We still clock in and out of work, we still tell stories in the break rooms and make fun of everyone and everything. Every morning I grab a few extra N95s and huck them on top of my box of gloves in the cab of the ambulance. There will be a new disease soon enough, evolution finds a way, so for now I take my mask off between calls, feel the passing breeze on my face, and wonder when we'll get hit with the next one.

There is a quote in David Quammen's *Spillover: Animal Infections and the Next Human Pandemic* that I typed up and posted in the locker room early in the lockdown days, when everyone was still scared instead of just tired and annoyed.

> . . . Ondzie's main job was to respond to reports of dead chimps
> or gorillas anywhere in the country, getting to the site as quickly

as possible and taking tissue samples to be tested for Ebola virus. He described to me the tools and procedures for such a task, with the carcass invariably putrefied by the time he reached it and the presumption (until otherwise proven) that it might be seething with Ebola. His working costume was a disposable hazmat suit with a vented hood, rubber boots, a splash apron, and three pairs of gloves, duct taped at the wrists. Making the first incision for sampling was dicey because the carcass might have become bloated with gas; it could explode. In any case the dead ape was usually covered with scavenging insects—ants, tiny flies, even bees. Ondzie told of one occasion when three bees from a carcass ran up his arms, under his hood flap, down across his bare body, and commenced to sting him as he worked on the samples. Can Ebola virus travel on the stinger of a bee? Probably, for at least a short period of time, if you're not lucky. Ondzie was lucky.

Does this work frighten you? I asked him. Not anymore, he said, Why do you do it? I asked. Why do you love it? (as he clearly did). "*Ça, c'est une bonne question,*" he said, with the characteristic bob and giggle. Then he added, more soberly: "Because it allows me to apply what I've learned, and to keep learning, and it might save some lives."

I look to Ondzie, again and again, throughout the pandemic. As fear and excitement give way to politics and exhaustion I wonder what Ondzie would think. I imagine he would smile patiently, bob his head, and get back to work.

"I'LL GO WITH YOU"

DAN QUINTO, RETIRED EMS SUPERVISOR;
FORTY-SEVEN YEARS IN EMS
SANTA CRUZ, CALIFORNIA

I always think about the amazing people I come across in this work. I have learned to never write somebody off in meeting them, ever. As you work with them, you often find out different things about them. I have learned to look at everybody's points of view, and it is really very humbling.

The last really, really good partner that I had was Shanoa. I've had maybe three or four partners in my career where we could communicate non-verbally and be completely on the same page. You form a true connection.

When my dad died, it was about six o'clock in the morning. My brother called me saying his heart stopped and they were taking him to the ICU. I told him I'd be off work in a half an hour and start down there. It's about a six-hour drive. Shanoa looks at me and goes, "We've been up all night. You're going to drive to LA?"

And I said, "Yeah."

And he goes, "Well, I'll go with you."

And he drove to LA with me. When we got there safely, he flew home. That's the type of bond that you can form.

03:16 a.m., Tuesday. We park the rig in front of an empty dental office and step outside into the warm desert night. We stretch out our arms and legs, cramped from hours in the rig. Before we realize what we are doing, we have both laid down on our backs on the gently sloping lawn.

The smell of the grass reminds me of Oakland, of childhood, of humidity.

We fall into the thin semi-sleep of a medic next to a radio—our thoughts drift and blur and darken but hearing the sound of the number "36" can slice through like a bright white razor and make us jolt upright.

Instead the sprinklers wake us up: I think it's rain at first, but Mikey shrieks like an elephant who has seen a mouse. We both grab our radios and sprint back to the rig, bowlegged and stumbling through the dripping grass.

FREEDOM HOUSE

Too many cigarettes, too little sleep

A state of strange lucidity

The mind outdistances itself and is forever doubling back to pick up stray thoughts

DR. NANCY CAROLINE, quoted in Kevin Hazzard, *American Sirens: The Incredible Story of the Black Men Who Became America's First Paramedics*

In paramedic school, we spent about an hour on the history of EMS. I struggled to pay attention as the instructor flipped through slides about what I saw as a bunch of white dudes with military boners trying to out-hero each other. Something about trauma medicine in Vietnam, a picture of a helicopter, some brawny moustaches in front a fire truck. I perked up for the part about funeral home ambulances, if only because the old Cadillacs caught my eye. But I mostly zoned out, thinking that I'm sure the guys in the pictures were very nice people but probably frowned on everything that I thought was cool about this job.

I found out a few years later that my teacher had skipped over the best part of the story. The nation's first true paramedics weren't military at all, or police, or fire. They were civilians, and they were from the wrong side of town.

I first learned about Freedom House Enterprises (FHE) from an old EMS chief, a thirty-year veteran who told me on hiring that I would need to find my higher power if I wanted to survive more than a week in San Francisco. He was tall and thin, with gangly arms and big hands that he threw up and down while he talked. He liked to lean against the railing of the warehouse stairs in our old station with his new hires gathered round like ducklings on the floor below. He would rail at the bosses of the Fire Department, or the fire commissioners, or the hospitals, or the mayor. Some days he talked about the decrepit ambulances from his early days, or would tell the story of the "Magic Bag of Destination": a blue velvet sack hidden on the back of his ambulance with wristbands from every hospital in the county. If a patient didn't know where they wanted to go, he would ceremoniously reach his giant hand into the MBOD and pick out a hospital.

One day he told me that if I really wanted to know my history, I should read about a group of young Black guys from Pittsburgh who changed everything. He said their story would blow my mind. Then he saw an alert on his cellphone, swore a few times, and ran back upstairs. I googled the name he had mentioned, "Freedom House Ambulance," and found an aging website with a link to a documentary that was currently unavailable. There was no Wikipedia entry, and no other easy lead. I tried to ask Chief about them a couple more times, but never really got a straight answer. I was still curious, but after a few more tries I lost momentum and let it go.

From time to time over the years I would stumble across a brief description of FHE in the back of a book or article. It was always the same, something about an early ambulance company that succeeded beyond anyone's expectations, then for some reason was shut down and lost to history. I spent years wondering how to find out more about what happened, thinking maybe someday I would travel to Pittsburgh and go door to door asking around.

As it turns out, I did not have to ring any doorbells. Or rather, someone beat me to it. In 2021 a paramedic and writer named Kevin Hazzard published *American Sirens: The Incredible Story of the Black Men Who Became America's First Paramedics.* The book is beautifully reported, and for those of us who have a personal relationship with the ambulance, it's a real page-turner.

The story starts with three men in a Pittsburgh neighborhood called the Hill. Actually, it starts before that, with the policies that created the Hill in the first place.

In the 1950s and '60s, American "urban renewal" and redlining strategies shattered the homes and professional aspirations of a generation of young Black men. Local governments destroyed entire neighborhoods in the name of progress, leaving their citizens either forced to relocate or homeless. The city of Pittsburgh, Pennsylvania, demolished the homes of eight thousand people, the majority of them Black. The government did not follow through with its promise of new housing, and the Hill neighborhood fell to disrepair. Thousands of local kids suddenly had nowhere to live, nowhere to safely hang out, and no job prospects. The roughest parts of town got rougher.

A preacher's son named James McCoy was doing his best to turn things around. McCoy had started a small program intended to help create jobs in his community. He named it "Freedom House Enterprises," and raised funds by selling vegetables off the back of a pickup truck.

Phil Hallen was a white guy working for a medical grant fund. He had worked previously as an ambulance driver, and noticed the emergency system in Pittsburgh was deeply segregated. White areas were served by police ambulances, volunteers, or local funeral homes, but all of these programs often delayed or outright ignored calls from Black neighborhoods like the Hill. Hallen thought that starting an ambulance service based in the community might help citizens get the emergency care they deserved, and that the jobs themselves were exactly the type of opportunity McCoy was looking for. After some convincing, McCoy was on board. Enter Dr. Peter Safar.

This was the same Safar who had arrived from Austria, revolution-ized rescue breathing and CPR, and kept trying to persuade the American Red Cross that teaching CPR techniques to laypeople was safe and effective. Safar desperately wanted to prove that "ordinary people" with no medical background could be trained in these lifesav-ing skills. Not only were Hallen and McCoy's people untrained medically, many of them had not even finished high school. They were perfect.

Safar, part Jewish, had survived Nazi-occupied Austria. He believed strongly in the ideals of the civil rights movement, and together the three men set to work. They secured money from Hallen's fund, found vehicles to outfit, and recruited students. The recruits—all Black, all from the Hill—were put through a demanding academy of Safar's design. They learned medicine that until then had been reserved for doctors: CPR, intubation, IV starts, EKG interpretation. They attended rounds in the hospital and practiced on real patients. At the time, the word *paramedic* was used in military circles but was not yet commonplace. The men of Freedom House would be a brand-new type of provider.

Their first call was a seizure on a city bus. The woman was treated appropriately and transported without incident. Before the arrival of Freedom House, the town's emergency services had been unreliable.

A survey in 1972 showed that the volunteer and private companies were generally providing terrible care, and the police weren't much better. The new standard set by FHE improved the quality of medicine being provided to the point that white citizens started to called 911 and specifically request "the Negro ambulance."

Over the next few years, Freedom House ran thousands of calls, proving its model could work. It could work medically, that is. Financially, they struggled. When the funding from Hallen's foundation ran out, it was hard to stay afloat. Politically, things were even more challenging. The police ambulances still provided coverage for most of Pittsburgh's downtown core, but their minimal medical training didn't even include CPR. The police furiously resisted any increased training requirements but also resented the idea that Freedom House could do the job better than they could. The city was loath to give FHE any more than a paltry $50,000 per year, despite happily providing fire with $12,000,000 and police with $19,000,000.

Freedom House had the same problem that had plagued emergency services since the Civil War days: Who would foot the bill? The city wouldn't pay. Their patients couldn't afford it. And when FHE tried to branch out into wealthier neighborhoods, where patients might actually have the means to pay, the private ambulances raised hell. Furious that FHE might step on their toes, they lobbied the city to put them back in their place, equating free ambulance rides with socialized medicine and calling FHE's very existence "unconstitutional." And the deeply racist city council was outraged that Freedom House would presume themselves so important as to take over 911 service from the police or privates, despite every evidence that they were doing a much better job.

My personal hero in the Freedom House story actually did not arrive until 1974. Despite political and financial troubles, FHE had been successfully operational for six years. By this point, other versions of paramedics had cropped up in several different areas around the country. The Department of Transportation was planning to choose an ambulance service on which to base a nationally standardized educational curriculum, and Safar wanted FHE in the running. He knew it would be a challenge, and he knew what it could mean if they managed to scrape out the win. Safar wanted to give the program to a resident who was up for a fight.

Dr. Nancy Caroline initially refused, knowing the job had come to her only because everyone else had turned it down. As the only woman in her residency program at Presbyterian-University ER, she had always felt like a misfit at the hospital and was sick of being talked down to by her colleagues. But Safar convinced her to accept a position as medical director of his fledgling ambulance program, hoping she could push FHE in the right direction. Caroline decided to give it a try. Her world blew open.

Caroline found the ambulance world intoxicating, as I did when I began. She slept on a cot at the station, consulting on emergencies all day and night through a two-way radio. She ran calls with crews, chasing patients through alleyways and arguing with cops. She instituted meetings to discuss patient outcomes with her medics.

Caroline was a dedicated swimmer, like me. She wrote poetry, kept journals, and chain-smoked. She nearly dropped out of medical school but stayed when an uncle convinced her it was the best way to achieve independence as a woman in her era. How could I not fall in love with her? When she was dismissed by the police superintendent after a confrontation about the dangerous treatment provided on police ambulances, she did what any self-respecting paramedic would do: she stole a police scanner and started jumping their calls.

The Freedom House story does not have a happy ending. The bad guys won. On October 15, 1975, FHE came to an end. The program ran out of money, and the city's efforts to give ambulance services back to the almost-entirely-white police department finally succeeded. The city did not appoint Safar as medical director, and in fact ignored most of his advice. They let the Freedom House paramedics apply for jobs if they agreed to take a first aid class—this to men and women who had completed hundreds of hours of medical training and run thousands of calls. Some applied, but between the working conditions and the racism in the police department, most left within a few months. But these guys completely redefined ambulance work in the United States. And they did win the Department of Transportation bid—Dr. Caroline's curriculum would become the national standard for paramedic licensure. Her textbook, now on its eighth edition, is still in print.

There are a few other locations that could rightfully make a play for the title of America's "first" paramedics. Around the same time that Safar was writing out Freedom House's curriculum, two doctors in Haywood County, North Carolina, designed a similar program. Their system was located deep in the Appalachians, in a community used to writing its own rules. Rather than waiting for legal approvals or defining an official scope of practice, the doctors simply got to work training their volunteers. Their team, the Haywood County Rescue Squad, hit the streets within a few months of FHE's first call. Miami, Columbus, Seattle, and Portland also introduced similar programs within a couple of years. And each of these services in turn owes a debt to Dr. Pantridge and his car batteries and his defiance of the Irish medical establishment. Still, Freedom House Enterprises remains by far my favorite ambulance origin story. It's a bunch of

Black dudes, an Austrian immigrant, and a Jewish woman versus the mayor and the cops.

Hazzard opens his book with an encounter between a Pittsburgh paramedic supervisor and a man having a mental breakdown. The patient, found shouting incoherently on a street corner like so many of ours in San Francisco, turns out to be familiar to the supervisor. In fact, they used to work together.

John Moon, the medic, and Ron Ragin, the patient, both started their careers as Freedom House paramedics. Moon stuck around, toughing out the frustrating transition and working his way up Pittsburgh EMS to eventually become assistant chief. Ragin didn't fare so well. Both these men withstood working conditions far tougher than what my friends and I went through—and I've felt on many days that while I hope to follow Chief Moon's path, I could just as easily end up on Ragin's. Moon acts as Hazzard's main muse throughout his narrative, and Hazzard includes a note of gratitude to him at the end of the book. I owe Moon my own thanks as well (and Kevin Hazzard, for bringing out his story). I found *American Sirens* when I was at my most bitter, my most burned out. Since then I have learned more about their work, as it seems they are finally starting to receive some fraction of the recognition they deserve. Freedom House represents the opposite of the militaristic, crew-cut American Hero attitude that turns me off about EMS culture.

Chief Moon didn't swing rescue axes, or jump out of helicopters. He wasn't a war veteran. But no matter what they threw at him, Moon put on his glasses, smoothed his hair, and went to work. As a nerdy, underweight Jewish girl from one of the blackest cities on the West Coast, I could never really relate to the blond guys standing in front of fire trucks in the history books. But Caroline, Safar, Moon,

Ragin; those are heroes I can grab onto. They were community oriented, medicine-first, and worked hard as hell to stay that way. It took me fourteen years in the field of EMS, but I finally figured out who I wanted to be when I grew up.

SAVE EDNA

We pull back into the parking at around 5:30 a.m. from a tough shift. While Jack is refueling, I grab the trash. We never seem to have proper trash bags, so we line our rig wastebaskets with disposable paper pillowcases. They tear easily, but they're better than nothing. When I get to the dumpster and heave open its heavy metal lid, I hear a yelp and the scurrying of paws. The sound travels around the backside of the yard towards my left. I chuck the trash away and drop the lid, then crouch down towards the ground.

"Edna!" I stage-whisper. "Edna, I know you're there!! I heard you on the dumpster!"

Jack looks over from the fuel pump and smiles. We both stop what we're doing and wait for a few moments until a scrawny orange cat slinks out from behind an oil drum.

Edna never seems to sleep. She was a street cat until some of the logistics staff started feeding her, and now she has a preternatural ability to know when your shift was a real ass kicker. Her fur is uneven and matted. She rubs against my boots and lets out a purr. I scratch her neck.

She's somewhere between a tabby cat and a calico, covered in patches of orange and black fur. A white stripe runs down her nose and up her chin, giving her face the angular geometry of a pharaoh's mask. When Edna first arrived, she was skittish and mean, and kept her distance from the crews. But over time she has warmed up to her new home.

On sunny days, we find her sleeping against an ambulance tire, back pressed up onto the hot rubber. Eventually she became so friendly that I am glad of the doubled material in my work pants to protect against her claws when she kneads on my legs. A few times we even catch her facing off against raccoons at our entrance gate, hissing and arching her back to protect her station from the masked intruders.

When the drama unfolds, it goes something like this: Someone submits a complaint. They believe Edna is gross, or unsanitary, or out of uniform, or something. She's been around for about five years at this point, but management finds an old city-wide rule declaring that no pets can live in government buildings. We point out that she lives in the parking lot, not the building.

Also, the firehouses get to have search and rescue dogs. And pet birds. And fish. Also, she chose us and we love her and could you please just let us have this one small piece of joy? The chiefs don't give a shit. The cat has to go and that's the end of it.

Except it's not. An anonymous employee uploads a bunch of photos onto an Instagram account with the handle #FireCatEdna and she starts getting clicks. The website *SFGate* picks up the story, writing an adorable human interest piece about hard-working paramedics trying to save their station pet from the pound. The department's leadership, famous for their strict management of the department's image, go fucking ballistic. A formal investigation is opened. We hear rumors that whoever started the Instagram is getting fired. Anyone who posted on the Instagram is getting fired. Anyone who looked at the Instagram, or thought about the Instagram, or thought about looking at the Instagram is getting fired. Then #saveEdna goes viral on Twitter. CBS News picks up the story, and BuzzFeed. Our cat is retweeted by @FDNY in solidarity, and a firehouse in Texas, and one in Australia. The papers quote a secret in-house source describing how stressful our jobs are, and how Edna has functioned for years as a de facto station therapy cat.

The chief doesn't budge. We receive a memo from operations reminding us that housing an animal on department premises is "not only a policy violation, but also a challenge to maintaining clean, sterile and allergen-free supplies and equipment critical to the Department's emergency services delivery." We point out that keeping all of our equipment in a decrepit, oil-covered garage without trash bags is also a challenge to maintaining cleanliness. We ask our captains to explain how exactly an ambulance that is covered in blood, vomit, and feces and has transported several live dogs and dead humans today is made less safe by the presence of an outdoor cat living in a parking lot. Our captains hold their heads in their hands and tell us they did not personally write the memo and could we please stop hassling them and go back to work.

A logistics staffer "borrows" Edna for the day and successfully gets her certified as a therapy animal. Doesn't matter. We learn that Tuesday will be Edna's last day at Station 49. I arrive at the station for work and find local news trucks parked up and down the street. I badge the gate open and drive in, watching in my rear-view mirror as some guy runs into the lot behind my car and ducks behind a Sprinter van. He's got a backpack and a camera. I walk into the captain's office, wondering if the cat will get some sort of last-minute reprieve, a pardon from the mayor or the president, and find my supervisor sounding exasperated on the phone.

"No, we are not providing comment at this time. Edna is fine. Yes, thank you for your concern. Please contact our public information officer with any more questions. No, thank you."

He looks up at me with *kill me now* in his eyes and hangs up. As soon as he sets the phone into the cradle it starts ringing again. He answers, has the same conversation again, and stares at the phone like it's a hand grenade. He puts it down. It rings again. He presses Mute and asks me if I need anything. I start to speak but am interrupted by the backpack guy from the gate rushing into the office. He starts begging my captain to hear him out, explaining he is so-and-so from the animal rights whatever, and he would like to offer to assist with—

Cap cuts him off politely but firmly and asks me to please escort our new friend out of this closed emergency facility. I gently take backpack's elbow and guide him outside.

We check our ambulance out and debate whether to stage a coup. We've been told that Animal Services are on their way. About an hour before they are supposed to show up, our equipment captain runs outside and grabs Edna, shouting something about how she will never go to the pound. Then she throws the cat into her Jeep and peels out of the parking lot. A picture appears on the Instagram of Edna craning her neck out of a cloth window, watching the station disappear behind her. Animal Services never shows.

I speak with the equipment captain a couple weeks later. Edna has settled into her house and appears perfectly happy snuggling with the dogs and watching TV. She seems to like sleeping inside. She even gained a little weight. A friend of mine points out that causing a massive, nationwide uproar just to upgrade her housing a little may actually be the most cat-like behavior he's ever seen. Back at work, we all keep showing up. No one ends up actually getting fired, but the chief still proved her point. Our emotions are no match for the Big Red Machine.

JOURNAL: AUGUST 6, 2016

"What are you guys, the sidewalk patrol?"

A long pause, then we all start laughing.

"You're goddamn right, brother," says my partner. "That's exactly what we are."

"WHAT'S ACTUALLY AT STAKE"

MICHAEL HAMILTON, PARAMEDIC/RN;
TWENTY-FOUR YEARS IN EMS
RENO, NEVADA

I had been an EMT for barely a year but still wasn't working on an ambulance. There was a big trauma symposium at the hospital that year, and it was all doctors and nurses. I thought if I signed up I'd be the only EMT there, and I really dug being the black sheep. I still had that punk rock ideal.

The first day of the conference went off without a hitch. The next morning was September 11, 2001. I found out about the towers while I was driving to the conference, listening to morning radio on 104.5. When I got there they had a big screen set up with a projector showing live coverage of the event.

I remember hearing about the firefighters and the paramedics and the police officers that went into those buildings and never came out. It was the first dose of reality for me. Up until that moment, I had a very hero-worship idea of EMS. I thought, *I'm going to be on the ambulance and I'm going to save lives.* And I bet that's what a lot of those people that walked up those stairs that day felt, too. I realized it's not all lights and sirens, and running around looking cool, and everybody loves you. At any given time, your life is forfeit.

I used to joke that when the zombies arise, the first wave will be wearing blue uniforms. We are the people that get sent into these events. Someday you might get called on to go up a tower and know that you're not coming back. You need to know that that is what's actually at stake. It drove me to be good at the job, because it forced me to take it seriously. It's not some nebulous philosophical idea of heroism. It's when the sky fucking cracks open, and everybody looks at you. It was a slap in the face.

BLACK WREATHS

(with credit to Kevin Hazzard, Ziwe, and several books of blackout poetry for concept)

> *The HIPAA [Health Insurance Portability and Accountability Act] Privacy Rule . . . creates national standards to protect individuals' medical records and other personal health information. . . . establishes appropriate safeguards that health care providers and others must achieve to protect the privacy of health information . . . holds violators accountable, with civil and criminal penalties that can be imposed if they violate patients' privacy rights.*
> U.S. Department of Health and Human Services, "HIPAA Privacy Rule"

In other words: the most dramatic stories are the ones we are not allowed to tell.

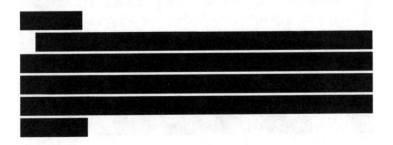

It was the last day of a short week and I was breathing in the sunshine and cool breezes of my last work day before a four-day weekend. We had the *mellowest* morning.

We'd run a few cancels, an easy transport, and now we're posted ████████ and the tones go off for another unit to respond to a victim of a gunshot wound. We drive around for a minute or two and hear some more radio traffic. ████████████████████

██

██

██

██

██████████████

The gunshot scene is "not secure." We have to stage about a block away while police check everything out. ████████████████

██

██

██████████████████████████

After a while we start to wonder why things are taking so long.

██

██

██

██████ a sudden commotion up by the ██████████████████

██

██

█ This is where it gets difficult to interpret the memory, what's real and what comes from other people's descriptions of events after the fact. █

████████████████████████████████████ I can't really see what's going on. ██████ leans against the driver's window and says something important that I can't quite hear. Then I'm getting out of the rig, and ██████ tells us ██████████████████████████████████████

█████████████ My stomach tightens back up. ████████
███████████████████████████ We pull out the gurney
and I look around. ████████████████████████████████
██
██
██
██
██
███
██
███████████████████████████ Cops are everywhere, with guns
drawn. Flanking us on all sides like we're in a drug raid on TV. I
think, *Oh, Christ. Here we go I guess.*

██
███████████ They wave us into a little alleyway off the main street.
They all have their serious faces on.

I'm not wearing a bulletproof vest. It had never occurred to me
to wear one at work, but now that I'm in a circle of jacked-up officers
and gunpowder my chest feels so bare, like I can feel a sudden breeze
against my ribs and heart. My back feels exposed. The stiff fabric of
my uniform has never felt so light.

████████████ when ██████████████████████ and active shooter
trainings become really trendy, we will practice this scenario once
every couple years, following line diagrams on stapled paper handouts. ███
██████████████████████ They have nicknames for the formations and
protocols describing what to do and say. The tactical EMS movement
always seems to have a bit of a blood lust to it, like it's okay if you
get half an erection as you put on your vest and helmet. We make
fun of it a lot, like, "If you get a tactical call-out, and you don't talk

to any girls on the way there, was it even a tactical call-out?" But this was ████████████████ and the trainings don't begin to capture the chaos of the real thing.

We hunch down in our uniforms, and follow directions. The police-gun-sweat-fear posse brings us through a driveway, and I focus on weaving the gurney between the edge of the cement on the left and the police SUVs parked on our right. My awkward gurney moments have been a running joke ████████████████ and I'm desperate not to scratch a car or stick the wheels in the dirt. Plus █ ████████████████████ seems cool, and I don't want to look like too much of an ass. He whacks the side mirrors in as we pass to make more room ██████████████████████ ████████████████████████████████ I desperately want to look up and see what the hell is going on but I'm just laser focused on the gurney and the skinny sidewalk and trying not to fuck that up. ██████████

██
██
██
██
██

██████████████████████ Then we get to the back of the alleyway and look around, the whole world freezes for a second. *Oh.*

████████████████ body on the ground in a large puddle of blood. At first █ looks ████████████ like a TV show crime scene. But the blood is deep red, and woven with thick rivers of coagulation, so instead of a smooth surface it looks more like a biological entity. Though ████████ is obviously dead, █ blood seems to still be a living substance; it has not yet become inorganic. █ hair is matted and wet on one side. ██████████████████████████████

denim wrapped tightly around this dead body ████████████
███ like
a nauseating punch to the gut. *You sick weirdo,* my brain says. *Don't*
think of that now.

██

██

████████████ "Look, we know what this is, but we need you guys
to pronounce. We have to be sure."

██

███ I don't
remember what color, blue, or black or something, ████████
█████████████ It made the scene all the more bitter, like suddenly
you were forced to know that ██ had been the type of person to █

██

██

██

██

█████████████ There's a tall brown fence behind ████████

██

██

███

So this whole time we're sort of jammed in this ████████████
███████████████████████ There's not great visualization
in any direction, and █████████████████████████████████
█ guns drawn. We're not sure what's going on, but something about
the situation obviously isn't right. ████████████████████████
██ the mood is aggressive rather than somber. People are jacked up.

As fucked up as everything is, I still want to get in close and see
our patient, help out, learn something if I can. My brain is doing

that surreal movie thing, where part of you is looking down on everything as if watching a film, being interested and taking it all in and asking questions, and whatever tiny voice in the back of your head that usually tells you that *this is real, this is actually happening* is completely drowned out by everything else going on. They roll the ███████ over onto █ back and ███ puts on the patches. I get close enough so that I can see the monitor, but I'm still not really able to get a good look at ████████████████████ I hear the phrase *gray matter*, and in a sad quiet sigh someone says ██████

The monitor shows a rhythm. ████████████████████

████████████████ the little green line ████████

██

██

████████████████ brain on the ground, though. ██████

██

██

████████████ phrases are quietly volleyed back and forth between the three or four people standing around. Gray matter. PEA. Pulseless. Nothing to do.

We're following our determination of death protocols, printing strips, fumbling with equipment, ████████████████████

██

████████████████████████████████████ There's too many people here, they're saying, *Get these guys out of here. We need to get these guys out of here. Get them the fuck out of here.* ████████

████████████████████████████ The ambient air temperature seems to jump a couple of degrees. It becomes clear that we need to leave. Everyone is yelling at us to be careful where to step, because there are casings on the ground and it's a crime scene. There are definitely too many people ██████████████████████

██ On the way out I am rolling the gurney on the skinny sidewalk again as best as I can. ████████████████████████████

██

██

██

██

██

██

██

██████████████████████████ Their bodies are tense as ████

██

I remember this image as the first time that day that I finally felt scared. As we stand around and try to figure out what to do, dozens of cars swerve into the street, doors open, and gun-wielding uniformed men and women multiply and swarm like bugs on a river at dusk.

██

██

██████████████████████████ We're all on edge, and confused. Finally it dawns on us that ████████████████████████████

████████████████████████████ I suppose there might be a gun-fight soon. Suddenly some of the ████████████ start moving with purpose in front of us. A couple break out into a trot. *Here it comes,* I think.

They shove us in the ████████████████████████████████

██

██

I'm not surprised to hear the first couple of pops, but then the sky lights up. It's like firecrackers, like a video game or a war movie. It's a lot of gunfire. Pop, pop. Pop. Pop pop pop, tch tchthchfhkaheka-kakakapapapkapa. █████████████████████████████

█████████████████████ It's loud. It's loud and it goes for really long. █████████████████████████

We can't really see what's going on. █████████████████

I can't stop laughing insanely and thinking about how hard my friends and I are going to make fun of this later. *If I live, I guess*, I laugh to myself again. I think about practicing soccer at Bushrod Park Field in Oakland growing up, and all the cancelled practices due to gunfire down the street. This memory reminds me of paletas, the frozen fruit popsicles sold by old Mexican men pushing carts along the sides of the field, which is absurd and makes me laugh even more.

██

████████████████

After some amount of time we are let out of the ██████████ ████████ and ushered down the street. ██████████████████ █ has been standing there the whole time, out in the open, looking calm. ████████ the stoic, placid expression of an old sea captain who had been perfectly willing to go down with the ship to protect his crew. ███ ████████ a supervisor you barely know is quite literally willing to take a bullet for you.

We end up standing in a little circle across the street, and then begin the old hurry-up-and-wait.

██ Helicopters circle overhead, like any big night downtown in a city. At first we're all jacked up and uncomfortable and even the ones who don't smoke kind of want a cigarette. We talk about how bad we want a beer. Everyone texts their loved ones. There's a lot of back and forth about what's going to happen.

██
██
██
██
██
██
██
██
██
██

Everyone's switching radio channels and calling around trying to figure out our next move; meanwhile, the street we are standing on is turning into a fucking war zone. Truck after truck is pulling up and vomiting out men and women in assorted badges. It looks like a black-and-white news video of a military coup. Armored vans, ████████████████████████ Guns strapped to every extremity and acronyms splayed across their backs. Cops, sheriffs, detectives. ████████████████████ This one guy materializes; tall and thin, with white hair and wire-frame glasses, and his face is a caricature of a gaunt, strange, high-level government official. He wears an ill-fitting suit jacket and his torso and head are cocked slightly sideways, and for the rest of the night we see him periodically walking back and forth talking on his cellphone or scanning his pale eyes around the scene. He never looks at us. He is the only one besides us without a vest.

████████████████████████████████

████████████████ After a while it becomes clear that as paramedics we are stuck in limbo. No one really wants us to leave, and the whole street is blocked in anyway. Our ambulances are stuck in the ████████ and have become part of the crime scene. A nearby ██ is being used as a command post but we're not really welcome in there. No one has time to deal with us or dismiss us. We settle in and take over a chunk of sidewalk.

As night approaches we start to get cold, but all of our jackets are stuck in the rigs, where we're no longer allowed, so finding some warm jackets becomes a good project. The conversation after a tragedy seems to go like this: *business, funny, funny, sad. Awkward pause.* Repeat. Someone says something relevant, about the radios or the jackets or whatever, then someone jokes, and everyone riffs and laughs for a while, then someone says something suddenly poignant about whatever just happened and everyone stops and stares at the ground. The silences are heavy, and breaking them with a joke seems disrespectful, so usually you have to wait until someone comes up with another logistical type of comment or question, and then you can start joking again. This is why the jackets thing is so useful: you need to have a point of conversation for the moments in between funny and sad so you don't just stare at each other.

After ██████████ the party breaks up and we all get sent home. ████████████████████████████████████ We head back to ████ ████ and debrief. I'm exhausted and full of shitty pizza and my menstrual cramps are back and the last thing I want to do is stay up all night running bullshit dizzy old-people calls, so when ████████ █ looks like he's thinking about it I nod, *Please say yes.* We all go home. On my way out the door, ██████████████████████████ █████████████████████████████ "Call me if you get weird," he says, and I know he means it. I think about how pissed I was at him all month and how instantly and completely it had all melted away ██████████████ Nothing like ████████████████████ ████████████████████████████ to make you forgive the little things.

██████████████ on the way home ████████████████
██
██
██
██
██
██
██

[redacted] barely put my head on the pillow before I'm asleep. I wake up early in the morning, buzzed, watch TV for a while, check the news about the incident, fall back asleep. Once I'm up I head straight up to my favorite beach for the whole day and just breathe in the joy of being alive. *I'll process later*, I think. Today is for waves. The sun shines and the wind blows and my muscles burn like hell and I stay out surfing until dark. It's one of the best days of my life.

They're making us do what's called a "Critical Incident Stress Debriefing." It's part of this big new push to get better PTSD intervention for first responders so that we stop killing ourselves so much. The idea is that we all meet and talk about our feelings within forty-eight hours of the Bad Thing, and then we won't sue our departments into paying for therapy later down the road. But [redacted] [redacted] and everyone feels pretty awkward about it.

We sit in folding chairs [redacted] [redacted] She takes turns asking us how it felt, how we were doing, and if there was a particular image that stood out for any of us.

[redacted] I'm struck that in the horror of our worst calls, the accessories stand out more than the faces or names. Little human details, clothing or jewelry or keychains. I think it is the act of picking them out, the choice of it. When someone is just a body, a victim of circumstances, it's one thing, but once you see a decision they made that morning it gives them a bit of personality and free will. It forces you to consider their humanity.

When it was my turn I said I felt like ██████████████. Then we ████████████ and ████████████████

██
██
██
██
██
██
██
████████████████████████████████████
██
██
██
██
████████████████

I go straight from the debrief to lunch, then get in the ocean ██ ████████████, and from that to the gym. I am working myself to the bone but there's still so much adrenaline pumping through me and I can't stop for hours. On ████████ I finally crash. I wake up feeling nauseated and tired and wrong. ████████████████
██
██
████████████████████ I feel these leftover waves of the energy I've been surfing off of all week, and I run around with the dogs, but in between it hurts. My stomach aches and I feel like I want

to pass out and throw up. People start showing up to hang out and I just can't do it. I go inside and lie on the couch on my back and Potato the cat comes and gets on my stomach and the heaviness feels good, like it's sinking into my nausea and grounding me. We lie like that for a minute and I stare at the ceiling letting the weight of everything sink in. Mostly it's the images from the scene, of ███ ██ I let myself ██████████, relieved that I'm human after all, capable of feeling grief after a tragedy instead of just adrenaline. The couch swims up and surrounds me, and the ceiling sinks down a little closer, and Potato becomes a thousand-pound weight that starts inside of my heart and expands out all around me. The heavy, warm sadness of a week's worth of pent-up trauma bleeds through me. ████████ ████████████ tries to chat with me about ██████ but I can't really figure out what's going on. It's so much effort to smile awkwardly and carry on this conversation with her, but I don't want to get up and go to my room because I like the couch and I like having Potato on my stomach. I think about what ████ had said a couple times about getting distracted after a bad call, and how it's hard to have normal conversations and you zone out a lot, and I think, ███ ██ here we are.

I drive up to to ████████████████ feel sick the whole way up. Like, carsick. By ██████ I feel like I should pull over or something. ██ ██████████████████████████████ It's like I can't wash ██ blood off of me, can't wash the sickness of the moment out of my hair. The freeway is starting to swerve. I think about all the advice everyone keeps giving me—*talk to someone, you have to talk to someone, don't ignore it, don't hold it in, just talk to someone, acknowledge it, let it pass.* I don't want to say it out loud. It's not the feelings themselves,

I don't even really know what it is that I'm feeling, it's just ███ ███
████████ blood on the sidewalk, ██████████████████████
███████████ the fear of my co-workers, my embarrassment
at what I'd said during the debrief, the heaviness of all of it. ██████
██
████████████████████████████████████ I try to breathe
through it. I try to cry but I can't, and it's not really what I feel like
doing anyway. I finally exhale audibly and pick up my phone and
call ██
████████████████████████

I tell ██ what's going on: what I'm feeling, the image of the ██
█████████████████████████ with the puddle of blood,
and the thickness and irregularity of it, and I tell him about the ██
█████████████████████ and how I couldn't really see
much but I was ███████████████ says, ██████████

And it's the funniest thing to me, because I've been so caught up
in the gravity of the whole thing, the tragedy and the hugeness and
my own ego in all of it, that I never stopped to realize that ██████
██
█████████████████████████ It's one of those
ridiculous things that only someone else that works in medicine
could possibly say, but the truth of it slices through my nausea like
a sharp cold knife. ████████████████████████ The sincerity of the thought brings me a wave of relief, like I understand a
little bit better what I'm going through. We laugh, and I laugh, and
it all starts to lift a little bit. Every giggle feels like taking a chunk of
that pile of snakes inside my stomach and letting it go.

██
██

▮▮▮▮▮ it all shatters when I have to acknowledge that this was a real person, which was something I'd been avoiding until today. I wake up at 4:30 so I have time to ▮▮▮▮▮▮▮▮▮▮

▮▮▮▮▮▮▮▮▮▮▮▮▮▮▮▮
▮▮▮▮▮▮▮▮▮▮▮▮▮▮▮▮
▮▮▮▮▮▮▮▮▮▮▮▮▮▮▮▮
▮▮▮▮▮▮▮▮▮▮▮▮▮▮▮▮
▮▮▮▮▮▮▮▮▮▮▮▮▮▮▮▮
▮▮▮▮▮

▮▮▮▮▮▮▮▮▮▮▮▮▮▮▮▮
▮▮▮▮▮▮▮▮▮▮▮▮▮▮▮▮
▮▮▮▮▮▮▮▮▮▮▮▮▮▮▮▮
▮▮▮▮▮▮▮▮▮▮▮▮▮▮▮▮
▮▮▮▮▮▮▮▮▮▮▮▮▮▮▮▮
▮▮▮▮▮▮▮▮▮▮▮▮▮▮▮▮
▮▮▮▮▮▮▮▮▮▮▮▮▮▮▮▮

▮ years later I still can't drive past that particular parking lot without picturing ▮▮▮▮▮▮▮▮
▮▮▮▮▮

▮▮▮▮▮▮▮▮▮▮▮▮▮▮▮▮
▮▮▮▮▮▮▮▮▮▮▮▮▮▮▮▮
▮▮▮▮▮▮▮▮▮▮▮▮▮▮▮▮
▮▮▮▮▮▮▮▮▮▮▮▮▮▮▮▮
▮▮▮▮▮▮▮▮▮▮▮▮▮▮▮▮
▮▮▮▮▮▮▮▮▮▮▮▮▮▮▮▮
▮▮▮▮▮▮▮▮▮▮▮▮▮▮▮▮
▮▮▮▮▮▮▮▮▮▮▮▮▮▮▮▮
▮▮▮▮▮▮▮▮▮▮▮▮▮▮▮▮

It is the first of many times that day when despite all our dark humor and awkwardness we are punched with heavy grief.

When we walk in and see the coffin

The ███ of the whole situation annihilates me again.

████████████████████████████████

████████████████████████████████

████████████████████████████████

███████████████████

████████████████████████████████

████████████████████████████████

████████████████████████████████

████████████████████████████████

                              The whole time ████
████ humanized, all day, again and again, and I can't stop thinking about ████ mangled body over and over and over again.

   I don't really remember the drive home but somehow we get back
to ████ and everyone agrees to meet for drinks in a couple hours. I
drive my car towards my house for a shower but end up parked in
front of ███████████████████████████████

████████████████████████████████

████████████████████████████████

████████████████████████████████

███████████████████████ I burst into tears. Suddenly
I can barely breathe. I spit out, "I just . . . I was at the thing. I just
needed somewhere to go."

   ████████ has no idea what I'm talking about but she takes me by
the shoulders and walks me into the back room. I sit down and cry
for about an hour. A woman I don't recognize walks back and stares
at me for a minute but I can't bring myself to explain anything to
her, I just keep crying. She ties a piece of yellow string around my
wrist, lights a candle, and leaves. Later she tells me she felt like I
needed a candle. I mean, she wasn't wrong.

After about an hour I get up and wash my face. I give ███████ a hug and go home for a shower. At the bar, all the guys are there. ██

A few days later I show up for my next shift and ███████████ ████████████████████████████████ ████████████████████████████████████ ███████████████████████████ we're going to try to get some coffee before we get a call. The wheels start moving and I'm in the ████████ ████ ambulance again, wondering what's happening outside. I guess I'll find out when we get there.

"STRENGTH AND HONOR"

DAN QUINTO, RETIRED EMS SUPERVISOR;
FORTY-SEVEN YEARS IN EMS
SANTA CRUZ, CALIFORNIA

My dad was a laborer. He made glass bottles at a factory. My mom and sister were nurses. We didn't have any money for college, but I grew up with an expectation that you were going to do something with your life that was of service to people.

I'm a huge movie buff. My son Connor was a film major, and we got really into how movies are set up and everything. When the movie *Gladiator* came out, before Russell Crowe would go into battle, he would look around and pick up dirt from where he was standing. He would rub it between his hands, and say, "Strength and honor."

I started doing that at work! Because you have to have strength to push you, and you have to be honorable about what you do. This one night, we were getting ready to pull a guy off of Highway 17. We had like ten people on this haul line, and this guy was pretty far down. I was at the front of the line, I don't remember why I was in front. I turned back to everybody, and I said, "Calfire is leading this. So when they say 'haul,' we haul." And I looked at the two guys at the front, and I reached down, and I picked up some dirt. I went, "Strength and honor."

And the whole haul line, everybody except my partner, went, ". . .What?"

And then one of them—Greg, he's an assistant chief now—he goes, "Huh! I get it. We're fighting death, right?"

I said, "Yeah!"

And so it became a thing that I did. After a while people just accepted it.

REMY

We're parked down by the Embarcadero on a beautiful spring day. I'm working with a part-timer I've never met before. He's nice but useless. I get a sticky rice from the teahouse inside the ferry building and we put our food and radios on the hood of the ambulance and eat standing up, trying to enjoy a little sunshine before night shift sets in. We chat about nothing for a minute. A homeless guy shuffles up to us and starts to ask for a blanket. Then I see his face and the edges of my reality get weird and melty.

"Remy," I say.

He startles. He's got a shoulder hunch and his neck bends upward like a turtle, so it seems as if he's looking up at me even though he's taller than I am. He's polite, a little nervous.

"It's Joanna." I say. "Do you recognize me? Do you know who I am?"

I didn't know Remy that well, and I can't pretend we were close after college. But we hung out together a bunch with my high-school boyfriend, Jeremy. After Jer and I broke up I stayed friends with Remy. I drank all night with him and Billy Cookie and a few other punkers at some random house a couple times; I remember him throwing up on the lawn at 8:00 a.m. in suburbia while the neighbors were walking their dogs.

"Jer told me you were out here, in the city. I've been wondering if I would see you."

He nods. His smile is strange and shy. I try to overcome the weirdness, give him a big grin, tell him it's good to see him. I give him a hug, pull his dirty clothes into my uniform to let him know I'm not going to be weird about it. The part-timer sits in the front of the ambulance. He doesn't say anything, but it seems like he's going to be cool. I lean up to the front, tell him I'm going to tell dispatch we have a walk-up patient, just go with it, I'll explain everything later. He nods, sure. I can't tell if he's being kind, or if he just doesn't give a shit. I think it's the latter.

I don't look at my partner. I try to talk to Remy, just, I don't know, be chatty. Get him on the hook. I want him to come inside, get in the rig, and stick around for a minute.

He looks okay. He's definitely sleeping outside. His hair is dirty. His clothes are stained but not torn, his boots dusty but dry. He's got a backpack in good shape. There's a folded flower sticking out of it, some pens. His hands are a little red and swollen but I don't see any sores. His skin is tough, a little greasy, but intact. He looks okay.

I ask where he's sleeping. He doesn't really answer, says "around." I tell him we have a lady who helps with shelters and food and stuff, would he talk to her, does he want to come hang out in the rig for a minute, anything to get him inside. He says sure. He seems a little suspicious, still shy, a bit of a puppy dog. His eyes dart around, not quite focusing on me.

I get on the radio and tell dispatch we've got a walk-up, then I pull out my cellphone and call our homeless assistance officer. It's Sascha today, thank fucking god. She says she's down on Market and she'll come right over.

Remy and I chat. The walls of the ambulance shift and breathe on me; the air feels heavy, like you have to push through it to get anywhere. I try to think of things to ask him, try to seem normal, casual. I remind myself that I'm probably more used to hanging out with homeless folks than rich people these days anyway.

I tell him I have something for him. I've been carrying around this little blue book of Baudelaire poetry for a couple months. I bought it ages ago and I had it on my bookshelf for the longest time. When I heard last year from Jeremy that Remy Moreau had fallen into schizophrenia, that it was getting worse, that he was out on the street homeless, on my streets—at the time I didn't really react. I tried to feel something but I couldn't. Instead I just stood dumbly in my living room staring at that book for fifteen minutes, then grabbed it off the shelf and stuffed it in my backpack and went to work.

There's this thing that keeps replaying in the back of my head. I have an image burned into the *who I was growing up* folder, etched deep into the grain. We're sitting on the back porch of Remy's house in the Hayward hills. It's shady, eucalyptus and oak and whatever else dropping leaves all over the porch. He's chain-smoking a huge pile of hand-rolled cigarettes, dropping the butts in a caked ashtray. We have some books of poetry out, and a couple bottles of red wine. I'm pretty sure it's just the two of us. He's not flirting, he's not asking me about myself, he's just talking. He's telling me about the French decadents, how they changed the use of symbolism in writing. He's discoursing on a poem from the book he's holding, *The Spleen*, and the poem's got a few parts, and he's explaining the symbolism and the layers and the darkness and what it all means and how he figured it out and he's got cigarette stains on his fingers and he's pointing in the air and the edges of the porch railings are starting to rot and the ash is snowing down onto the table and the words of the poem are sucking off the page and dancing through the afternoon. It's making sense, the way he's teaching it, and it's better and more interesting and beautiful than anything I've learned in school, and I wonder if maybe I would like learning literature more if all my teachers weren't idiots. I don't know how many times I went over there, how many times we smoked cigarettes and drank red wine and spun webs out of untethered pretentiousness in the dusky evening light. It could have been a dozen times; it might have been only once.

But the point is I can smell the eucalyptus oil and feel the splinters of the table while I'm sitting in this ambulance with him now, and he looks like my last thousand homeless patients: sweaty, tired. I keep telling myself he looks like he's eating; he might be using some but his arms don't look like junkie arms. He's moving his limbs okay, he's walking okay, he's holding up his head okay, he's not limping and stumbling like a lot of people I see in the streets. He doesn't have obvious track marks or skin-popping scars.

He can hold a conversation, almost. He tries to tell me a funny anecdote about the Catholic homeless shelter free dinner versus the Protestant one. I can tell it's supposed to be political and irreverent and reference history a little, the type of thing Remy used to love, but the words don't really make any sense on the way out and so I just laugh and pretend I get it. I ask if he has a phone and he says no and looks at me and says, "Do you know about cellphones?" Do you *know* about it, like he's asking if I understand this important thing and I think *oh*, and I ask what, and it's like the shelter dinner story—he starts rambling and I can tell it's more or less about cellphones and the government, tracking, cell towers, whatever, but the words aren't in the right order and it's not even the right words so I just let it go for what seems like an appropriate amount of time and then make noises like I understand.

Jeremy said Remy has been on and off of medication. His dad and sister have tried to help, his friends have tried to help. He's been in and out of treatment facilities but the schizophrenia is ravaging his brain and his street punk childhood keeps taking over somehow and he keeps alienating everyone and disappearing.

I bring up Jeremy a couple times so that he'll make the connection and he says, "So you guys are still . . . you still know each other, that's great." I say yeah, it's really great, we're still friends, he's married now, she's awesome, and he says "Layla." He remembers her name, and Jer made it sound like they met only once or twice. I barely remember people's names, so I get excited that he can put that together.

I ask him again where he's sleeping. He dodged the question before but now that we've been talking a bit he opens up, tells me outside. I ask about shelters and he shakes his head. I know what he means. I've been in those shelters a lot; they're crowded and buggy and full of bad smells and bad vibes. It's hard for folks with mental illness in there. It's hard for anyone.

I pull the poetry book out of my backpack and show it to him. I open the front cover and write Jeremy's phone number and mine in Sharpie across the inside of the jacket and tell him to call us if he ever gets a phone. I write "WE ARE YOUR FRIENDS," then underline "FRIENDS." When I hand it to him he cradles it in his hands, tells me over and over again that it's really sweet of me, that it's nice, and he smiles when he looks at it. So that's good.

I ask him about the flower sticking out of his backpack, made of a folded dried leaf. It looks like something you'd get at an Indonesian tourist market. He says, "Someone . . . Someone made it for me," and smiles a little. Maybe he's got a lady friend. That's good too.

Sascha shows up. She's perfect. Dispassionate, knows exactly what to ask. A bunch of yes or no questions, jams through her usual interview. He answers yes to the yes questions and no to the no questions, like it all makes sense. He tells her his full name, and that he's been sleeping outside. He has a medical diagnosis of "aphasia." He had told that to me too, that he has aphasia. It's why he can't find a job. He says he doesn't have schizophrenia.

She writes some phone numbers and addresses onto a business card and hands it to him. She tells him where to go for what. She makes a couple calls and gets him a shelter bed for the night. I offer him a ride in the ambulance, which I'm not allowed to do, but he says he can walk there. It's early afternoon now, so he's got plenty of time. I ask him which street he's going to walk down. I try to convince myself that he's actually going to go, that he will be safe for one night, but I can't really hold the idea too tightly.

When Sascha leaves, Remy and I chat for another minute. I'm trying to make it normal, our homeless assistance officer telling you how to find a bed for the night, you can't make a full sentence, your hands are swollen, and I'm in a uniform with a badge, and we're just hanging out, just ran into an old friend. When I forget that it's Remy it does feel normal to me. I spend so much time hanging out with homeless folks, up all night, bullshitting with overdose victims and kicking around cardboard and blankets, and people are people in the end. It's as weird as any other social interaction with someone I don't know or haven't seen in a while, just people trying to find connection. Remy sleeps outside now and wanders around with his backpack on; I show up to work and drive my rig around the same neighborhoods. There but for the grace of God go I, you know? It wasn't so long ago we were all choosing our paths.

Words toss back and forth between us. We look at each other. Eventually I feel the walls of the ambulance closing in and my watch ticks and my radio gets heavier and I guess I should go back to work. I say something, he says something, I don't know. I tell him I should get back on the clock. I know he doesn't want to ask me about the blanket again so I say, "You still want some blankets?" He says yeah and I give him as many as he can carry. I ask if there's anything else he wants, bandages or hot packs or whatever. He says no. We don't have any water bottles to give out today, which makes me curse a little in my head.

Eventually we make it out back out onto the sidewalk. I give him a few hugs. I tell him I'd love to see him again soon, he should call me or Jeremy any time. "*Any time,*" I say, "I stay up nights, don't worry about it." He does the little tucked-under sideways nod again. I tell him we should just get a burrito some time and he perks up a little, seems to like the idea. He says it's great to see me. I hug him again.

Eventually I hop back into the ambulance and we drive away. I tell the part-timer what it was all about. The part-timer asks me if I need to have a minute or whatever. I say yeah, that's probably a good idea. I make a joke about not wanting to cry at work. I start to dial Jeremy's phone number; I haven't called the guy in years but I know it by heart. He picks up, he's in the middle of his workday. We talk for a while. I jump down out of the rig and walk over to the water to cry but it won't really come. I'm still in uniform, in public. I'm hiding behind a building, against a railing looking out at the bay and it feels like a private spot and I start to well up a little but then a couple comes around the corner to steal a kiss and I'm out in public again, on the streets of San Francisco, at my goddamn job, in my office. I shake my shoulders and fix my radio. I stuff it all down and walk back to the rig.

That night I squeeze myself between Kyle and the dog and tell him I had a tough day at work. I talk it out and he listens, he says nice things, but it's not the running into Remy I can't describe, the ambulance, the homelessness, whatever; the part I can't seem to communicate to Kyle is the cigarette stains on our fingers and the smell of the eucalyptus and a Baudelaire poem about how *February, peeved* at Paris, *pours a gloomy torrent on the pale lessees of the graveyard next door* and a *mortal chill on the tenants of the foggy suburbs* too and how Remy's aluminum voice had woven it all together in the night. And now he's out there and I'm in here and it's still foggy and the mortal chill is pushing at the cracks in your door. And if I squeeze myself up hard enough against you and the dog I can feel warm for now but I know he's still out there and these clean bedsheets can't wash away the smell of sidewalk in the rain.

Author's Note: I have changed the name of the friend in this story to protect his privacy, but I think he would have liked it to be French. I ran into Remy two or three more times after this, and he looked rougher each time. Eventually, I received a text from Jeremy with the inevitable news: Remy had been found dead, most likely a drug overdose. I found some relief in knowing that he was no longer out there suffering, but mostly I felt anger. My years in the city taught me too much about the byzantine and failing mental health system in San Francisco. I realize that the medical treatment of schizophrenia in the past was often horrifying, but I still find myself wondering if he might have found a healthier life had he been born in a different place or a different time. If there is an afterlife, I hope that he has plenty of tobacco and lots of good books to read up there. He was thirty-six years old.

MAGIC ERASER JUICE

Author's Note: This essay was first published in September 2019. At the time, I had been working in San Francisco for three years. Many of the details in the piece were drawn from my time on the "QRV," a quick-response medical unit dedicated to the Tenderloin neighborhood.

In the years since the story came out, fentanyl overdose deaths have skyrocketed not only in San Francisco but around the country. I have come to see my experience on the QRV as a canary in the coal mine: an eerily accurate warning of what was yet to come. I had originally intended to update this piece to reflect a more current experience, especially following the COVID-19 pandemic. Unfortunately, the stories relayed then now seem to be more relatable than ever. The omnipresence of fentanyl has made an old-fashioned heroin overdose seem almost quaint to the average EMS worker. I've changed a couple of sentences to reflect my own improved understanding of the crisis, but have otherwise left the original essay untouched.

I hope that someday soon this piece will become irrelevant.

There is one particular alley in San Francisco that is policed by a local little person on a scooter named Leticia. She sports a stylish short haircut, heavy makeup, and a shoulder bag with a large handmade pin that reads "I have narcan." She has to reach up above her head to the handlebars of her scooter, and she can dart the thing through traffic with breathtaking agility. I've seen her screaming at a guy to put his dirty needles in a sharps container instead of leaving them out on the sidewalk. Last time we ran into her she asked if we had any gloves. We went into our ambulance and gave her our last box. We figured she'd probably have more field saves than us by the end of the night anyway.

An opiate overdose kills you by first lulling you to sleep and then slowly suppressing your respiratory drive. You breathe ten times a minute, then eight, then four. You turn blue. Your breathing stops, your brain begins to die, and eventually your heart stops pumping. Fentanyl is faster. A fentanyl patient will "fall out"; that is, take one big hit and topple over dead.

It looks like a pretty good way to go—until some over-caffeinated paramedic like me stabs you with Narcan and ruins everything. Narcan (generic name: naloxone) is a competitive opioid receptor antagonist, which means that the Narcan floods into your bloodstream and bonks all the opiates off their receptors. This ends both the overdose and the high. So, with a cartoon-zombie exaggeration, quite literally back from the dead, the patient sits up, gasps, cries, sometimes vomits, and almost always looks around with wide, sweaty, who-the-fuck-are-you confusion.

"Good morning!" we say, way too casual. "Welcome back."

It's pretty common in my city to have a dose of Narcan drawn up and rubber-banded onto the rear-view mirror of the ambulance. We keep the rest of our gear all the way in the back of the rig, but we run so many overdoses that it's just easier to have the Narcan ready to go. We're lazy that way, I guess.

You remember EpiPens? You probably knew a kid in your elementary school who had to keep one in his backpack in case he was attacked by a peanut. They make something like that for Narcan now, and they give them out at clinics and the needle exchange. It's a little plastic device that contains a single dose, quick-release Narcan shot and can be given with little or no training. They're all over the street.

"We gave him Narcan already!" a homeless man shouts as we pull up. "I gave him two of the thingies, the ones they gave us!"

Police carry them, social workers, other drug users. Often a patient will get far more than the recommended dose before we arrive, and we will step carefully through a pile of used needles and tin foil and Narcan packaging on our way to the patient. I've Narcan'd the same guy twice in a shift. Some days everyone is just dying and coming back left and right like junkie whack-a-mole.

Fentanyl is quick, beautiful, and cheap, and it kills you.

What does it mean to drive around with an antidote? It's a strange feeling, knowing that there's an oops button on an overdose. We don't always get there in time. If you're by yourself, or if you took a particularly strong blend, or if your friends suck at calling 911, sometimes you die all the way. But a lot of the time, you die most of the way, and then we pop you full of magic eraser juice, and you come stumbling back from the edge.

There's a range of reactions on waking up. Some patients are upset, some surprised, some nonchalant.

"Oh, I've OD'd a bunch of times."

One patient walks away as soon as we get to the hospital. We pull the gurney out of the back of the ambulance and he casually undoes his seatbelts and gets up. We ask where he's going and he tells us he's going to walk back down the hill and buy another hit. I ask if there's anything I can do to change his mind and he laughs and says no, but maybe you can try again next time.

We bring back a woman wearing matching mittens and a hat who is confused, then starts to cry. She's been using meth every day but has been clean from heroin for twenty years. I arch an eyebrow. She sobs, then screams, then grabs my arm.

"How did this happen? Who did this? I have to know what happened." She repeats herself, panicked, still high on the meth she was probably shooting before she took the dirty dose by mistake. "Where was I? Who did this? How did this happen? I could have died! I could have died?" We try to calm her, but she's so far gone into her own circles that it's difficult to get through. We wake up plenty of overdoses who claim they're clean, but she's so up front about the meth use that I start to believe her story. Once she slows down a little we determine that she shot up what she thought was her usual meth dose and woke up to a team of paramedics pressing a mask to her face and hauling her off the ground into a gurney.

She was going to dose her friend next, the man who called us, and when she realizes that if he had gone first he might have died she starts sobbing again. "It could have been you! If it wasn't me it would have been you! Oh my god, how did this happen?"

We found her lying in a puddle behind a gas station, with a pile of so many scattered needles that we had to pull one sideways out of her thigh. Here you are, Miss Mittens, at two in the morning, lying in a fentanyl-riddled alleyway, in a fentanyl-torn city, in the fentanyl-soaked night, you've lost half your friends to ODs, and you're tying off your arm and pumping your vein full of some sketchy meth that you bought from who knows where, and you're, what, surprised that things went badly? We could lecture her, or be mean about it. On the other hand, fuck it, you know? It was an honest mistake. She's not taking it out on us, she's just plain scared. I unpackage a disposable blanket and wrap it around her. "I'm so sorry this happened to you. We're going to take really good care of you. Just focus on your breathing, okay? We've got you now."

We wake up a guy in his thirties who says, "Shit . . . Did I OD?" "Yeah, man, we gave you Narcan. Welcome back." He sighs, leans his head back, and looks defeated. "I was clean for seven years." He shakes his head. We close the charting computer and talk for a while. He tells us how he got clean, put his life back together, even worked in a drug counseling clinic to help other addicts get off the street. He's a young white guy with a beard, flannel shirt, and torn jeans. He's wearing a T-shirt from a band I like under the flannel. He tells us he hates the failure but he's been slipping lately. His voice is soft but he holds nothing back. A brush with death always brings closeness with it, but to be brought back from a death that was caused by your own greatest personal vice, to have lost your greatest struggle, and then look up from the depths into the eyes of your witnesses— there's nothing left to hide.

"Is there anything, you think, that anyone could do for you? A program, a counselor, a friend? Is there anything that we could do? You seem like someone who could fight this. What would work, do you think, for you?"

He stares at his hands for what seems like a long time.

"No," he says finally. "I don't think there's anything that would help. It's a hell of an addiction."

They say heroin is amazing. It's a cheat code. That it's better than any other feeling that you've ever had up until that moment. Everything you've ever tried for, every challenge you've failed or risen to, every struggle and every injury, it all just falls into place. It was all worth

266

it, every minute, every gasp, to bring you here to this moment. It's meditation, it's orgasm.

I'm not a heroin user, but I know what it feels like to search for something and think you've found it. I know that aching, dark emptiness of an addict, and the feeling that one more step, one more grasp, and it's just within reach; that thing you've been hunting for, the thing that has kept you up at night. It's right there, right beyond your fingertips, just stretch a little farther, escape a little more. I can't begin to know the pain of a true opiate addiction, but I have no judgments for those in the struggle.

A lot of people blame the Sackler family for the current American opioid crisis that has swallowed cities like mine; immigrant pharmacists turned CEOs turned opiate drug kingpins, the Sacklers created OxyContin. Released in 1997, Oxy was stronger, purer, and more addictive than any prescription pain pills that came before it. Its "time-release" formulation made for easy crushing, snorting, and shooting. The soul of the poppy flower wove its way from opium in Turkish smoking dens, to morphine for Civil War soldiers, to laudanum for menstrual women, to the heroin of jazz musicians, and found its home in orange pill bottles across every strata of the American experience.

Purdue Pharma, owned by the Sacklers, marketed the drug so heavily that they were eventually convicted of felony "misbranding." They said it was nonaddictive, abuse-proof. (So did the first doctor to inject morphine with a syringe, incidentally; he said the addiction had been caused by eating the drug, but injection was safe.) Purdue bought and sold doctors to overprescribe the medicine across America, bringing in billions of dollars in profits. Purdue Pharma bought lunches and dinners and weekends on yachts for the doctors who prescribed the most pills to the most humans, rich and poor, black and white. Reps were given bonuses for getting doctors to prescribe more pills and higher doses.

Long before the Sacklers, before time-release capsules and hydro-morphone isomers, the British went to war with China over opium. Europeans wanted Chinese tea and silk and couldn't find enough silver to pay for it all, so traders flooded China with opium from India instead. The addiction spread quickly, the need grew, and soon Southern China began to writhe and cripple under the poppy flower's curse. The Qing dynasty tried to outlaw the drug and stop the influx. The British drug suppliers, with profits burning in their eyes, sent war ships into Chinese ports to blast their way to their opium riches. Two separate wars followed this plotline, only twenty years apart.

Historians still debate the long-term effects of it all, but a thin, sticky, tar-colored thread runs itself across an ocean and two hundred years. There was a dusky evening, once, in Southern China, say 1842. Gold would be found in California in seven years' time. Maybe it was late spring, maybe the crickets hummed as the nights began to warm for the season. Maybe a shorebird cried out, a wave slapped a wooden dock, a rope sagged heavy with moss against a boat. A man leaned on the rotting wall of a shopfront and sucked opium through a pipe. The smoke burned his lungs and filled his head with warm clouds as war raged around him. His life melted, his worries faded, the creases in his worn face relaxed and lay open to the last of the evening light. The money he would pay for this feeling, the unlimited resources that could be torn from his hands to fulfill this need. Men in parliaments would curse and tear up trade agreements, fire would be set to ships, borders redrawn, before he would give up that dope. There's a diagram to be outlined, somehow, between that tired Chinese pipe and the needle in the sidewalk under my boot. That man, if he could pick himself off the storefront wall, walk a few steps, peer his head through the filmy curtains of time, what would he say to my sidewalk junkies on the downtown streets? My twisted, bleeding twenty-five-year-olds, sleeping on cardboard, scratching at infected sores, poking needles in their battered arms. Would he nod, half asleep in the fog? Would he pass the pipe?

So I'm driving around the city at one in the morning, seeing street folks wrapped in blankets dancing to a boom box, milk crates full of crack pipes and diapers, scarred arm veins waving up at the city lights, sleeping bags pushed against the forced-air heat vents of a sewer grate, and I'm listening to the radio, to politicians and talking heads discussing what to "do" about it, how to "fix" it, with policies and regulations and focus groups, addiction, trauma, law and order, enabling, decriminalization, buzzword after buzzword coming down like rain. And I can't stop reading about the Opium Wars, how humankind found out just how beautiful and deadly this shit was, just how far humans would stretch their misery to fulfill the need for smack.

I've had a lot of non-medical folk ask me about fentanyl. What's it like? It's awful, isn't it? They should do something about it, and right away! Well, sure, I guess. Who's they? I love that you're sitting at a mahogany table on the thirty-fourth floor trying to double-click a solution out on your laptop, I love the effort, I really do, but I'm watching Leticia the scooter mayor wearing the gloves we gave her dig through her purse and the ghost behind her plunge the needle into his vein and lean his head back and exhale, just close his eyes and breathe the syrup into his blood and give a little shiver and his whole world gets soft and you're up in your apartment and I know you can hear the sirens but we look like ants from where you are.

THE HOSPITAL REVIEW.

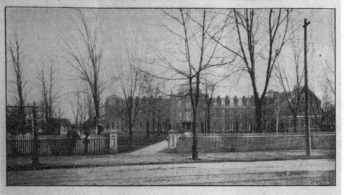

DEVOTED TO THE

INTERESTS OF THE SICK AND SUFFERING

AT THE

ROCHESTER CITY HOSPITAL.

| TELEPHONE 696. | " I WAS SICK AND YE VISITED ME." | AMBULANCE CALL 656 |

| VOL. XXXVI. | ROCHESTER, N. Y., MARCH 15, 1900. | No. 8 |

Hospital Notes.

The Out-Patient Report for February shows a record of 185 patients who made 351 visits to the hospital and received 410 prescriptions, treatments, dressings, etc.

The recent storm brought few inconveniences to the hospital, all things considered. The failure of the milk supply would have proved a serious annoyance had it not been for an abundant reserve stock of malted milk, and various food preparations, upon which it was possible to subsist during the state of siege. For two days the milkmen were not able to reach town, and the advantage of being "fore armed" was practically demonstrated.

The laundry women were not able to go to their homes on Thursday night, and remained at the hospital until Friday.

The first physician to reach the hospital on Thursday, March 1st, was a woman, who arrived before 9 A. M., coming from a great distance to visit a patient.

During the height of the blizzard on Thursday evening, March 1st, a "hurry call" for the ambulance was sent in over the telephone. The case was reported as one of morphine poisoning, and the victim, a woman, was to be called for at a factory in a distant part of the city. The ambulance was sent out, the horses struggling with difficulty through the drifts, but the surgeon found, on arriving at the place designated, that the call had been sent at the instigation of a young woman who thought free transportation in the ambulance preferable to making the attempt to walk home in the storm.

"Hospital Notes," *Hospital Review* (Rochester, NY), vol. XXXVI, no. 8 (March 15, 1900)

"911 HAPPENS"

JAMIE PREDMORE, PARAMEDIC/FIREFIGHTER;
EIGHTEEN YEARS IN EMS
NINILCHIK, ALASKA

A few months after I got hired, when I was getting used to working in an emergency system, a co-worker of mine asked me, "So?"

I said, "Yeah?"

"What do you think?"

I answered, "I don't know, this is . . ." and trailed off.

He said, "You were expecting everybody to be so sick, right? You don't know what to do when it's not a true emergency every time?"

And I said, "Yeah, exactly!"

It's actually really challenging as a new provider, because you expect to be only responding to cardiac arrests, and heart attacks, and serious motor vehicle collisions. Then you get on scene, and everyone's fine. You go into their house, pumped full of adrenaline, ready to help, and they look totally fine. You think, what am I missing? What's really going on? In what surprise way are you going to be sick? Because you look fine. And then at some point you realize, "Oh. It's because you are fine."

I work in a very rural community in Alaska now, and I thought it would be different in an area like this. It's a small community with a deficit of resources. Just something like going to the store looks vastly different than it would in an urban setting, and when I moved up here I assumed that it would make folks better at prioritizing. But people still don't have the information that first responders have. When they get out of their comfort zone, they will call us. The first call I ran up here was for an old man who wanted to go out for a walk. He'd had a stroke recently, and his niece was very nervous about his behavior. When I spoke to him he was very lucid. But she was playing worst-case-scenario games in her head. She had gotten herself panicked because of her own emotions, and what happens? 911 happens. It's the same wherever you go.

Part III

BIRD'S-EYE VIEW

BURNOUT

MICHAEL HAMILTON, PARAMEDIC/RN;
TWENTY-FOUR YEARS IN EMS
RENO, NEVADA

Your partner on the ambulance is your homie, right? And then you see your other homies at the hospital when you're dropping off patients. We would all congregate in a circle, talking trash and eating pizza at three in the morning. Somebody would be smoking a cigarette. It was a fellowship, and it was hard to imagine life outside of that. These jobs become your identity.

When you've been doing this work for a while, it changes you. I don't mean to be melodramatic or hyperbolic, but I have seen some of the worst shit that a human being can see. And some of the worst things that human beings can do to other human beings. What else can I do for a living now?

I was a high-school dropout. I had no college education. I had a certification that allowed me to do one job, and that job paid my bills. I had no other usable skills. I think that is the story for a lot of paramedics. Once you get into the career, and it really starts to mess you up, you don't have a plan B.

Every paramedic is dealing with some kind of pain. You see it with the overcompensating fire bros; you see it with the "paragod" who has to be the smartest person in every room; you see it in the female paramedic firefighter who has to get really aggressive in order to be taken seriously. But on top of that, you throw in tons of mental and emotional trauma. We are placed in high-stress situations over and over again, our alarm response is all messed up.

I never really had any nightmares. But I had waking terrors for years. My therapist called it the 8mm slideshow. Visual and auditory flashbacks. Screams. There was no trigger; they were random. Just flashes of things.

I don't get them too much anymore. I cope with things quite a bit better now. I'm in a much healthier relationship and I have a lot less stress. I've been sober for five years. I'm no longer engaging in risky behavior to cope. I'm not smoking cigarettes, I'm not constantly fighting with a romantic partner. I get lots of exercise, I snuggle with my dog. I have a supportive partner.

I joke with my wife, Rosie, about what it's like to try to feel normal. At three o'clock in the morning, you can wake me up out of a dead sleep and have me run a neonate arrest. And I can do it. I can make split-second, life-changing decisions at the drop of a hat. I'm comfortable working on very, very sick children. But I had a full-on panic attack and had to leave the grocery store because I was trying to decide on one out of several brands of ketchup. It became overwhelming. I had to leave and I couldn't bring myself to walk back inside. My wife had to go to the store and buy the ketchup. She was very kind about it.

WHEN ELEPHANTS FIGHT

Our clients are not the "deserving poor"; they are just poor—undeserving in their own eyes and those of society. At the Portland Hotel there is no chimera of redemption or any expectation of socially respectable outcomes, only an unsentimental recognition of the real needs of real human beings in the dingy present, based on a uniformly tragic past.
GABOR MATÉ, *In the Realm of Hungry Ghosts: Close Encounters with Addiction*

In 2021, there are rumors of a new program that has something to do with mental health and street medicine, but no real details about what the teams will do or when they will start. After eight years on an ambulance I am ready for a change, so when I receive an internal email one afternoon advertising positions on the "Street Crisis Response Team," I am intrigued. The flyer is vague: special squads will be formed by the fire department to "respond to behavioral and social calls for service and . . . assess community members for medical, behavioral, and social needs."

I know what this is code for. Mental illness. Drugs. Poverty. Patients who set up camp in doorways of businesses and refuse to leave. Patients who scream on the sidewalk and take off their clothes and throw trash at cars. Patients who die on the street because they can't pay for bus fare to the hospital. When I apply to the program,

I have no idea how exactly the teams hope to remedy these situations, but I think to myself: *Well, anything's better than what we've been doing.*

I apply, interview, and am accepted into a six-week training course for my new job. I learn that the program was conceived in response to the Black Lives Matter protests, the activist movement that erupted across the United States during the summer of 2020. Instead of sending police or ambulances to calls involving mental illness, our leaders want to try something new. They have imagined teams of unarmed, specially trained behavioral experts who will offer alternative solutions. In theory, the roles are defined like this: a paramedic, to assess for medical need; a social worker, to navigate behavioral issues or access to food and housing, and a trained peer counselor, to use their lived experience to gain rapport and advocate for the patient. We're supposed to be a sensitive, sympathetic alternative to a traditional police response.

Our van is red, with fire department logos on the sides. It has sirens and a light bar, though we are told not to use them. We carry basic medical supplies but no gurney or restock. The most exciting difference between an ambulance and a Street Crisis van, for the paramedics anyway, is our new ability to transport to what are called "alternate destinations." A traditional 911 ambulance crew is only authorized to bring a patient to one location: a hospital emergency room. As a community paramedic, thanks to my extra training, I am suddenly allowed to drive folks anywhere I'd like. An urgent care, a rehab facility, a homeless shelter. It's an intoxicating idea for someone who has spent a decade wondering if there was a better way to help my people.

The goals of the program are admirable. But by the end of our first month, we are confused and overwhelmed. Ambulance crews and firefighters call us for patients suffering from all kinds of mental health and economic issues. Police call us for homeless folks they have known for years, hoping we can offer something besides jail or an ambulance. Locals see us and say, "I'm so glad to see you guys, there's such a need," with a knowing sigh. People tap our shoulders in Starbucks and tell us about a particular homeless man who has been living in their neighborhood for months. Shopkeepers point at someone sleeping on their step and grunt as though to say, "Here's one. Deal with this." A young lady leans out of the rear window of a still-moving Tesla and tells me to "check" on someone a few blocks back who "looks like they really need help." No description, nothing further. She waves and shouts "Thank youuuuu" as the car speeds away.

In reality, we have a limited skill set. The peer counselors are excellent at leveling with folks in crisis. We have snacks, clothing, and water. But most homeless shelters and rehab facilities in San Francisco are difficult to access. They have few beds available and communication is challenging. We have entry to one or two mental health programs, provided that they have a space and our patient is calm enough to get through their intake process. And almost all of these resources are closed after 4:00 p.m. or on weekends, which means that our night shifts crews are forced to turn almost everyone away. And even with my newly expanded transporting capabilities, I am still bound by my paramedic scope of practice. I cannot refer my patient to a therapist, prescribe a psychiatric medication, or make the kinds of decisions that will provide long-term support with housing or mental health. Usually all I can do is take them to an entry point to further care and wish them well.

Both business owners and homeowners imagine we will "clean up the streets": that we will sweep away all of the poverty and addiction on the sidewalks with our calming words and our six-seater van. The

Street Crisis units are a fantasy, I realize, about protecting our mentally troubled patients from police while at the same time making them gently disappear.

We do the best we can. It is frustrating work, and I'm not really cut out for it. I have always loved solving puzzles and having answers. The immediacy of emergency work is my favorite part, the need to problem-solve in real time using my hands. Give air. Stop bleeding. Assess for trauma. This new job is the exact opposite, and I hate it at first. Problems are slow, complicated, and usually not fixable by our team. We are a point of contact; sometimes we can nudge someone in the right direction, but more often we simply give a kind word and an empty promise. Our job, as it is originally laid out for us, is not to fix problems but to react to 911 calls with calm voices instead of fists or guns. I can do it—after a decade in EMS I am even good at it—but I struggle to find meaning in the work.

We recognize her from previous interactions; she's going by the name Waterfall today. She's wearing white go-go boots with a torn sarong at her waist. On her chest is draped a loose scarf that doesn't seem like a shirt until she lifts it up to shimmy at us, or to press her ribs against the window of a nearby restaurant. One of the social workers is pretty sure she uses female pronouns, so that's what we're going with. We try to ask but she's way too high to understand the question.

I'm staring at her. My social worker is asking what I want to do. All I'm thinking is, *Honestly, I'd like to go home.* It's not that I don't want to help this person. I want desperately to help this person. It's just that I don't have that ability right now, and I didn't yesterday, and I won't tomorrow, so at this point I want to leave. I want so badly to help but I can't, so please, just let me go home.

I stare at Waterfall's meth-torn eyes, flying around the sockets, up and down, and back and forth. Her hands are shaking. She's talking gibberish a mile a minute with newspapers stuffed in her shoes to keep her feet warm, now turning her back to the restaurant, now crying, saying how much it hurts, now grabbing her scrotum and waving it at us, now dancing again.

We have no way to help Waterfall today. She's too much work for any of the understaffed mental health facilities in the city to take care of. She needs someone to sit with her, tell her not to run into traffic, not to lick the sidewalk, not to pull her hair out. She listens when we coach her about these things but we don't have the staff to watch over her for two, six, twenty hours while the meth runs its course, and neither does anywhere else. Not to mention the months or even years of medical intervention that her brain needs to recover from such heavy methamphetamine use.

So here's what we can do for Waterfall: we can leave her be or we can tie her up and take her to the emergency room. If we let her go she will dance around, pulling her clothes on and off, digging through trash, and trying to rub herself on strangers. If we take her to the ER they will lock her in a room alone with no cords or sharp objects for a few minutes or hours until the meth wears off a little, or until they need the bed, and then they will discharge her back to the street. I am not a big fan of either of these solutions, so I just look at her and then I look at my social worker and then I look back at her. I respect this social worker and I want her to like me and I'm pretty sure right now she thinks I'm either lazy, disinterested or both. I tell her I don't know what to do. I can write my chart to make it sound like we had to force Waterfall to the hospital because she was too altered to make her own medical decisions, or I can let her walk away. I will myself to come up with something. *Come on, Sokol*, I tell myself. *Sound smart and compassionate. Say some shit about her mentation or whatever that sounds medical and thoughtful.* I try to make my mouth move but it won't.

Now Waterfall walks out into the street, cars are swerving, and the social worker says, "Okay, fine, we're writing a hold."

She's not wrong. We can't have people getting hit by cars. So now we're writing an involuntary psych hold and we're calling an ambulance. This will temporarily lift the problem and place it behind the sliding door of an ER room for a couple hours so the good people of the neighborhood don't have to look at it.

We call for transport but it's level zero and the city doesn't have an ambulance available for an hour and a half. We keep almost getting one and then a cardiac arrest or a stroke or something pops and we get bumped to the back of the line. Initially there are only three of us on the call: a social worker, a peer counselor, and myself. But our captain stops by to check in, and he has a trainee in tow. Then the police show up to help with crowd control. Now we have eight of us fanned out around Waterfall in a loose circle. We've taken over about a thirty-foot area, and every time she gets close to the street we all jostle our positions like a soccer team's defensive lineup and shuffle her back towards the sidewalk. It's a lot of personnel, to be honest, all of us paid for by the city and all of us feeling pretty useless at the moment. She sings a little, gyrates her hips, lays down, stands up, screams, talks to us, dances some more. An hour and a half is a long time, as it turns out. At one point a woman in a designer jacket walks by us looking angry and says, "Why haven't you fucking taken him yet? He's been out here for an hour and a goddamn half?!?" She's pissed. She looks at me with disgust and waves her hands to demand an answer.

———

We are not the first city to use EMS for something other than traditional ambulance work. The phrase *community paramedicine* is an umbrella term. In 1995, a rural area in New Mexico with a desperate need for primary care doctors temporarily gave its paramedics additional training and responsibility to fill the need. Since then, community paramedicine projects have been created for all kinds of initiatives. Paramedics have been trained in pediatric asthma prevention and care, and then sent to houses to educate families about how to use an inhaler. They've been given portable lab value machines and sent out for post-surgical follow-ups. They meet with opiate overdose patients to start medication for withdrawal symptoms and help folks into addiction treatment. They work with geriatric fall prevention. Congestive heart failure. Diabetes.

The thought process generally goes like this: Medics are already out there in the communities. We are cost-effective. We are ready to help. And most importantly, if these issues don't get addressed, we are going to be the ones dealing with them anyway. Why not give us the tools to try to nip some of this stuff in the bud? But getting community paramedicine programs off the ground is difficult. They encounter problems with political will, funding, staffing, and often face opposition from nursing unions and physicians. And they are almost always providing the type of care that, while saving money for communities in the long run, does not collect an immediate paycheck. They tend to rely instead on grant money and can struggle to stay afloat.

In San Francisco, for the time being at least, the programs remain funded. The SFFD has in fact run its own form of community paramedicine for two decades now, since way before the Street Crisis teams. Back in the 1990s, an EMS captain from our fire department helped author a series of studies showing that a high percentage of

911 calls were actually made by a very small cohort of people. He wondered if there was a better way to address their needs. Over the next twenty years, the SFFD built out a team of EMS professionals who purposefully engaged with these folks instead of waiting for them to call for ambulances. The captains, who go by the radio call sign "EMS 6," follow certain patients through the 911 system, meet with them in their homes, talk to their case managers, and fight to get them placed into rehab facilities or nursing homes. The media-friendly description of the goals of the program says the EMS-6 team aims to "break the cycle," get people "the care they need," and "help decrease the strain on the 9-1-1 ambulance and hospital systems." In other words, try to get them to stop calling 911 so damn much.

By the numbers, EMS-6 is a success. The program has bridged some of the deep gaps in the San Francisco health-care system. It has placed patients into care homes or back home with their estranged families. We had callers with annual counts in the four hundreds who use 911 once or twice a year now. I'm not sure anyone has bothered to add up the actual money saved for the city and local hospitals but the guesses are usually in the tens of millions of dollars. But the work takes a toll. It can take months or years to get a particular client placed into a facility somewhere, and even after all that they can get turned back out if one administrator in an office somewhere is having a bad day. I've watched my EMS-6 friends arguing on the phone with nurses, case managers, public health officials, insurance companies, and local politicians. I've seen them with their heads in their hands at 3:00 a.m., a client on speakerphone, taking notes and holding back tears. They work with the most difficult minds, the sickest bodies, the most exhausting crevices of our broken system. Their people die a lot. One captain shows me a series of poems written by one of her favorite clients and asks if I could put them in my book.

He was young when he passed, born with severe disabilities and made sicker by years of heavy drinking and drug use. The poems are beautiful and surprising. He has no family we can contact for permissions and a lawyer tells me it's not allowed.

And the calls don't stop. No matter how many mountains they move, no matter how many people they help, the EMS-6 team is not going to wake up one day and find their work complete. Every time they knock a client off of a high-volume caller list, three more appear in his or her place. The names on the list change, but in a city as large as San Francisco, there will never be a shortage of heavy 911 users. As hard as they work, my friends do not have the ability to fix a national crisis in elder care or opiate addiction from a small office in the back of a warehouse in southeast San Francisco.

The Street Crisis Response Teams are created as an offshoot of the EMS-6 program, and run by the same managing team. We go through the same training program. We are taught to use the term *client* instead of *patient*. This leads many of us to believe that we will be participating in the type of long-term case management that the EMS-6 captains have shown can be effective with some of our frequent callers. I think I might finally be able to help some of my most challenging mentally ill patients, and then observe them over time to see what works and what doesn't. But unfortunately, this isn't at all how the Street Crisis teams are designed. We are simply a point of contact for calls that had previously gone to police. We have no mechanisms in place to provide long-term follow-up or track our clients through the community. If we are not able to get our people accepted into a facility that day, we take down their name and leave.

Our bosses keep putting out media releases about how successful our program is. They cite how frequently we are able to "resolve" a situation without violence, even if the resolution is that we leave without doing anything to help. Less than a year ago, the brutal murder of an unarmed Black man named George Floyd galvanized the protest movement that had led to the creation of our teams. In the context of his death and the politics surrounding it, any interaction of ours that does not end with a knee on the neck suddenly counts as a win.

I don't remember how we first encounter Jeremiah. He might just walk up to the Street Crisis van and ask us for some water. We chat while the social worker digs around the van looking for supplies. He is relatively calm and lucid, but we guess from his speech patterns that he's usually cognitively disorganized and seems to have been given some sort of sedative or anti-psychotic, probably Zyprexa. We wonder if he was just released from a hospital in the neighborhood. We find paperwork in his coat pocket confirming our theory: he has a history of schizophrenia and bipolar disorder. The emergency room found him in crisis this afternoon, gave him a single dose of anti-psychotic medication, and kicked him out. This means we have four, maybe six hours if we're lucky before he starts to escalate into his illness again.

He wants help. He says he's alone, he's scared of being out on the streets, and he's scared that things will ramp up tonight. His manner of speaking is melodic if confusing. He's able to answer simple questions. We call Angel Wings, a mental health respite facility that we are supposed to be working with closely. The clinic at Angel Wings is subject to the same paradox as the rest of our mental health and addiction resources: you've got to be sick enough to qualify but calm and coherent enough to get through their intake interview and take care of yourself in a group setting. There simply isn't enough staff to babysit everyone or provide a safe environment for someone who is in severe crisis. If we can get this guy inside before he starts to ramp up, maybe we can actually get the ball in the goal this time. They tell us they have an open spot tonight, and based on our description are willing to let him inside.

We drive him over there. It's a peaceful drive, joyful even. We're all pleased with ourselves and our luck. The guy has a sweetness to him, a heartfelt affect, and between murmuring and gibberish he thanks us for taking him in.

When we get to Angel Wings they give him a rapid COVID test. He's positive. They do it again. Positive twice.

So now he can't go inside.

He doesn't understand why, and there's no option B. He has no symptoms and was cleared medically at a hospital about three hours ago. He asks why he's not being allowed inside; he tells us he'll be *good*, he promises. I try to explain to him what COVID is but he doesn't understand. Now he's even more scared. "I'm sick?" he wants to know. "Like cancer?" "No, buddy, not like cancer. Basically they're not going to let you in today but you can try back in a couple of days, I promise. Just go back in two, three days." I keep telling him this but we both know that by morning the meds will wear off and he's going to be way too escalated and confused to understand any of this or to be let back inside. When he goes back to shouting, or twitching, or when paranoia or confusion sets in, he won't be allowed into this facility anymore. Once he elevates back up he'll either be restrained and back at the hospital (probably the same one he just left) or, more likely, he'll be stuck out on the streets. There is a tiny sliver of just-sick-enough-to-qualify-but-not-too-sick, and for once our guy is square in the middle of it. Except for the damn COVID test.

None of that matters in this moment though, or rather all of that matters but none of it does. Right now it is my solemn duty as a heroic mental health hero to kick him out into the night, alone. There's no other option. The only other place we would be allowed to bring him, a twenty-four-hour mental health urgent care, has only eight beds, and in the nine months I've been working this unit they've had an opening twice. There's literally nothing else. We had one shelter bed this morning, but they stop intakes at 4:00 p.m. It's 5:30 now, and he wouldn't have been stable enough to be allowed in there anyway. I call my supervisor, I call my chief, I call everyone I can think of. During the height of the early pandemic the city had some "isolate and quarantine" sites, hotels for COVID-positive folk, but those are either long gone or long full, nobody knows how to access one anyway, and nothing takes intakes past 4:00 p.m. So he's just getting put out on the street.

The head of Angel Wings tries to get in a fight with my immediate supervisor. Everyone wants this to be someone else's fault. The health department wants an ambulance called to take him to an emergency room, to which the EMS supervisor says absolutely not, he has no medical complaint, he was just released from an ER, every ER in the country is desperately begging people to stop coming in to get COVID tests, what the fuck are they going to do for him there anyway? With the brand of test we are using, people can come up positive for months after their illness is gone. And hospitals don't "treat" asymptomatic positive COVID tests because there's nothing to treat. Angel Wings says that since he was brought by our unit, he is our responsibility.

While the supervisors are fighting it out on the phone with each other, I let the guy back into the van. I'd rather hang out with him than a bunch of angry bureaucrats anyway. An Angel Wings aide who has the same tired body language I do says, "I'm gonna go heat him up some food, let's give him a meal at least." I nod my thanks, our faces mirrors of the same exhausted shape. I help Jeremiah into the passenger seat and sit with him while he eats. After the meal, he asks me if we can go inside now.

The budget of the San Francisco Department of Public Health this year is just shy of $3 billion. And somehow there is nothing to do with this young man besides give him a blanket and kick him out into the cold, wet night. He realizes what's happening and looks afraid, starts mumbling faster and faster about the night and the dark and the snakes and the birth and death and circles of night wrapping into and out of the rhythm of his disorganized brain, speeding up and up and even though the medication keeps the volume of his voice muted, the patterns of his sentences tighten and the words run together. His eyes widen with fear and he says, "It's so cold out there, cold, cold, cold." "I know, bud, I'm so sorry. I really wanted to help you." I give him two blankets, three. I want to throw the box of blankets out the fucking window, honestly, and drive over it with this stupid ineffective red van full of lies.

He eventually stumbles down the street, gripping his blankets against his chest like a child with a stuffed bear. He sits on a street corner about a block away from us. We stay parked and argue with each other and our supervisors for about another thirty minutes. Nothing changes. He's alone, confused, and cold, and he's going to spend the night that way.

We drive home in silence. I drop the crew off and then call my mom to cancel the coffee we had planned after work. I have a pit in my stomach and I can't escape the dark shape of his silhouette walking away, holding the blanket, hunched in the cold.

———

Every time I am tempted to give up and stop trying completely, my team pulls me back from the edge. The schedule rotates, but I am placed most frequently with the same two women. The social worker, Sofia, is young. At first I'm annoyed by her inexperience, feeling as though I shouldn't have to explain every aspect of the 911 system, how our job works, who our patients are, and what they have been through. But her non-stop questions and genuine optimism wear down my defenses, and after a few months I find myself appreciating her earnest attitude. My peer counselor, Jaya, has been through homelessness, addiction, and multiple hospitalizations for psychosis and suicide attempts. She found her way into activist communities, put herself through university, and is easily one of the most well-read members of our whole program. She is a persuasive speaker, able to build unrehearsed thoughts into an eloquent crescendo and unafraid of embarrassing our management. The three of us form a tight bond, our conversations swerving from public health initiatives to revolutionary political movements to Korean soap operas.

One evening we're parked in front of St. Matthias. Sofia and I walk inside to pee in time to see an older Black woman being removed from the emergency room. She screams at security, kicking at their heads and clawing their uniforms, but gets face-slammed into the floor. She pees herself during the process, then gets thrown out onto the sidewalk in her wet pants. The medics step out of the way and the hospital social worker doesn't even look up from his clipboard. Sofia looks like she's going to cry.

I give her a look and walk towards the bathroom. We see this type of thing a lot at this particular hospital, and none of us feels like getting into it with them today. But next thing I know Sofia is walking straight up to the security guards like she's facing down a pride of lions.

She leans in. "So how do you guys feel? That was a lot, right?"

The guards look at each other. *What . . . is happening right now? Who even is this chick?*

"It's a lot to hold," she says softly, unironically. "That kind of interaction. How are you guys feeling right now?"

At first I can't handle how awkward I imagine the confrontation will be so I start to walk away, but after a minute I find myself turning around. Before I can comprehend what's happening, they're having a quiet heart-to-heart with her. One of the guards says, "Everyone is always telling me to go back to Africa, and that really hurts. No one ever asks how *we* feel, you know?"

He leans down slightly, so Sofia can hear him better. She nods, holding her hands in front of her. "Wow, yeah, that must need some support." I shake my head, laughing to myself, and walk out of the ER. Over the years I have hated these security guards, been grateful to them, rolled my eyes at them, and wrestled a patient alongside them. But never once have I thought to ask about their emotional state. Sofia can be naive at times, and frustratingly cheerful, but I will never again doubt her commitment to the cause.

Most of our clients are too confused to achieve a meaningful interaction. When we write up our medical charts we use phrases like *hyperverbal* or *tangential*. We might write, *The client was disorganized and hyperverbal but directable.* This means that although he was too out of his mind to answer questions or have a coherent conversation, when I gave him a water bottle, he took it from my hand. When I asked him to sit down, he sat.

They speak as though they are unable to control the words as they come out. Individual pieces of coherent grammar railroad together in a chaotic rhythm, an endless parade of commas, a waterfall of speech bouncing down rocky ledges of half-thoughts.

*I have the lord as my savior? Okay? I don't even want to actualize.
I've been way the fuck too long to understand why the fuck this
city, like, why they put these two retarded motherfuckers, like, its like
a kick in the vagina, like, i'm just trying to self actualize, i'm seeing,
i wouldn't even really claim your husband and your children, like, i
stay with them or not, i can't im 31, i'll never even be 32, i don't wanna
fucking, theyre trying to call me out, if you're, like, some kid and
they're trying to call you out like you've doing something wrong—*

    *That's gonna be my whole life? No that's crap! I don't want to
see that shit.*

    *It's one thing or whatever to see it like that, but i see other
people driving around, other times of days—*

    *You're my elders, okay? Even you. I know you're an elder. You
need to be available because i don't want to need to tell you a
fucking thing. I don't want to be someone's throwaway kid, you
know? Butthole surfers and shit. Trying to surf someone's butthole.*

    *You try. Sour, you ever have sour cake before? Not my, for me,
its like, let em get all, i'm like, that's exactly what i'm gonna do.*

In December 2021, a few months into my time on the Street Crisis
unit, I come across an article in *The Atlantic* about methamphetamine.
The journalist, Sam Quinones, describes a profound change in the
American drug trade over the last couple of decades. For the next
several weeks, everyone I know in EMS passes the article around,
muttering *Holy shit. Holy shit.*

For most of its history, methamphetamine was synthesized from
the ephedra plant, a pretty flower used in Chinese medicine for
thousands of years. But when the U.S. government clamped down
on production and imports of this key ingredient in the 1990s, the

illegal meth trade set to work finding another way. Quinones describes how in the last decade or so a few international groups of chemists finally figured out how to easily synthesize methamphetamine from simple chemical precursors without needing farmed ephedra at all. No longer constrained by weather patterns and trade routes for an agricultural product, they are now able to use widely available household ingredients to make astonishing amounts of product at rock-bottom prices. This new meth has exploded across the United States and Canada, leaving a trail of mental illness in its wake that is hard to comprehend. It is usually nicknamed "P2P meth," a shortening of its chemical designation. The newer production methods are cheap, fast, and easy, and they make a breed of methamphetamine that destroys the brain in ways that are unrecognizable from most of known neurology. Quinones outlines how, in city after city, the post-2010 meth is a completely new and unbelievably destructive influence.

I've read so many news stories, since I was a little kid, about the next Scary New Thing: razor blades in the Halloween candy, serial killers in the supermarket, kidnappers around every corner—and most of it has wound up amounting to TV ratings and hyperbole. But now, when I read descriptions of this new meth psychosis, my hair stands on end. I've been a paramedic since 2013, and the timeline of my own career followed the proliferation of this new brain-melting chemical so closely that I wonder how different a person I would be today if I had gotten my license just five years earlier. I reach out to Quinones eventually, and we speak a few times. He asks me if I've seen the influence of methamphetamine in my work on the ambulance, especially as it relates to mental illness. I tell him I have a hard time even imagining what my job would be without it.

When I first started as an EMT, I remember running calls on meth users who would talk really fast, scratch at scabs, and take radios apart. But you could still converse with them most of the time, assess them, put them on the monitor to see their rapid heart rate. These days it is so, so normal for six of us to have to fight a guy who is completely covered in feces, screaming gibberish, and fighting a storm of attacking demons. When I pull up to a scene it doesn't take much for me to sigh and get the sedatives out of the lock box. I'm not a particularly muscular person, but there is kind of a sweet spot in the crevice between a person's knee and their lower thigh where, if I get right in the dent, I can control the legs much more effectively than you would think no matter how hard they are kicking. It has become so unbelievably mundane for me to be just sitting on a guy, exhaling slowly while I jam my shins into his legs as hard as I can, throwing my whole body weight into my legs and using my hands to try to hold myself in place as six or seven of us ram ourselves onto this guy, and he sweats and screams and tries to buck us off like a rodeo bull. I nod at the firefighter next to me and he meets my eyes with a slow blink as if to say, *When did this become our job?*

Quinones expands on the magazine article in his book *The Least of Us*. In it, he quotes Dr. Rachel Solotaroff, the director of a sobering station in Oregon that was forced to close in 2020 due to increasing violence and psychosis in their clients. Before the arrival of P2P meth, the station had been operating for thirty-five years. Solotaroff tells Quinones, "The degree of mental-health disturbance, the wave of psychosis, the profound, profound disorganization [is something] I've never seen before. If they're not raging and agitated, they can be completely non communicative . . . I've never experienced something like this—where there's no way *in* to that person."

A Los Angeles Police Department officer, Deon Joseph, spent twenty-two years on skid row. "They'd be okay when they were just using crack," he tells Quinones. "Then in 2014, with meth, all of a sudden they became mentally ill. They deteriorated into mental illness faster than I ever saw with crack cocaine." Quinones travels the country to interview drug users, dealers, law enforcement, neuropsychologists, homeless shelter employees and advocates, and every type of recovery and addiction medicine specialist. Almost as though rehearsed, they describe similar changes in their community since the introduction of new synthetic meth. Dr. Jennie Jobe, the leader of a Tennessee drug court, describes the process of getting to know her residential clients. "It takes longer for them to be here mentally. Before, we didn't keep anybody more than nine months. Now we're running up to fourteen months, because it's not until six or nine months that we finally find out who we got. It's not unusual for them to ask what they were found guilty of and sentenced to."

When Quinones and I talk, he explains that when he began his research for *The Least of Us*, he wondered if there was something in the chemical make-up of P2P meth that was affecting the brain differently than ephedrine-based meth. Several years later, he has come to believe that the impacts of these new drugs may be less about their chemistry and more about their volume and potency. Quinones explains that the new cooking process is so much more cost-effective (and difficult to regulate) that the market has been flooded with a seemingly unlimited supply of incredibly pure meth. He emphasizes the price drop: between 2003 and 2013, rather than rising with inflation, the cost of meth fell by 90 percent. His research found huge volumes of meth pouring into communities which had previously been sheltered from the drug. He tells me that we are witnessing a large-scale unofficial experiment in real time: what happens to the human brain when exposed to previously unheard-of amounts of unadulterated speed. "These changes in people that used to take seven or ten years," he tells me on the phone, "now you see them in a week."

We commiserate about how challenging it can be to apply traditional harm reduction strategies with someone who is in this type of psychosis. During our encounters, many of my patients are so mentally altered that attempting to talk about shelter or addiction counseling seems absurd. All of the techniques I have learned as a paramedic in verbal de-escalation, trauma informed care, and compassionate counseling are totally useless if my patient is hallucinating so violently that they can't even hear my voice.

People start using meth for all kinds of reasons. For many decades it was the drug of choice of the American working class, used to stay awake at factory jobs or prescribed by doctors for everything from nasal congestion to narcolepsy. Historians blame the rise of meth use on all kinds of factors: World War II, industrialization, the North American Free Trade Agreement, class struggle in the American Midwest. But in academic conversations, methamphetamine is almost always treated as an unpleasant side effect of the opiate crisis. Newspaper articles, public health programs, and addiction medicine innovations all seem to focus on opiates and sideline or ignore the effects of meth. And while it is true that fentanyl kills a far higher percentage of people, I sometimes wonder which drug is responsible for a greater overall decline in quality of life.

When they are coherent enough to speak with me, I often ask my patients why they began to use or what they like about meth. Folks with schizophrenia often say it soothes their moods and quiets the voices. Working parents use to stay awake at two or three jobs. Homeless patients, both women and men, tell me that they were raped while sleeping outside and now smoke all night to keep vigilant and stay safe. It's not that all homeless people use meth, or that all meth users are homeless. It's just that in the year I work on a street mental health crisis team, I have very few clients for whom meth is not a factor. Almost all of our patients use some amount of meth, and the most severe cases—the folks who shout incoherently, take off their clothing, run into traffic, and soil themselves—are almost always on a bender.

When I start to bang my head against the steering wheel and rant about how impossible and stupid this all feels, Jaya tells me I'm flat-out wrong. She quotes Frantz Fanon, the Caribbean revolutionary philosopher, to remind me that small failures on the front line of a movement do not negate its global need. She tells me that the work we're doing as the first point of contact is valuable and important, and that every day matters. I try to believe her.

We had been called yesterday for a gal who was lying at the entrance of a kids' museum. At the time, she was too confused and sick to qualify for any of our mental health facilities. She shook her head back and forth, rolled on the ground, and had trouble walking without our help. She couldn't answer any questions other than her name. We had accepted that there was nothing we could offer and requested an ambulance to take her to the emergency room.

Now, maybe fourteen hours later, she is lying on the sidewalk in front of the ER doors. We have just finished a different call and had parked in front of the hospital to take care of some paperwork. Jaya was the first to notice her, but soon all three of us step out of the rig and walk over. She makes squeaking noises when we try to talk to her and sticks her tongue out. There is something childlike in her demeanor, like a toddler who has learned to make eye contact and reach for things but not yet begun to speak. We walk inside and find out that last night the hospital gave her a sedative and kicked her out. We poke a straw into a juice box and hand it to her. She drinks. We still don't have anywhere to take her. She's too fucked up for Angel Wings, and apparently not fucked up enough for the emergency room. As we're talking, she vomits up her juice and begins blowing vomit bubbles and getting it all over her face and tie-dyed sweatshirt and staring at us with a little tilt in her head, like a puppy. Sofia visibly stiffens and says, "I think I'm going to put her on another hold."

When we met her yesterday I had thought that she was simply high on meth, but today it seems more clear that she has some sort of developmental delay. She holds the juice box as though it's hard to grip. She seems totally unaware of the vomit covering her face and chest. I had thought yesterday that she would come around a little bit once she sobered up. But it's been almost twenty hours since then and her mentation is still just as confused. As Sofia and I debate how to break the fewest number of rules, Jaya lies down on the sidewalk next to our patient. She looks into her eyes, then sees the juice box. She begins to tell a story.

"You're walking through the forest, and you can feel the warm sun on your shoulders." The patient leans her head in, face still covered in vomit and apple juice, and smiles. "The leaves crunch under your feet. The branches stretch out over your head. Do you want to keep walking?"

The patient nods eagerly. Jaya tells me later that she was trying to create a sensory experience, a technique she had learned to use to help ground an anxious patient into reality. She said that she could not stop thinking that, left alone in the streets, this person would not survive the night. She continues to talk to our patient, guiding her through the forest and out to a summery beach.

Sofia and I call for a second ambulance and I prepare to explain to the crew why I have asked them to literally meet us at the ER doors. Usually this would be a ridiculous request, because a patient located within 250 yards of a hospital emergency room legally still belongs under their care. The crew steps out of the ambulance with their eyebrows raised, but when they hear my explanation and look at our girl their demeanor softens. They agree to transport her to a different hospital, hoping that maybe she will have a better outcome the second time around. We follow them there in the van, which I will get a phone call about later—the higher-ups will remind me not to waste our time doing follow-up when there are more calls pending. But in the moment we all agree that it's worth a slap on the wrist to feel that we've done everything we can for this woman. We talk to the social worker at the new ER for a minute when we get there and he seems more receptive to trying to figure her out, to see if she belongs anywhere or has a place in a program or something instead of just medicating and discharging. But he could be just trying to prove a point about being better than the other guy, and if she doesn't already have a bed somewhere it's hard to imagine she'd win that lottery today.

When I'm cleaning up the rig after, I find the juice box we gave her. It's got writing on the back with a cartoon illustration, where they sometimes put lost children or jokes. This one has a drawing of some animals, and the text of an old African proverb: "When elephants fight, it is the grass that suffers."

I read a ton of fiction growing up, and science, and math, and politics. But the first big, dense, nonfiction history book I ever finished was Paul Starr's *The Social Transformation of American Medicine*. Years before I joined the Street Crisis team, I was a young medic increasingly confused by the systemic failures that we battled against every day on the ambulance. I pestered my dad, the history buff, with questions about why things worked the way they did and how it all got so messed up. Eventually he told me that if I really wanted to understand, I'd have to read Starr.

I found my dad's old paperback copy on the bookshelf in Oakland. The pages were soft and worn, all 514 of them. As I made my way through the last couple hundred years of American medicine, economics, and labor history, I underlined page after page of events that may have seemed inconsequential at first but had ballooned over time. I searched for a root cause, a single theme that would help point me in one direction or another. I wanted good guys and bad guys. I wanted a story. Instead, I found a massive, geographically and culturally diverse nation filled with thousands of communities that were each doing what made sense in the moment. There were moments of greed, of course, and cruelty, but I also found efforts at altruism and collaboration. By the time I began my work on the Street Crisis units, I had come to see our history not as a deliberate descent into evil but as a big fat mess of imperfect humans trying their best.

As I stumble through my shifts on the Street Crisis team, one detail from early in Starr's book keeps jumping out at me. In pre-industrialized societies, a "hospital" was not somewhere one might visit to be cured of a disease. Before the discovery of antibiotics or modern surgical techniques, hospitals were full of sickness and death, and to be avoided by all those who could possibly manage without. If a family member was injured or fell ill, those who could afford it would pay a doctor to make a house call. There was one main route to ending up in a hospital: you needed help surviving, and you had nowhere else to go.

Starr tells us how in early Colonial America, religious and charitable orders established public hospitals to house the "aged, the orphaned, the insane, the ill, the debilitated." He writes, "hospitals had been formed mainly to take care of people who did not fit into the system of family care." He goes on to explain how these "alms-houses" slowly transformed over the next several centuries. By the late 1800s and early 1900s, developments in hygiene, anesthesia, and antibiotics shifted the role of the hospital from a place to live into a place to be treated and sent back home. The work I do on the Street Crisis teams places me square in the middle of the community that was left behind by this shift.

It's not so simple, of course. Nursing homes still exist, as do psychiatric facilities and public housing. But as I walk through the sidewalks of downtown San Francisco, talking to client after client facing severe mental and physical disabilities, I often find myself daydreaming about the early colonial almshouses. Wondering if we are fulfilling some piece of their legacy.

In winter the rains come. Sofia, Jaya, and I spend hours standing around encampments, helping our people sort through their sopping-wet belongings and determining who is hypothermic enough to require ambulance transport and who we can put in our van. One afternoon we are pulled out of service to join a Zoom meeting about program logistics, and we take the opportunity to turn the heat all the way up in the van and dry out our own clothes. We idle the engine in the far corner of a parking lot down by the water, and the windows quickly fog. Jaya realizes that with our phones balanced on the headrests just so, we are only visible in the meeting from our shoulders up. Working quickly, all three of us pull off our soaked pants and lay them on top of the dashboard vents to dry out, holding blankets on our laps and grateful for the clouded windows.

About twenty minutes into the meeting, I peek outside the van to make sure that no one has gathered to take photos of the Street

Crisis Underwear Team, and realize that our parking spot has flooded. The rain is coming down so hard that the sidewalk drain has clogged and water is partway up the tires and rising. I shout to the girls and hop into the driver's seat, still in my underwear. Jaya tosses me a blanket. Sofia interrupts the meeting to blurt something about a mechanical emergency and then mutes all three of our phones and throws them on the center console. The girls squeal as we peel out of the parking lot in a spray of floodwater, with gray felt blankets held at our waists and wet uniform pants flying across the dashboard. We make it out of the lot just in time to see a clot of leaves burst out of a nearby storm drain and release another gush of dirty water.

It's a deep, wet cold, two weeks of storm on and off. Everyone on the news is excited because California needs the water and there is finally snow on the mountains. But the city runs out of shelter beds quickly. The mental health facilities are full, the hospitals are full, the urgent cares are full. There's one sleeping site left, an "interfaith" winter program that rotates between churches every three weeks. You line up between 6:30 and 10:00 p.m. for drop-in to see if you can get a bed. Most nights they fill up and lock the doors by eight or nine o'clock.

A few days after our parking lot excitement we are called by an ambulance to Lucy's Place, a simple drop-in shelter in a rough neighborhood, for a man outside in a chair. He was discharged from a nearby emergency room and given a taxi voucher to their address with no other plan. Lucy's Place is full, obviously, and the sleeping area is up a flight of stairs. This guy can barely walk on his own. He is elderly, with back and leg injuries, and pees into a catheter bag. The shelter staff called an ambulance as soon as he showed up and put him in a chair outside to wait. Now the ambulance has called me, wondering if we have access to a bed somewhere so they don't have to take him back to the same ER he just got kicked out of and watch him get kicked out again. The ambulance medics are tired, their shift having ended about half an hour ago. They don't want to get stuck for three hours past the end of their shift, babysitting the man at an overcrowded emergency room until a nurse can finally take his blood pressure and then wheel him right back outside. We put the patient in the van while we figure things out and I tell the ambulance crew to go home.

He's in his sixties, with dark skin and a short afro. He's wearing thin hospital scrubs and a blue sweatshirt and both are wet from the rain. I can feel the catheter bag tied around his left leg inside his hospital pants. He reeks of damp clothes and ammonia and the smell is strong when we shut ourselves inside the van with him. The social worker puts on an N95—it's not Sofia today; we have a part-timer named Linda instead. We ask the patient how he's doing and try to assess his needs. The responses we get from him are single-word shouted demands: "Cold!" Or "Food!" Each word he spits out looks like it takes effort. He draws a breath, pauses, flexes each individual mouth muscle, shouts the word "Water!" and then immediately goes slack in his head and neck. His bottom lip juts out like the effort of it all was just too much and he can't be bothered to pull it back in.

We give in to the demands that we can. Once he's in the van we peel off his wet clothes and slip him into a new sweatshirt that almost fits. We cover him in thin felt blankets and jack the heat all the way up. This makes the urine evaporate off of him in such a thick cloud that Linda coughs a little and has to step out for a minute. The paramedic in me can't help but snicker at her. *Ha. Wuss.*

Jaya and I leave him in the warm van to sleep for a minute and join Linda outside in the rain and get on our phones. No room at Angel Wings. The Mental Health Urgent Care has been full for weeks.

No more shelter beds. It's too late for an intake, but we could try to pull a few strings and see if there is still a bed at South shelter. The only one left yesterday was a top bunk. "Can he climb up a ladder if that's all we have?" God no, of course not. "Eh, never mind, the bed is gone anyway." Do any of the supervisors know him? He seems like he gets transported a lot. Linda finally gets hold of his case manager and puts him on speakerphone. We all listen in. "Oh, Theodore? No. Absolutely not. He's been kicked out of every goddamn shelter in the city, a couple of nursing homes, a couple of SNFs [skilled nursing facilities]. He's got no more bridges left to burn. You guys do whatever you want with him."

Click.

Linda looks at me. She says, "Did a case manager really just hang up on me?"

The night is closing in. It's growing darker, and wetter, and colder. We're down to two options: call another ambulance to take him back to an ER, which will kick him back out into the cold after an hour or two; or we drive him over to the interfaith temporary winter sleeping site, which isn't open for another couple hours but theoretically might have somewhere indoors for him to stay for the night. We all stare at each other, our phones glowing, droplets of wet light in a storm.

We're picking between garbage options and we know it. Taking this elderly, disabled man somewhere safe and warm, for just one night, simply is not possible. We decide anything's better than the ER that just kicked him out. We try to explain the plan to Theodore, but he's got too much dementia to really understand; he keeps just saying "warm" and "food" and "water." His words come out staccato and demanding. Angry, spittle-coated echoes of the three most basic human needs.

I drive us all the way out to the church where the winter storm site is located this week. It's about six miles away, almost an hour in traffic. Every single one of these cars is on their way to somewhere, from somewhere. Lit-up little boxes of moving rain protection, every one of them. When we get to the church, we circle it a few times trying to figure out the entrance and find an iron gate with some guys gathered outside. The doors open in an hour and a half and there are maybe fifteen or twenty guys milling around. All men, all between thirty-five and sixty, mostly white. Why this demographic in such a diverse city? I have no idea. We try to decide where to put Theodore, and I desperately wish we had a chair. He needed so much help getting out of the van. I'm pretty sure he could get up from a seated position by himself, but I'm worried he'll be too weak and stiff to get all the way off the ground on his own. Plus the body can lose a ton of core heat on the cold wet ground, especially for someone as bony and elderly as this guy.

We settle for a patch of raised curb with a pole he can lean against. It's a little too close to a group of guys I'm not sure about, but as we get closer, one of them shouts, "Hey, ambulance lady! I know you! You guys helped me out one time!"

It's Jaime. I spent a whole day with him once, trying to get him into a "low-barrier walk-in" mental health urgent care facility. That day ended poorly, but that's another story. Fortunately Jaime remembers me for the day of trying, not the failure in the end. I ask how he's doing and he says pretty good and I believe him. He looks pretty good. I point at Theodore, who has become a sagging, damp pile of blankets against a pole.

"Hey, Jaime," I ask. "Would you mind keeping an eye on this guy when they open the doors? If he doesn't get in, could you call 911 for him? He doesn't walk so good."

They nod and wave at me, *You got it, sister!* I get a couple mock-salutes from hands holding cigarettes or blunts. Ha. I guess that's something.

We walk back to the rig and slowly drive out of the parking lot. Everyone is a little over it. No one is proud. We haven't saved a life. We've witnessed a cold, damp tragedy and prolonged it for one more night.

I want so desperately to blame this on something or someone. To find the reason that no skilled nursing facility will hold Theodore, that we don't have enough shelter beds, that people end up in his position in the first place. Lately, my personal punching bag has just been this city itself. I've given her personality traits in my head, origin stories, motivation. This patch of land and buildings has become a cartoon villain casting a deep foggy shadow over a forty-nine-square-mile peninsula of evil. It's good to have someone to shout at, to focus my rage. Anger is much easier than grief.

When I walk away from this man's bony, elderly knees buckled against wet cement, it's much easier to give in to simple fury at the system that put him here, rather than accept the whole reality of where we are in this moment. I know that humans have always lived with disease, and old age, and sorrow. I know that no one person or entity or system of government is at fault for this man's trauma. But as I leave an old man alone in the rain, my mind strays. I think of angry speeches I will never give in air-conditioned offices, emails I will never send to hospital administrators, things I will never say to overworked charge nurses who discharge patients without a plan. Metaphors, corruption, politics, history, anything, *anything*, to release my mind from the searing pain of the present moment. Whoever said "live in the now" has never worked in medicine.

We look up Theodore the next day and find out that he was transported by ambulance from the shelter first thing in the morning. The church staff wakes everyone up around six and kicks them out to make room for visitors during the day, so they must have called 911 when they couldn't get him out of bed. The ambulance crew's chart isn't finished when we read it, but it says he was picked up from a cot inside the church, so we figure at least he made it indoors for the night. It's a tempered relief. I'm glad to know that we made the right choice, that he got warm, slept for one night on a cot instead of the sidewalk. But I still find myself wondering how things are so messed up in this city that *that* feels like a success.

I have a good friend who has been working at the intersection of EMS and social programs in my city for longer than me, and at a higher level. We sit with my parents at dinner one night and they pepper us with questions about work. Sam peels the label off of her cider and says, "Look, all these new programs are great. I'm glad they're trying new things, trying to fix gaps. But I would trade every single one of these programs, and all of the people in them, for five new long-term psych beds in the city. Five."

The lack of resources is everywhere, all day, every day. The number of humans in need vastly overwhelms the amount of help. A simple math problem with a thousand incomplete solutions. It is easy for me to see hospitals as the enemy, but I understand their plight. In many ways, urban emergency rooms have become de facto homeless shelters, and they do not have the resources to adequately feed, clothe, and house every sick person in the city any more than we do.

For some reason, building long-term mental health facilities seems to be much harder than creating flashy new "linkage" programs and bringing in the news to cover their success. An old supervisor of mine who helped pave the way for programs like this says, "Everybody wants to do outreach. Outreach is exciting, it's sexy, you're out in the streets, in the photo op. Nobody wants to do long-term care or follow-up, or build and staff the facilities farther down the path." This sentiment is echoed by almost every worker I talk to in the industry. Mike tells me you can't just "slap up new programs," you have to fund the ones you have, you have to pay the employees enough that you actually retain some of them, so that everyone with enough education and skills doesn't leave for a better job. A peer counselor I work with spends one frustrated night shouting that our team is basically the *Pimp My Ride* of social programs: all sparkly paint and flashing lights, no engine work.

But there is another issue complicating even the best-funded mental health outreach programs. Most of the people we speak with do not want our help. In some cases they are so out of their minds that we will force them into an ambulance to receive care, but usually they are just barely oriented enough to tell us to leave. I think the public has this idea that if someone is behaving irrationally or looks out of place, we will swoop them into our van and remove them. Or that if we offer a shelter bed to everyone who sleeps outside, they will jump into it gratefully. But determining how or when a human is no longer allowed to make their own decisions is problematic, scary, and comes with a deeply complicated legal and political history.

The criteria for a true involuntary hold are very specific and (despite what many of our well-intentioned 911 callers believe) "being super weird at a gas station" simply does not fulfill them. Most of the clients we wrestle to the emergency room will be released within hours and be right back as they were. A lot of the time we simply offer people water or food, ask if they need anything, and walk away, leaving the 911 caller disappointed that we have not made the "problem" disappear. During the year I spend on the Street Crisis Response Team, San Francisco is finding itself at a cultural breaking point. Whole city blocks are covered by tent encampments. Many of our calls are placed by locals who are increasingly hostile to this community, and we find ourselves in the middle of an emotional tug-of-war. I often stand on the sidewalk between a furious shop owner and a homeless client, unsure of who I am supposed to disappoint.

We are not alone. Every couple of weeks, we pass around a news story about a similar program cropping up or expanding in another city. They are spreading across the United States, and the media coverage tends to be positive. Of course, most of the quotations given in the news are provided by people who have an interest in seeing these programs succeed. Not included: hundreds of paramedics spitting a mouthful of dip into an empty 7-Eleven cup and saying, "Waste of fucking money, that's what it is."

I try to learn a little bit about some other systems. The COVID-19 pandemic is releasing a lot of funding for community paramedicine projects—for ways to use EMTs and paramedics outside of the ambulance. Some cities have set up programs like the Street Crisis units, run by police departments or activist groups intending to help mentally ill clients. Others, like our EMS-6 teams, work with high-volume 911 users. Still more are run by health departments or fire departments and focus on public health initiatives or COVID testing and disease prevention. Like the cholera epidemic that inspired the nation's first municipal ambulance service, the specter of disease once again scares everyone into action.

I visit the Sacramento Metropolitan Fire Department and learn that their battalion chief does not use the term *community paramedicine*. He prefers *mobile integrated health care*, to reflect that their team also uses nurse practitioners or physician assistants to assist with primary care. The program sounds promising—a paramedic riding with an advanced provider and looking for any opportunity to relieve the stress on the overburdened ER system. The team—one paramedic, one advanced provider—drives around town in an SUV filled with medical supplies. On the day I tag along, we monitor 911 radio channels and send messages to ambulance crews or fire engines to let them know that we are available to help. I watch a nurse practitioner write a prescription for a girl with a sinus infection, allowing her to stay home instead of taking up an ambulance and an ER bed. We check in on a woman who usually calls 911 a lot and see that she is doing a little better after a change in caregivers. In the afternoon the chief buys me tacos and asks what I think. I tell him truthfully that the program looks impressive, but I think they are taking on a lot. I am worried about the sheer volume of work they are inviting on themselves. The chief chuckles. He does not disagree.

News coverage of Sacramento Metro Fire's program has been favorable. One local reporter says the number of frequent 911 callers dropped by 43 percent over two years. Another estimates that the program has saved the county over $2.4 million in only one year. As a Santa Cruz ambulance supervisor says to me over coffee, "We started talking about community paramedicine over twenty years ago. It's the answer to everybody's problem. But there's been a zillion pilot programs, and once they run out of money, they go away."

But although programs like EMS-6 and the Sacramento Metro Fire team are making progress in some areas, the issues we face on the Street Crisis vans often feel insurmountable. I have *no idea* how to help the decimated brains of P2P meth users. I have no clue as to how a van full of non-violent do-gooders armed with sweat pants and snack packs can hope to make a difference in the grand scheme of things.

When I find someone whose brain is so far gone on meth that they don't remember their name, shivering and ducking their head and flapping their arms at the tornado of black helicopters they see swirling around the street corner, I often stand limply, wondering what if anything might help. I wish for tranquilizer blow darts that came with a magical additive that would kill not only the high but the rest of the addiction also. There has been modest success for opiate users with methadone and Suboxone, drugs that ease the pain of withdrawal and help guide users back to some neurochemical normalcy. Unfortunately, there is not yet a medication like this for meth users. What hope can I find in writing involuntary psych holds on the same clients, over and over again, dozens of times, just to watch them released back out onto the street, using again within days or even hours?

In the first twenty years after surgeons invented anesthesia, surgical outcomes worsened. Surgeons were trying longer, more daring surgeries now that their patients could be put to sleep, and they were killing more people than ever. As modern medicine prevents more and more heart attacks and strokes, cancer rates go up—all the people we saved from an early death have lived long enough to die later from a different disease. Perhaps we are trying things today in mental health that are failing terribly, miserably, but I hope against all odds that we are failing usefully. I want to see this thing work; I want someone to fill in the gaps, pull down the barriers, see which parts of the story we are missing and why we are messing up so badly. What Suboxone has done for opiate addiction, what radiation has done for tumors . . . I want *someone* to figure out *something* to do about the P2P-scarred screaming naked humans sprinting through the streets.

My time on the Street Crisis team is tough. In attempting to improve a narrow but real issue facing American EMS and police work, we find ourselves butting up against profoundly big questions about human rights, the role of government in a society, and the ability of individuals to determine their own fate. Can we "fix" the challenges faced by modern paramedics without systematically solving every single social determinant of health? Do we have to cure poverty? Is that where this conversation is ultimately headed?

Let's take Theodore. Elderly, cold, sick, and alone on a rainy night. No one likes that image. For a writer, to be honest, his story is a bit of a cheap shot. But remember his world-weary case manager on the other end of the cellphone call? Multiple city agencies had already tried to place Theodore into, if we are to believe the case manager, literally every care facility in the county. He has left or been kicked out of all of the services that we have tried to provide. At what point do we force him to accept care? Do we tie him to his bed, if that's what's required, and lock the door, and tube-feed him twice a day and tell ourselves we have saved a life? Or do we let him shiver outside in his urine-soaked hospital scrubs? Which, in the end, is more cruel?

Many of our clients are accepted into a facility only to set fire to their room, overdose, refuse their meds, tear the plumbing from the wall, and end up back on the street. In order to place (or not place) this one particular patient into one particular shelter on one particularly rainy night, we have to agree on some of the most fundamental philosophical questions humans have debated since language was invented. Where is the line between mental illness and personality? Who decides what constitutes "normal," and what is allowed in public view versus private? What role does the government have in all of this? What even is free will, anyway?

As a medic, I run into ethical questions all the time, but on some gut level I always believe that the concept of medicine itself is a solid enough foundation. If a fellow human is bleeding to death, you stop the bleed. Sure, you can debate the ethics of preserving life in a world where overpopulation poses the greatest threat of all, but on a day-to-day basis helping folks who are hurt and sick feels like a pretty reasonable way to check the "I'm a good person" box. That guy was sick; now he's better. Good job, me.

But parsing through a seething metropolis of millions of people and figuring out who gets to decide what about where and how others can and should live, what the difference is between helping and condescending, when which humans should lose their freedoms . . . A few hours on the crisis response team makes me feel like I've lost all semblance of right and wrong. There is something vague and gaseous underneath the whole entire concept, and the further up the thought experiment you get the more wobbly it all feels. I read hundreds of pages of opinions about personal responsibility versus societal commitment to change, about homelessness versus criminality, about whether harm reduction policy ultimately hurts or helps. I respect my colleagues' commitment to the cause, but after a year of the work I am ready to get back to the ambulance.

I have always loved the lack of moralizing in emergency medicine: I don't care why this person overdosed, or crashed, or found themselves at the wrong end of a shotgun. I hate feeling like the arbiter of other people's life choices. I've argued more than once about how many times we should Narcan the same person before saying, "Sorry, punch card's full," and my perspective has always been the same: You're missing the point. My job is to save first, ask questions later or not at all. Airway, breathing, circulation. Nowhere in the ABCs is there a line about good choices and social contracts. *Theirs not to reason why/theirs but to do or die.*

Most of the men in that poem did die, for the record. They charged ahead on a famously mistaken order and lost the battle and their lives. So maybe they should have reasoned just a little.

WHAT I WOULD HAVE LIKED TO WRITE IN MY CHART NARRATIVES

1. Nursing home tried to kill rich old lady. We did stuff that definitely didn't help and took her to the hospital. She will receive all sorts of expensive medical care to prolong her suffering until the inevitable. Death gets us all in the end.

2. Called lights and sirens for a lady being homeless and loud in a fancy neighborhood. Cops were going to put her on a psych hold but when she agreed to go with us they peaced-out immediately and moved on with their day. We transported her non-emergent to a hospital in a shittier neighborhood, who put her in the waiting room without even speaking to her. Circle of life.

3. Called for a low-speed Uber accident. The driver is young, pale, and sweating too much. He says his shoulder hurts but mostly speaks Arabic and can't really answer many questions. He seems to have real pain in his shoulder. He seems to trust that going in the city ambulance is the right thing to do; that this government service was designed to help him. I don't know how to say "two thousand fucking dollars" in Arabic, so we buckle him up. I pray silently that he has insurance, or has given us a fake name.

4. Code. Guy was dead as fuck. We broke all his ribs and pumped him full of epi until his tired, dead heart shuddered and squeaked

a little and we called that a pulse and took him to the hospital. The pulse came and went; the ER put him on a drip to trap his corpse of a heart in a lifeless electrical shiver.

5. Otherwise healthy thirty-one-year-old activated 911 for wrist sprain. Young white guy. Parked ambulance on street and wove gurney through driveway filled with three brand-new cars. On arrival, patient found in living room sitting upright on couch. Several family members present, each of whom possessed a driver's license and keys to said vehicles. Ambulance crew evaluated patient and explained that while the ambulance is always an option, he may want to consider self-transport or requesting a ride from a family member to avoid an unnecessary bill and release our ambulance to respond to other emergencies in the community. Patient responded "Nah." Patient climbed onto gurney and waited to be carried down his own driveway like Aladdin during the "Prince Ali" musical sequence.

"TRAIN WRECK"

JODY GEARE, EMT/FIREFIGHTER;
TWENTY YEARS IN EMS AND FIREFIGHTING
APTOS, CALIFORNIA

I want this story to reach other people that are survivors of trauma. I want them to know that whether it is professional trauma or personal trauma, there is a light at the end of the tunnel.

I want to educate people to understand what happens when you go through something traumatic. You are having a normal reaction to an abnormal event. If you mitigate your symptoms you can still have a normal life. That is something that I didn't have, so I just thought I was weak. I thought I was broken, and unlovable, and a terrible firefighter. And it was just all bullshit. The trauma was playing tricks on my brain. I had to be quiet about it for so long. It didn't even feel like it happened. So to be able to get my story out, and acknowledge that this happened, and maybe help some other people through it, that is healing for me.

I got my hormones checked a few years ago, when I was thirty-three. The doctor sat me down and told me I was infertile. She said my stress hormones were jacked up and that I was suffering from adrenal fatigue. I was low on testosterone, estrogen, progesterone, everything was low. She gave me some medication to help out, and said that with the right care I could heal. It was validating, because

I was always taught that I was just being weak. To have a doctor say that my bloodwork was all fucked up was actually reassuring somehow.

For the first ten years of my career as a firefighter, I was a number. I was meat in the seat, replaceable, and I bought into all that. I was in the middle of the pack. My job was my whole self-worth. It wasn't "Hi, I'm Jody, and I'm a firefighter." It was "Hi, I'm a firefighter and I'm Jody."

Eventually it all blew up on me. I had some very significant personal trauma when I was younger, and for ten years I held everything down and didn't deal with it. I just muscled through. But then there was an incident that threw all that in my face. I was supposed to get off work that morning. We got called for a structure fire at three or four o'clock in the morning. It was just myself, an engineer, and a volunteer, and we could see the fire from station. You know when the adrenaline's really pumping, and you can feel it in your ears? And you're going through all your steps, like, *Okay, what am I going to do?*

We pull up, and there's a woman with a T-shirt on and no underwear. Screaming. It was a hoarder house, which is the worst. With a little white picket fence. We get out, and my engineer goes to set up his side of things. He was obviously stressed out. There was one police unit on scene already.

I pulled the hose line to the door, and I remember it being a pain in the ass to get over the fence. I get to the door with my mask on, and the cop says, "There's a guy in this room."

We don't go inside without two of us unless there is a confirmed rescue. But by this point I don't even know where my engineer or my volley [volunteer] are, so I think, *Well, I'm fucking going in.* I tell the cop to break the window with his baton.

I jump in the window. I get down on the floor. It's pitch black, there's smoke everywhere, and I start crawling around. I feel a bed, and

I move past the bed. I feel this guy's body. He's naked, and he's on the floor. And I was just like . . . I got him. I'm going to get him out.

And I drag him out. He's a really big guy. I get underneath his arms, I drag him to the window. The woman is still screaming outside. Keep in mind, the window was broken by a baton, so there's a bunch of jagged edges. I remember this specifically because I thought I screwed up by not clearing the window.

We're dragging this guy over the glass. My engineer is running around. By then another engine and EMS has shown up. We carry him around to the back of the engine. I remember thinking I am weak because he's so heavy. But in hindsight, he would have been heavy for anyone, you know what I mean?

It's all reasonably fast. EMS gets him. We start on overhaul, which means digging and sorting through everything to make sure that the fire is out.

A little while later, one of the other volleys comes back and tells me that the guy didn't make it. I just look at him. I can't wrap my head around it. Do you know how rare it is to pull someone out of a fire like I just had? In today's day and age? It just doesn't happen. I don't work in New York; you don't just run around making saves. I just went into this burning building, *Backdraft* style, through a broken window, and dragged his heavy ass out of a burning fucking building, and you're telling me he's dead?

Within two minutes, the battalion chief asks what happened. I say, "I don't know, I pulled him out." I don't know what to say to him.

He says, "As soon as you got him out, did you start CPR?"

And I think . . . "No?" I had my mask on still. I had my gloves, and everything. I'm wearing a fifty-fucking-pound SCBA [self-contained breathing apparatus] and a helmet. When I got him out,

I just handed him to the rest of the crew. I didn't think to take my gloves off and check for a pulse. I just pulled him out. I didn't, I couldn't . . . and then I start spinning.

Whether the chief intended it that way or not, all I hear as a twenty-six-year-old little firefighter is "You fucked up. You killed that guy. Why didn't you start CPR?" And I'm like . . . *EMS was here! And the BUILDING'S on fire!*

But as soon as he says that to me, I feel a chemical rush. I walk up the driveway, thinking, *I just fucking killed somebody. I didn't start CPR. Maybe if I had been faster, I would have saved this guy's life.*

We still have to do overhaul for about six hours. You're supposed to be masked up, but all we had was shitty N95 painters' masks, so all of us get sick. We go back to the station and one of the volleys goes to get breakfast burritos, but we can't eat. I put the engine back together and go home.

I fucking lose it. I drive home thinking I killed somebody. I go home and get in the shower and start throwing up. I've got black, bloody shit coming out of my nose, and I'm fucking crying, and spiralling. I'm thinking, *Why am I even a firefighter? I'm a piece of shit. I just fucking killed somebody.* It starts a physiological and emotional spiral. Even worse than when I went through my personal stuff when I was younger. Over time it had all added up. For months I wake up at 4:30 every morning with diarrhea, crying. I can't sleep, I can't eat. I call in sick to work a bunch.

The long and short of it is, I was a train wreck. I wasn't sleeping, I wasn't eating. The guy I was dating ended up breaking up with me. At work, the bosses were pissed at me. I remember one guy said, "Jody, you have the ability to change your mind and stop being sad about this." He thought I was just freaking out about the breakup.

I remember looking at him and thinking, *I'm shaking. I'm having panic attacks. I'm dying on the inside.* But I thought I was weak, because if he could do it, why couldn't I do it?

We never did a debriefing or a discussion. I found out years later that one of the other guys actually ended up cussing out the chief that day. He said it was a gnarly fire and the chief shouldn't have said that to me. The medics told me at the time that the guy was dead way before we got there, but I didn't believe them. They said his lungs were charred. He said I had actually done everything right. It was textbook, what the fuck I did.

After a couple of months, my captain pulled me into the office with the chief. He said, "We have an issue." He told me that it was brought to his attention the number of times I had called in sick. And others had noticed that in the station, any time I wasn't on an assignment I would just wait in my bunk. He tried to have a big intervention talk with me, but I ran to the bathroom and lost my shit. You have to remember that my entire identity was being a firefighter. I believe now that he was actually trying to help me out, but all I could think was that if I was a bad firefighter, then I was a bad person.

Eventually I told them, "That fire fucked me up."

They were surprised. They thought it was the breakup, or my personal issues. Once they realized what was happening, their whole tone changed. We talked for four hours. Each of them told me about their worst calls. I asked what they did after theirs, and my captain said, "Well, I got divorced." The other guy said he ran a call on a SIDS baby and then became an alcoholic for six months during the off-season. There was no mention of PTSD, or ways to process trauma. We were just each telling our stories. Even after the whole conversation, I still thought that they had found ways to get through their trauma, but I couldn't get over mine. I thought I couldn't be a firefighter anymore. I quit the job for two years that day, and they let me walk away. They didn't try to stop me.

I don't blame those supervisors at all. There was a completely different culture back then. There was a lack of education. It takes people dying in order to make change. In 2015 we had more suicide firefighter deaths than line-of-duty deaths. But change is happening! We have critical stress debriefing now, and peer counseling. Now we have pamphlets and seminars, and all kinds of shit. Back then it was like, "No, we don't cry. We just drink it off."

For me, I don't feel the way I did five years ago. I don't feel the way I did one year ago. With therapy, and peer support, and medication, I'm not having nightmares anymore. I'm sleeping through the night. They refer to trauma treatment as recovery now, like an alcoholic. It is a lifelong thing that you will have to deal with.

You have to have people that you can talk to and vent to. You can't work it off, you can't sleep it off, you can't drink it off. You have to process it. Everyone has weird details that stick in their head from the bad calls, whether it was the way they smelled or a teddy bear in the corner.

My whole thing was "There's nothing wrong with me. I can go to work." My psychologist diagnosed me with depression, and I told her I wasn't depressed. But she asked if I felt empty, and I said yes. Hopeless? Yeah.

I'm available for peer support now. I got a text about one today. A six-year-old kid got run over by a family member, and the entire volunteer company knows the family. And knew the kid. So I'm going over there tomorrow night to run a debrief.

I love being available for them. And using what I know now to help prevent someone else from getting as bad as I did.

The first time we did something like this was recently. The process is so new that we don't have an official policy or chain of command yet. I just got a phone call from a captain. He said, "Hey, my station had a rough call today. Do you think you could come by and talk to some of the guys?"

I said, "Absolutely. When and where?"

We set it up for the next night at 6:30. I looped in my chief, and my assistant chief. Within an hour we got a hold of everyone, and everyone said yes, we want to do this. It was really cool to watch that come together. And it was great. It worked. I have a little flip book that we talk through. There's a lot of evidence that these types of interventions have a huge effect on preventing future PTSD symptoms.

Weird shit goes through your head when you think you're going to die. When I was in the worst of it, I remember thinking, *I'm not ready to die, I'm gonna save the world.*

"SO, DO YOU LIKE BEING A PARAMEDIC?"

WHY I HATE MY JOB

Because when I try to get follow-up information on patient outcomes so that I can learn what to do better, I am met with rolled eyes and unanswered emails. After ten years as a paramedic, I have no idea if I am any good at this job.

Because even on a slow night, even after fifteen years in this industry, I have to beg a dispatcher for permission to go home like a third-grader asking for a bathroom pass.

Because my shift ends at 0200, and it is 0158 and dispatch just sent me on a

WHY I LOVE MY JOB

Because little kids crowd around the ambulance and look in the windows and ask us for stickers. And one little girl was upset about the bullies at her school so I let her hit the airhorn and she screamed and fell off the driver's seat she was so excited.

Because I can wear cargo pants and boots and cuss like a sailor and I am still somehow considered a professional adult woman.

Because when private ambulance companies instituted drive cameras, a policy they said was to

run that will take three
hours.

Because my supervisor,
who has less field experience than I do, is insisting I
sign on early without
checking out any of my
equipment because "ambu-
lance levels are low." I
refuse, telling him that I
don't want to go out with
missing or broken gear. He
tells me to just sign on and
look through my stuff later
when I have some down-
time. I tell him all of the
restock is located here, and
we haven't had "downtime"
in months; he says I probably won't use any of the
rare equipment anyway; I
tell him last week I signed
on early to jump a call for
an off-going crew and it
was an infant who was
barely breathing, and if I
run on her again would he

protect us but was obvi-
ously for their own insurance liability, the medics
responded by recording so
many clips of themselves
telling jokes, singing along
to the radio, dancing at
stoplights, and generally
being idiots that the companies had to change the
entire way the videos were
stored so that the system
could still function.

Because there is this
moment when you first
enter a patient's home—
when they are terrified and
awkward and unsure if calling was even the right
thing to do or how this
works or what will happen
next. And you walk in
calmly with just the right
amount of ease and ask
"what can we help you with
today" and then the ten-
sion deflates instantly and

like to explain to little
Carlita's parents why I'm all
out of pediatric breathing
masks? And we go back and
forth until we've wasted
more time than it would
have taken me to just go
check out my gear and sign
on in the first place.

Because we are begging,
begging our supervisors for
more training and more
ways to advance our skill set
but the answer is always the
same: not enough staffing.
Shut up and do your job.

Because I can feel the wet
spittle landing on my chin
and neck as this engine
captain screams at me for
taking so long to get to a
call when I've already run
eight calls in seven hours,
haven't stopped moving
since I signed on this
morning, and just drove

suddenly everyone is glad
you are there.

Because an old partner who
was mean and cranky for
years pulled me aside in a
hospital parking lot and put
his hand on my shoulder
and gave me a slow, heartfelt apology about what he
was going through at the
time and how he has figured
out how to move forward.
And now, two years later, he
is stuck behind the desk for
the day so we are racing
against the clock to surprise
him with a carton of his
favorite pastries and get
back to post before dispatch
notices that we were gone.

Because my buddy
Thompson, who carries
himself like a six-month-
old golden retriever
puppy—gangly and floppy,
all limbs—is learning from

WHY I HATE MY JOB

forty-five minutes through
rush-hour traffic to get to
him—and when I check on
the board later I see that it's
his second run in a forty-
eight-hour shift.

Because I tried *really hard*
to calm this patient down,
earn her trust, do a complicated assessment, make sure
I ruled out everything I
could, and figure out a
decent idea of what was
going on, and this nurse
cut me off three words in,
threw my EKG in the trash,
and told me to put her in
the waiting room.

Because this firefighter is
telling me how high the
expectations are for cooking meals in the firehouse,
how it's actually really
stressful because the chiefs
expect you to make all your
own sauces and desserts, no

WHY I LOVE MY JOB

Tasha, the gymnast, how to
do a handstand in the hallway outside the weight
room. She shows him how
to hold his legs up and he
slips and slams his butt into
the wall and there is a perfect, round, Thompson-ass-
shaped hole in the drywall
and he sees it and sighs and
walks straight over to the
man sweating on the
Stairmaster and hangs his
head and says, "Chief, I
done fucked up." Chief
walks outside, howls, and
tells Thompson he's going
to frame it. A week later,
the hole is still there, with a
cute wooden picture frame
and a label hanging on the
wall: "Thompson, 2018."

Because of the grandmother
in Reno, an asthma attack,
who began to feel better
after treatment and insisted
on walking us out to her

326

store-bought salad dressing, and lunch always needs a chopped fruit, and dinner always needs a salad. He has been teaching himself to make little chocolate spiderwebs and candied bacon to decorate their Halloween cake. It's all very cute, except I keep wondering why these guys have time to plan, shop, cook, eat, and clean up such elaborate meals on the clock when I and every other medic and nurse I've ever met is wolfing down a cold burrito with one hand while typing up a chart with the other.

Because as frustrated as I get in San Francisco, I know that paramedics around the country are working much harder for a fraction of the money and I can't fix their situation any more than I can fix my own.

garden so that she could pick us two ripe peaches off of a tree planted by *her* grandmother, and give them to us for our help. They were sun-warmed and soft and the juice dripped all over our gloves.

Because one minute I'm in the back corner of a giant commercial kitchen, stainless steel ladles and spatulas hanging over twenty-quart pots, orders flying out around us as I wait for a family member to answer the phone and translate Swahili or Tagalog or Nahuatl, and the next minute I am looking out the window of a penthouse suite. I have seen the newspaper-collaged attic of a conspiracy theorist, the windy deck of a fire boat at sunset, and the inside of a hidden ridgeline ranch

Because so many of my friends are trapped in this life: they believed stories of altruism and hope when they were young and now they are stuck with aching knees and bills to pay and no hope of further education or career advancement.

Because our protocols are written by a group of doctors and administrators who have never worked a day in the field.

Because sometimes it's not even about the money. We just want to be treated like adults.

Because our most challenging patients are cycled through the system over and over and over and over, and as a street paramedic there is nothing I can do but keep on spinning the wheel.

twenty miles off road in the Nevada desert plastered with signs telling us to *keep out* and *stay away*.

Because of Sarah Zhang, who made a gingerbread ambulance for the station for Christmas, with a tiny gingerbread patient on a tiny gingerbread gurney, and a little melted candy light bar, and two tiny cookie paramedics and a little gray blanket and a miniature bottle of Taaka vodka on the ground.

Because when we are getting hammered, like really non-stop brutalized by calls, the crews all start texting back and forth to figure out how to jump each other's runs and grab each other's restock so that folks can get to the bathroom or eat or have half a shot at going home.

WHY I HATE MY JOB

Because my back hurts.

Because my shoulder hurts.

Because my wrists hurt.

Because my stomach hurts.

Because my neck hurts.

Because I'm so, so tired.

Because this patient's pain is legitimate but I am so exhausted, so burned out, so bone tired that I simply don't care anymore. I can hear how flat my voice sounds when I speak, and I can tell how shocked my patient is that someone could act so inhumanely, but I simply have nothing left to give.

WHY I LOVE MY JOB

Because no matter how much I resent the suppression guys for all their job perks, on a difficult call they will back me up, jump in front of a violent patient, help me make a difficult decision, or literally reach down and pull the backpack off of my shoulders and carry it down the stairs for me.

Because when someone posts on our station Facebook page about designing an official EMS mascot, the two winning ideas are a black sheep and an enormously fat raccoon.

Because even when you don't save a life, you can make people who are very scared and very alone feel just a little bit safer.

NIGHT SHIFT

We're trying to catch a nap, is what we're doing. We've been running calls back-to-back for nine hours and some heaven-sent dispatcher has finally seen fit to post us down south for a minute. We hop on the freeway and get out of downtown as fast as we can drive.

I'm back on the ambulance with a new hire named Jack. I'm driving at the moment, which means it's my job to show him around town. I head to the community college, empty and dark at this hour of the night, and weave through campus into a large parking lot in the back. It is a perfect EMS secret spot—no people, no lights, no security, no tourists with cellphone cameras. And against the very back of the lot a smooth dirt hill, sloping up out of the concrete like it was made for us.

The seats on most ambulances only recline an inch or two, if at all. So if you want to rest your back muscles even a little bit at any point during the shift, options are limited. You can crawl in the back and throw a sheet on top of your god-knows-what-soaked gurney and try not to think about the body lice crawling all over your last patient or the fact that the radio's probably going to beep just as soon as you lie down. You can try to spread out on the narrow bench seat, which is only slightly less gross than the gurney. If you'd prefer to stay in the front seat, the closest thing to comfort is found by parking the ambulance facing up a steep hill. You can't lean back exactly, but you can feel the weight shift off your sit bones for just a few minutes, and that little hint of relief hits you like a cool breeze on a hot day.

So I'm the big sister tonight. I'm proud of my superior napping knowledge, and I'm letting Jack in on a well-guarded SFFD secret. He earned it. We've had a busy shift, and he is proving to be a hard-working and entertaining partner. I'm going to try to catch us a couple minutes of rest. What I do not realize is that in the older diesel ambulances that I was trained in, the undercarriage sits quite high off the ground. Not only that, but the box on the back is shorter, so the rear wheels are proportionally closer to the back bumper. In Medic 88, our shiny new gasoline rig, the box is longer and the clearance is much lower. Low enough that as soon as I rev up into the dirt hill, we both feel the back bumper of the ambulance grinding against the cement of the parking lot. Weird.

Jack looks concerned. I chuckle and roll my eyes. I put the rig in reverse and press down on the gas to get the bumper off the ground and get us settled. The truck shudders a little but doesn't move, and the grinding sound is louder. I pump the gas and brake a few times, feeling out the situation. The rig rocks back and forth but still doesn't shake out of its spot. Feeling like I'm stuck in the snow, I step harder on the gas to try to get some momentum. But the force only seems to shove us farther into the hill. I realize my mistake too late. Oh, no. Oh, no, no, no.

"Are we . . . *stuck?*" Jack asks, eyes wide. I shake my head.

"No, of course not. I'm gonna take a look. Stay put for a sec."

He doesn't. We both jump out of the ambulance to look around. The back wheels of these new rigs are located so far from the end of the box that there are almost five extra feet of truck and bumper behind the rear axle. What this means is that when I gassed it up on the hill in the first place, I managed to wedge the ambulance in at such a steep angle that the back bumper is now jammed into the concrete of the parking lot. The back wheels are spinning in the air about an inch off the ground. In other words: we're fucked.

Jack panics. He is on probation, which means that he is in a very vulnerable position should we have to explain to management why exactly we were trying to drive up the wrong side of an unmarked dirt hill on private property at three in the goddamn morning. I reassure him that I will take the blame for this; I'll tell them I was driving, I made the decision, he didn't want to but I forced him into it, he was so busy memorizing the fire department mission statement and saluting that he didn't even realize what was happening until it was too late. Jack can barely hear me because his life is flashing before his eyes. We both start frantically digging in the dirt with our hands, trying to get something under the back tires that they can push off of. If we can get unstuck before we get a call, no one will ever know. I pray silently to the EMS gods—*Please, cut us a break, just this once, do it for Jack*, I ask them. It's a race between us and the good people of San Francisco.

I pull my phone out. Kyle keeps late hours. More importantly, he has driven dirt trucks for almost a decade and knows more than anyone I have ever met about getting vehicles unstuck. He picks up after a couple of rings. I explain exactly what we've done, and when he is finished laughing he asks me for photos. I switch to FaceTime and show him the whole scene—the stuck ambulance, the hill, the parking lot, Jack pacing in circles. I learn that no, actually, he is not done laughing.

But he is not without ideas. At his instruction, we start gathering rocks. Is there anything flat in the ambulance we can use? Wait, of course there is. So now Jack and I are shoving two long plastic back-boards under the back tires, one on each side, wedging them between the tires and the rocks. I hop in the driver's side and Jack climbs up onto the front bumper. With Kyle on speakerphone Jack jumps on the front of the ambulance as I gas, trying to bounce the thing off of the hill. We succeed in carving a deep tire-shaped groove into one of the backboards, which will remain in that particular board for the rest of my career at the SFFD. The rig is still stuck. Unfortunately, our luck has run out. We hear the radio page our unit and look at each other.

"Maybe they just want us to move," I tell Jack, just as he is hoping the same out loud. "Maybe it's a code two. We still have time." But no. We do not. It's a code three cardiac arrest, about a mile from our current location. In addition to all the guilt I now feel about potentially getting Jack in trouble, I also feel guilty about missing the call. This seventy-four-year-old man will receive an ambulance from farther away because my dumb ass doesn't know how to drive. I'm forcing another rig to run what should have been my call. I might get Jack in trouble. I'm an idiot. I close my eyes, swallow my own panic, and get on the radio.

I tell them that we are "out mechanical," which is shorthand for a broken rig—actually a pretty common occurrence with a fleet that is driven twenty-four hours a day, in rough city traffic, for ten or twenty years. Ambulances aren't traded in or sold when they start to have problems—they are driven until they are either totalled in a wreck or are so broken that the city mechanics finally put them down like elderly animals. Dispatch quickly assigns another unit to the call, but now I have to phone someone and explain myself.

The night shift supervisor is some fire suppression guy, in for the day, who does not know or give a shit about the details of ambulance operation. I gamble that maybe, just maybe, this guy cares so little about EMS and wants so badly to go back to sleep that I can get him to roll his eyes and hang up the phone without bothering to write us up.

"Look, this is really dumb, Cap," I explain. "The rig is fine, we just need a tow truck. We are fine, the rig is fine, I'm just an idiot and we need a tow truck."

I hear a long silence at the end of the line. I wince.

"You and your partner are both safe?"

"Yes."

Another silence.

"Do I want to know what happened?"

"No, sir. You really do not."

"Fuck it. Call BOE, they'll get you a tow. I'm going back to bed."

"Thank you, Captain. Yes, Captain. We will do that right now. Thank you. Please have a nice night." I look at my phone. He's already hung up. One down, one to go.

I call the Bureau of Equipment, a station full of mechanically inclined firefighters who work twenty-four-hour shifts changing flats, jump-starting batteries, and generally keeping our rigs as alive as they can until the city's central shops open in the morning. The BOE guys are cranky about being woken up. I go into a little bit more detail with them but not much. I promise them the rig is in perfect condition; I was just an idiot and parked stupidly and now we need a tow. I don't say anything about the hill, figuring maybe they'll think I accidentally put a tire in the gutter or dropped into a pothole or something.

We are not actually allowed to nap in the ambulances, despite the fact that we work all night and don't have sleeping quarters. These guys are not technically my supervisor, but anything they write up will end up on someone's desk at some point, and I don't want any part of that paper trail in Jack's employee file or mine. They consult with each other—I can hear pieces of their conversation. They can call a tow service to pick us up, but they are required to come take a look at any ambulance that gets towed just to give it a once-over. Their station is pretty much all the way across town, though, and, well, it's still three in the morning. Actually, by now it's closer to four. They debate with each other. The one on the phone with me sighs as he says that unfortunately they have to come out and check. He sounds just as upset about it as me. I tell him no worries, we're not exactly going anywhere. He says he'll see me soon.

I hang up and turn my attention to Jack, who is holding his head in his hands. I tell him that I was driving and promise him again and again that I will take the heat. He smiles politely and tries to crack a joke but I can tell he's still sweating.

We kick some more dirt around under the tires, but we both know it's not helping and realistically the jig is up. Finally, we both lean against the dented bumper to wait it out. My phone rings again. It's the Bureau of Equipment phone number.

I answer. A gruff voice says, "Okay. Do you *promise* that there's no damage to the vehicle?"

I tell him absolutely not. The vehicle is perfect. Scout's honor. I hear a long sigh. "Look, we had a long night. We're just gonna say we came out and it was fine, sound good?" I tell him that sounds great. He tells me the tow truck's on the way.

A few minutes later we hear an engine rumble and spot headlights on the other side of the parking lot. We expect to have to direct them where to go, as we are tucked all the way in a corner in the back, but the truck drives straight to us. The driver looks like he's in his twenties. I'm ready to explain the situation but he hops out, shakes his head, and starts chaining up the tires. He asks me why we all keep parking here if we just keep getting our rigs stuck. I cough and Jack's eyes widen.

The driver laughs. "This is like the third one this month. It never used to be a problem."

I blink. I ask him if the calls started right about when we got a shipment of the new ambulances. He nods. I look at Jack. We both blink slowly.

Jack and I spend the next week or so walking on eggshells, scared we're going to be called into someone's office for a meeting. Every time a supervisor says my name I jump, expecting a write-up, ready to fall on my sword to defend my partner. But we never hear a word. Jack makes me promise that I won't tell a soul until after he has finished his probation. I keep my vow until the day he is cleared.

AMBULANCE LADY

*It was heavy, grueling work at that time but I would not have
had it otherwise, for this intimate daily and nightly contact with
the old Bellevue brought me closer to the very heartbeat of my
native city.*

EMILY DUNNING BARRINGER, M.D. *Bowery to Bellevue: The
Story of New York's First Woman Ambulance Surgeon*

One hundred and eleven years before my first day as a full-fledged
paramedic, a woman named Emily Dunning Barringer stepped, no,
jumped, onto the back of a horse-drawn carriage in New York City.
There was a bit of skill required to get your legs all the way over the
wooden step on the first try. She wore a thick wool coat with plenty
of pockets, specially designed by a local tailor who had written a
letter requesting the honor of creating a uniform for the nation's first
female ambulance surgeon.

*My first ambulance call was set for the evening of June 30th, and
they made it a transfer of a patient from Beth Israel hospital up to
Bellevue hospital. I telephoned my family that I had received my
first orders, and was ready in my uniform with the ambulance bag
in my hand when Dick Bateman who was the driver on duty
backed the ambulance in. He quickly jumped down and ran
around to me saying: "Doc, I want to show you a trick or two, how*

to get on the bus, if you want me to." Did I want him to! Good,
kind Dick Bateman; in a five-minute demonstration he showed
me just what and what not to do, and I have been eternally grate-
ful to him. He showed me how to sit up on the seat and with one
quick bounce swing both feet up from the step of the ambulance
over the tailboard and so into the "bus." He made me rehearse this
three or four times and I soon found it was not unlike mounting a
horse. When once you were on the seat, a sense of balance helped
you keep it and there were two solid leather hand straps that I
gratefully relied on at first. I have always felt that this careful,
thoughtful instruction gave me a good start and as soon as I had
the proper technique, I never knew what physical fear was in our
roughest and hardest driving.

By the time Barringer had picked up her patient and transported
to Bellevue, the word had gone out that the ambulance carried a
woman doctor. Barringer tells us that when she arrived at the hospital the walls of the entrance were lined with onlookers, including
crowds of young boys shouting, "Get a man, get a man!"

Over the next eighteen months, Barringer braved the streets of
New York City to treat fevers, broken limbs, gallstones, and stabbings. She had five minutes to get from the hospital dorm to the
ambulance for an ordinary call, three for a "hurry call." She describes
people attempting suicide by drinking carbolic acid, and men hallucinating from alcohol withdrawal. She writes of her ambulance
time with love and humor—around the station today we would call
her *a real medic's medic*.

Barringer's out-of-print autobiography is an amazing read if you
can find a copy. At the time of her training, women are allowed to

practice medicine after attending an all-women's medical college, but are limited to treating women and children. After a political fight, she applies to a medical university that until this point has only admitted men. She places first in their entrance exams only to be denied placement due to her gender. The next year, with the backing of a progressive new mayor, she retests and places highly again. The staff of five local hospitals petition against her appointment, saying that the idea of having to take orders from a woman would be "decidedly distasteful." But with the mayor's insistence, Bellevue Hospital is forced to allow her in.

On her first night she is told to go change out all of the urinary catheters on the male ward. "I felt as though a stick of dynamite with a burning, sputtering fuse had suddenly been placed in my hands," she writes, realizing the men have specifically contrived a test that they believe she will fail. They think that she will surely refuse, or the patients themselves will revolt at the thought of a woman completing such an intimate task. Understanding the cruelty and importance of the moment, Barringer nods curtly to her orderly, rattles off the equipment needed, and heads out into the ward.

She eventually works her way through every hazing ritual thrown at her and earns the respect of the hospital staff, but no part of her training is more hotly anticipated than her time on the dirty, dangerous ambulance. At Bellevue, ambulances are staffed by a driver and a surgical intern. Newspapers follow Barringer out on her routes, calling in fake hurry calls just to get a photo of the woman surgeon. The ambulance drivers take a liking to her and defend her from drunks and rowdy lookie-loos. Barringer describes her fears, excitement, and eventual confidence on "the bus" as she is forced to work more hours in worse conditions than any of her male counterparts.

Some of Barringer's calls sound exotic and old-fashioned to me. Babies and children falling off fire escapes in a world before air conditioning were "among the most usual of hot weather emergencies." A frozen stowaway found tangled high in the rigging of a sailing ship down on the waterfront, recognized by locals only as a nameless "little wharf rat." A colleague is sickened by typhoid contracted in the hospital.

But I'm far more surprised by how familiar most of her days feel. She describes poverty, cold, and addiction. Overcrowded tenements, babies left unfed by alcohol-soaked mothers. Suicides, infections. The sinking feeling knowing that a pre-dawn pneumonia call is usually serious. The way that the city rumbles itself awake at sunrise after the long dark quiet of night. Even a gambler poisoned by a gangster's "knock-out drops" turns out to be an opiate overdose, kept alive by rescue breathing all night until the opium's grasp wears off and the man begins to breathe on his own.

I laugh out loud when Barringer describes "Beckie," the "prima donna of malingerers . . . [with her] amazing ability to simulate almost any known disease and get away with it." Other than describing her patient as a "squat little Jewish woman," I believe you could take Barringer's telling of her story and transpose it into any modern firehouse locker room without changing a thing. She says Beckie could fake a more complicated disease when she wanted longer board and lodging, could suss out younger doctors and ply them for more treatments. Barringer describes a street corner scene, with Beckie appearing as though dying, drawing a crowd, and pulling a hurry call from police. A rumor even circulates that Beckie once faked appendicitis so skillfully that a top physician operated to remove a perfectly healthy appendix.

That last trick might be harder to get away with these days thanks to bloodwork and lab tests. But the way that Barringer writes about Beckie—with frustration, compassion, and even endearment—reminds me of my most frequent regulars.

Of course, Barringer is eventually allowed to deal with Beckie in a way that is prevented these days by lawsuits and camera phones: by giving her some "straight talk." That is, by threatening to arrest her if she ever "throw[s] a fit on a street corner again."

There is romance for me in Barringer's hand-sewn cloak. She describes the ambulance house as smelling of oats, and hay, and horses, which sounds so glamorous compared to the diesel and Lysol I walk into at the start of shift. She writes of the red brick and wood of the carriage house, the personalities of each of the horses, and the pot-bellied stove that politicians and reporters like to stop by to sit around for a chat on a cold morning.

Ambulance work is not a career for Dr. Barringer. She eventually completes medical school, marries a handsome colleague, and becomes a prominent gynecologist and leader in women's medical training. Dr. Emily Dunning Barringer does not write her memoirs until 1950, when she has a long and impressive career to look back on. And yet about a third of the book focuses on her brief eighteen-month stint on the ambulance way back in medical school. The title of the book, *Bowery to Bellevue: The Story of New York's First Woman Ambulance Surgeon*, promises the reader a window into what I suppose she must have believed was the most exciting part of her career.

I have sworn to myself many times over that I will not become one of those old war vets who defines their entire life by the one tour they served in the seventies. I don't own any EMS coffee mugs; I don't go to the gym in my station shirt. I tell myself again and again that although my time on the ambulance will one day end, I can have an important second career, as a physician assistant or teacher or writer, and won't spend the rest of my life defined as someone who "used to be a paramedic." But I must admit that I don't really believe I will ever do anything else quite as exciting as 911.

> *Our usual route was west across Grand Street to the Bowery, then up the Bowery and Third Avenue to Twenty-sixth Street, and east on Twenty-sixth Street—that street of ambulances, for ambulances from hospitals all over the city would bring patients to be admitted to Bellevue. If that old street could speak, what tales it could tell of the freight those ambulances carried of human suffering and heartache; of terror and pain; of warmth, protection and help; of the wealthy banker, officially on his private yacht cruising in Southern Seas, but in reality on his way to the Observation Ward for the testing of his sanity; of the criminal, heading for the prison ward to heal his wounds so that he could face his trial; of the alcoholic too befuddled and incoherent to know his own name; of the tragic amnesia case unable to account for himself, who must be added to the ever-swelling list of lost persons in our great city. Ceaselessly, on they came, those ambulances, and poured down Twenty-sixth Street, across First Avenue to Bellevue Hospital.*

"SUPERHUMAN"

JAMIE PREDMORE, PARAMEDIC/FIREFIGHTER;

EIGHTEEN YEARS IN EMS

NINILCHIK, ALASKA

If I could tell the world something about being a paramedic? I think there is a perception on the outside that you should be some sort of superhuman. That you should remain professional and respectful while being called a fucking bitch, or being told that you are doing a shit job. And I'll tell you, I can let things roll of my back like water off a duck when it's just one time. It's not that difficult. But when it happens every single day, call after call, at what point do you turn back into a human being?

It's not personal—I know that whoever is treating me this way would treat any person this way, but it's being directed at me. When it happens so often, it's hard to put up with.

I can think of a recent one. It was back when I worked in a city, a call to a grocery store for an interaction between a customer and a security guard. We go into the back of the ambulance, and I do my assessment, and the patient starts becoming more animated. He is upset that we aren't tearing away to the hospital, lights and sirens. I'm not finding anything abnormal about the assessment, and I'm trying to explain that it is in his best interests to wait a moment for the police officers to complete their report. They actually thought that the security guard was in the wrong, not the patient, and they were trying to review the footage to help him out. But nothing I could say was satisfactory to this person.

He started making these really ugly comments, calling me names, digging into me harder and harder. I looked up, and sure enough, he was filming me. He wanted me to say something incriminating. I went to give the radio report to the hospital, and I felt myself starting to cry. I was so frustrated.

It's like a housewife that gets abused. Again and again, every day, every day. She doesn't, like, build up her emotional muscles. It just beats her down until she eventually breaks.

When we got into the hospital with this guy, I asked him, "Sir, could I take this monitoring equipment off of your body?"

He said, "Fuck you, don't touch me." So I told my partner to do it. And as soon as we got to the hospital I just jumped out of the ambulance, because I knew I was going to fucking lose it. I was going to either punch something or burst into tears, and I didn't want him to see me cry. I ran ahead and gave registration his name and birthday, and then went around the corner. There were other ambulance crews at the hospital, and everyone was super understanding. They've all been there. They took care of the patient for me and let me have a minute. Depending on where you work, this type of thing happens every day.

Everybody starts their EMS journey under the feeling that they want to help. And if you do this job long enough, in a context busy enough, you will lose a lot of your compassion. Our old chief used to give a speech about "curbside prejudice." He thought it was the single greatest danger to the urban paramedic. Not gunshots, not physical danger. The loss of your humanity.

If you do this job long enough, you will start to feel like you are a monster.

No. You're not. You're not a monster.

You're a human being that is exposed to very atypical human situations. Everything that you're feeling is normal. I want this book to give a sense of comfort and camaraderie to paramedics. A reminder that everyone feels this way. If we're lucky, maybe this book can provide that for a lot of people. That would be amazing.

For the non-paramedics reading this, I would just want them to be able to relate with us and understand the sentiments that we are talking about. I want them to see us as people.

PRIME RIB

0435: First alarm goes off. No.

0436-0453: More alarms, more snoozing. I listen to the pattering of the rain against the window and think of the way rainwater pulls urine all the way up the pants of homeless people and penetrates the smell through the back of a wet ambulance.

0455: I crawl up to a sitting position and say out loud, "Fuck."

0515: Make coffee, fry an egg, wrap it in a tortilla and throw it in my backpack. Put some ice packs in my lunch. Grab the bag of leftovers to take to the station tonight.

0545: Pull into the parking lot. I'm later than I like but whatever. Ambulances are driving in and out, cars try to park, voices sound muffled against so many idling engines. Headlights shine prisms through the rain. I change in the locker room, run upstairs and throw the leftovers in the fridge, grab my lunch and zip it into my backpack with the ice packs.

0600: Change into my uniform in the locker room and sneak into Sara Petersen's locker to borrow her jacket for the day. She's not back here until Thursday.

0603: Maggie is already outside at the ambulance. We say good morning/good night to our night half. Together the four of us hand equipment back and forth, restock supplies, wipe down surfaces. Everybody is getting rained on every time they step in and out of the ambulance or walk back into the garage for more supplies. We tell them to go home and get some sleep; they say to have a good shift.

0630: We sign on and get posted downtown, which means not that far of a drive. I pull out my fried egg wrap.

0638: Code two to Blue Star Motel for someone who called 911 and said they were "sick." I hate the Blue Star. It's full of rats and bugs and nightmares and I can't even walk inside without feeling itchy for an hour after. I'm still complaining about it and putting my gloves on in the front seat when Maggie points out that our patient is outside walking towards the ambulance.

It's a regular named Stardust. Today she has sparkly painted nails, a men's jacket, torn leggings, and a large straw sunhat. She wants to go anywhere but St. Matthias. Sure. Me too, lady.

0745: We clear from the hospital and head code three to a man "slumped over at a bus stop." Dude's trying to sleep. We offer him a blanket again and leave him be.

0755: We clear from that and drive back downtown, then sneak up to the closest emergency room to use the bathroom. While I'm peeing I hear a code two go out for us.

0814: He's trying to break into stores, throwing trash, talking in circles and singing. We work with police to coax him onto the gurney but as we're doing the seatbelts he spits at Maggie and a cop yanks him onto the ground. Now we're fighting a twenty-five-year-old who looks like a child, tying him to a backboard. People are staring. *Merry fucking Christmas*, says the cop.

Once he's in the back of the ambulance I look at him again. He starts to slam his head onto the hard plastic backboard, gnash his teeth, click them together, and bite at his shoulders. I hate the sound of the enamel grinding down. Maybe this poor kid's front teeth will be my big field save for the day. I get out the sedatives and give him a shot.

0912: We steal cookies from St. Matthias and post downtown again.

0914-1155: More calls. An old guy with pneumonia, an overdose, another homeless man trying to sleep. People always call even more of those in on holidays. Maybe they feel extra guilty or something.

1157: We post near the park and try to track down some food. We find a coffee shop that's open and I get in line, but we get a call before I make it to the register. As we leave, I glance back inside the shop: three or four people drinking coffee, looking peaceful, staring at their phones. Twinkly lights, tinsel, paper snowflakes in the windows. It's nice.

1158: Back south again for a code three: a man on the sidewalk. His hospital gown and scrubs are soaked through with urine (there's that smell I was dreading). An empty bottle of Taaka vodka lies next to him. Stable vitals, no signs of trauma. We code two him to the hospital and the triage nurse looks at his feet and says, "I picked out those shoes! That was the first thing I did this morning!"

"They're pretty sweet kicks," I say. "You did good."

The nurse says, "We only let him out a couple hours ago. How do you even get that drunk that fast?"

1241: I tell dispatch to delay us for a few so we can wipe up the pee. I refill my water bottle at the hospital water cooler while the gurney is drying. There's a group of ER techs wearing ugly Christmas sweaters and ribbons on top of their scrubs, all posing for a quick group photo in the ambulance bay before they run back inside. Cute.

1256: I find a police station to pee in. A couple of tired-looking cops are holding down the fort; when they first see me their eyes widen, looking for a patient, but when I ask for a bathroom everyone relaxes. I chat with the sergeant. They have a tiny dog sleeping under the desk who shuffles over to me for a head pat and I tell her she's doing a great job running the station. When I leave everyone says Merry Christmas again.

1301: More calls. We hear the radio page out a big bus crash on the freeway; they send tons of resources over there. Sounds like a shitshow. Not us, though; we get sent to a shooting instead. A police officer is doing chest compressions when we get there, panting and smashing down onto our patient's ribcage. We can see the blood dumping out of the guy with every push. The cops have placed tourniquets on both arms and cinched them down so tight that his biceps look like water balloons. I know what I'm looking at, but we attach the cardiac monitor to confirm. I touch the cop's arm and shake my head. He swears. I tell him he did everything he could.

While I'm cleaning blood off our equipment, I briefly wonder if I should be feeling more emotional about what I've just witnessed. But before I can wax too poetic, I hear the ding of a message coming through our dashboard computer terminal. Dispatch wants to know if we are going to transport or not. They are wondering if we can take a code two call down the street. I read the address.

I lean out of the ambulance and shout to Maggie.

"Hey, dispatch wants us to go deal with Big John. Code two. Should I tell them we need a minute?"

Maggie squints at me.

1322: Big John's house. Booze, dizziness, liver pains, the usual. Today he's stuck on the floor behind the bathtub.

1435: It's too busy to let us back to station for food, so a supervisor drives around the city bringing around plates he boxed up. The portions are small but good. I never ate a prime rib until I worked as a medic on Christmas, and now I seem to do it every year. I wonder if good red meat will always remind me of tinsel and cold weather and hospital parking lots and diesel engines. I stuff my slice between torn halves of my Hawaiian roll and eat it like a lopsided sandwich. The food is warm even in the front cab of an ambulance and it cuts through the weather a bit.

1455: Flowers Gate care home, code two. It's a Brazilian Jewish family, which is cool to me. Not a lot of Brazilian Jews in this city. I can't figure out a polite way to ask their family history. The staff says that Regina had two, wait, maybe three episodes of dark and tarry stool today and her blood pressure has been dropping. I flip through her paperwork. She's on blood thinners. Goddamn it. The dark and tarry stool means she's probably bleeding, and the thinners mean she could be bleeding a lot. They tell me she's usually perky if confused, but today she's weak, lethargic, and doesn't seem like herself. She grimaces when I feel her abdomen. Her family is really sweet, calm but concerned. The home said an inter-facility company would send an ambulance within an hour, but they wanted us to come faster. I tell them they were right to call us; the other company probably would have waited an hour and then turfed it to us anyway.

"The blood thinner was for a pulmonary embolism," the son says, like he's reciting a book report.

GI bleeds are tricky. Sometimes you're overblowing it and they're totally fine; sometimes they lean over, puke a gallon of blood, and then die. We get her downstairs to the ambulance and check her blood pressure again. 88/40. "Yeah, this is code three. Lemme grab a line." On the way over her pressure drops down, seventies, then sixties. Okay, well, shit. I was right to be worried, unfortunately. I have a twenty-gauge catheter in a fragile hand vein and I spend most of the transport trying to get a larger bore IV. I fail. As I blow my last attempt at a second line I grab my last pressure, 63/37, and I watch her heart rate speed up to the 130s. *Don't brady down, don't brady down, don't fucking brady down,* I think. For Regina, a fast heart rate is bad; but a slow one is much worse.

We're on the freeway. I'm by myself in the back, and we're going to a hospital I barely ever go to. I don't want to roll into the emergency room doing goddamn chest compressions on the gurney. I stare at her.

"Regina," I say.

"Yes?"

"Stay with me, please."

I never say cheesy shit like that to my patients. I tell myself I'm not being silly, I'm just trying to tell her to stay awake, that I'm checking her mentation, that I'm trying to keep her engaged. I stare at her. *Don't code, lady.* I pretend to be Matilda and shoot eyeball lasers at her that control life and death. *Fucking don't code, Regina.* She doesn't code.

As we pull in, I lean up front and tell Maggie quietly, "Hey, when you get out we're going to move fast." I think it's the first time in a while she's seen me this jacked up about a patient. While we're unloading the gurney and pushing it up the driveway I tell the son, "Sir, I'm concerned about your mom's blood pressure. When we get inside, we're going to move very quickly. Once she is settled in someone will explain everything to you, okay? Just let us do our thing. Someone will talk to you as soon as we have time." He nods and says okay. He looks scared but he's trying to keep it together.

At the hospital they put on a pressure bag and start dumping saline in her, and I'm not a doctor but the whole thing seems like it's going to end badly. I think, *Well, when I dropped her off she was alive.* As I get my signature from the son and wish him well, he puts his hand on my shoulder and looks at me and says, "Thank you." Then looks a little embarrassed. It's a quick gesture but it actually means a lot.

I didn't do much, I think to myself, *and the hospital might kill your mom now, but hopefully you know that someone cared today. Someone tried real hard. I hope that means something to you.* I think he's trying to tell me that it does.

1543: We clear the call and wait for another. Usually this time of day would be busy, but big holidays can be surprisingly quiet. We get sent all the way across town to cover a different zone; we drive through the city slowly, looking for decorations on buildings as we pass by.

1601-1714: A woman faints into her spaghetti at family dinner. We get her cleaned up and take her to get checked out.

1735: Dispatch wants to get us home in time to enjoy Christmas dinner. They say hopefully the citizens of San Francisco allow it. We start driving back towards station.

1750: We get a run, but a nearby night crew offers to take it for us so we can make it home. We text them a thank you note and say that tomorrow's coffee is on us.

1800: We get off on time. It's a Christmas miracle. We clean out the rig, refuel, and then go upstairs to find the supervisors' kitchen smelling like maple and herbs and chocolate. There are mountains of cookies. Someone brought in a vat of tamales and each is wrapped with a little ribbon. Maggie makes me try a mince pie, which is a tiny fruit pastry, apparently a tradition back home.

1815: The conversation ebbs and flows, mostly shop talk.

"Oh, the choking? First time I've used Magill forceps in eight years on an ambulance. Eight years! Yeah, they all thought they were getting their inheritance for Christmas, cut the meat into big pieces for Granny, right?"

"So I'm standing there, just totally fried from getting held over four fucking hours late, holding my Costco card against the lock instead of my badge and wondering why it's not opening—"

"They're up right now, just have to beat the Lakers tomorrow and they're in."

"Yeah, at that time of night you are not getting my A game, right? You are getting, like, my C game."

"What the fuck, man, yeah, it was like a 'near drowning.' They got there, the mom said he'd been in the tub, and he was pale, unresponsive, just shitty, shitty. They said when they transported he was pinking up and coughing."

"I mean if he keeps nailing three-pointers the way he did last week—"

"Yeah, the dude was sitting in his car, and the girl was just walking her dog and gets shot in the leg, what the fuck?"

Some of the folks eating are night crews who came in early and haven't started yet, some of us are day crews winding up. There are decades of experience in this room right now, decades of days and nights filled with the most desperate moments of people's lives and deaths, Russian doll nesting inside the memories of every medic and EMT in this room. Stories and jokes and echoes of tragedies bounce around the room.

Bits of radio traffic pop through the conversation. Anyone who is still on the clock is listening with half an ear and when a call goes out we all twitch a little, hoping it's not ours. Hoping to enjoy the warm food and family for just another minute before heading back out into the shit of it.

On my way out I weave through the parking lot, saying *Merry Christmas* to the night crews who are only just starting. *My shift wasn't too bad, hopefully things stay mellow out there. I'll see y'all in the morning.*

"DISPOSABLE RAZORS"

MICHAEL HAMILTON, PARAMEDIC/RN;

TWENTY-FOUR YEARS IN EMS

RENO, NEVADA

As paramedics, we are disposable razors.

We are cheap to manufacture and produce.

We do one job, and we do it well, but we can only do it for so long.

When our edges are blunted and we are no longer able to do that one job, we are thrown away.

SIDE EFFECTS

This is the key difference between writing about a far-flung community and your own. The decision to wield a pen rather than, say, a hammer gets increasingly hard to justify. At various points over the years, I have vowed to stop trying to describe things and start trying to change them, but each time, I've concluded that words are the only tools I know how to use.
STEPHANIE ELIZONDO GRIEST, *All the Agents and Saints: Dispatches from the U.S. Borderlands*

In many cases the damage was done long before I'd been called, and there was little I could do to reverse it. I was a grief mop, and much of my job was to remove, if even for a short time, the grief starter or the grief product, and mop up whatever I could.
. . . [M]y problem was that I had collected all this grief and had no place to put it. I was filled up, and every call I went to just poured over the top.
JOE CONNELLY, *Bringing Out the Dead*

I used to race downhill mountain bikes. One day, before a race, one of the guys looked at me very seriously and said, "Okay, Jo, here's the best advice I can give you. If you ever think you pissed your pants, and you look down and there's no piss, you have to go to the hospital. That's internal bleeding and you *have to go*." He nodded slowly and finished his beer. *Um, thank you, Davie. Good to know.*

The disc injury doesn't feel like I peed my pants, exactly, but there is something *wet* about it. Something cartilaginous, an almost electrical buzz. My knees are bent, hands waist-high gripping the rail of the gurney. My partner and I count to three like we have ten times today, a hundred times this week, a thousand times this year, and on three I look up and push my legs and feel the weight of the patient transfer to my own body as I heave him into the back of the ambulance. Only this time, as I shove the bed up, there's a slipping feeling. A dark wet zap bursts out of my low back and down my legs. *Shit.* My partner tells me later that he heard me make a sound, not a cry or a yelp but more like a little groan of disappointment. Once we get the guy loaded up I give my partner a look and say, "Hey, buddy, I think we have to do an injury form when we get back. I'm really sorry to make you do paperwork."

"Did that lift pull your back out?" he asks.

"Yeah."

"Shit."

"Yeah. Shit."

Most paramedics injure their backs sooner or later. It's like crane operators and neck pain, or restaurant chefs and forearm burns. We knew this when we signed up, of course. Everyone told us, over and over again. But I was *twenty* when I got into this. I thought my back would hurt the same way I'd eventually wear diapers in a nursing home—a blurry line in the fine print miles away. I scrolled past the warnings, clicked "accept these terms and conditions," and went on my way.

Ten years later I'm lying on the couch, watching other guys surf the first big swell of winter and squeezing a hot water bottle against my back. This isn't the first time I've hurt my back and it won't be the last. But this is the second year in a row that I've missed the opening month of surf season due to back injuries, and I'm way less Zen about it this time. The weeks crawl by. My life becomes an injury character arc from a movie, only I don't get to skip the hours between camera cuts. I have to drag myself around the whole damn time. I lie on the couch, walk to the fridge, lie back down on the couch. I watch a TV show about a figure skater who hurts herself on the ice and then gets a bunch of badass music to train to and then cries and practices and heals and wins the contest in the end. The whole time she is montaging around onscreen overcoming things, I have to just lie there.

Once I can walk, I start back in the gym, running through the same exercises I've done for a decade now. Warm up on the stationary bike, then planks, crunches, side planks, thrusts. Lat pull-downs, back flexion raises, one leg sits. It's boring. It's so fucking boring. I wonder how many minutes of my life I have spent holding a plank on the floor with tears in my eyes.

I still remember my first adrenaline rush. I was eight or nine years old, downhill skiing with my mom, traversing a particularly steep patch of sheet ice between two rocky chutes. I lost an edge. As the mountain rushed towards me, I felt a fierce and sudden wakefulness. I flew headfirst down the hill, my legs splayed out behind me with skis jackknifed against the slope, and I spread the fingers of my gloves out as wide as I could. I watched my hands in awe as I pressed my snowy arms down to the ice, trying to collect resistance and slow my slide. I remember the sight and the feel of the snow flying up over my gloves and into my face. I remember trying to steer myself to the right, into a stand of trees, as my fall accelerated. And I remember smashing against them, curling into a ball as best as I could and crumpling to a stop. As my mom and I collected ourselves in the trees, gasping for air, I was scared and overwhelmed, but mostly uninjured. I cried. I felt amazing.

They say the worst thing that can happen on your first trip to Vegas is winning big. After the fall, my mom helped me back into my gear and gave me a parental speech about picking oneself up, dusting oneself off, and getting down the rest of the hill. When I reached the bottom of the mountain that day, and felt the last shivers of fear bouncing themselves out of my knees, I tucked my chin into my jacket and smiled. I wasn't sure why or how, but I knew in that moment that I was probably immortal.

I was moody as a child, and restless. My teenage journals are filled with imagery about boiling black rivers, twisted veins, strangling, clawing beasts. These days it's all very embarrassing, but back then I felt constantly claustrophobic and full of rage. One way or another, I became addicted to emergencies.

The taste of adrenaline feels to me similar to the way I've heard alcoholics describe their first drink. "For the first time in my life, I felt like I *belonged*." I felt like a real person, like I knew who I was and what my body was supposed to do. I felt this way when I first started snowboarding, when I discovered downhill mountain biking, and again with surfing. When the adrenaline kicks in I feel suddenly clean, focused, and awake. The darkness evaporates. The ambulance is the ultimate expression of this discovery—not only do I feed my adrenaline lust, but I do it in the service of others. It's all the fun of extreme sports with the self-righteousness of a noble cause. When I zip up my work boots and get on the ambulance I know where I am. Or I used to, anyway.

———

My first real panic attack was in the bathroom of my friend Jessie's house on a weekend trip to Seattle. We'd had a couple of shots earlier in the afternoon on a touristy distillery tour and then ate some fancy chocolate back at the house. I checked my phone idly and found an email from human resources informing me that my paramedic license was up for recertification three months earlier than I'd thought. I called the office and had a panicked conversation with an administrator who confirmed that I had to complete six months' worth of continuing education credits by the end of the week. In the moment, I didn't actually feel any emotional stress at all. I felt calm, knowing that I would do what I had to, stay up all night, and get the project done one way or another. But I went to use the bathroom and sat down uncomfortably, feeling as though the whiskey had not mixed well with the chocolate. Things started to spin and I felt suddenly sick to my stomach. I wasn't thinking at all about the paramedic license or my own emotions. They were the farthest things from my mind. All I knew was that my stomach did not feel right, and I was terrified of the nausea.

I felt overwhelmed by adrenaline, by fear, by sickness. My hands and legs started to shake—a stiff, seizure-like muscle spasm that I could stop if I flexed tightly but would start again as soon as I let go. I kept trying to breathe slowly but soon the bathroom kept spinning and the shaking got more violent. For some reason the muscle spasm seemed to clear the nausea. I felt like the sickness was escaping my body through the fear, like it was releasing some trapped awful feeling from me. The harder my hands and legs shook, the more the release valve opened.

As the bathroom walls closed in, I let the sound of my own breathing reverberate around me. My deepest fear in that moment had nothing to do with work, or life, or love, but was instead that I might somehow lose my lunch. I pulled a trash can forward, just in case, but I kept breathing and shaking and trying to send the discomfort out into the air somehow. I walked back to the TV room to distract myself and then back to the bathroom. Eventually I went into Jessie's bedroom, holding his bathroom wastebasket at my chest, still shaking and panting, and said, "Hey, Jessie? I think I'm having a panic attack."

A few years later these episodes become familiar. But never again does one associate so cleanly with a particular event. Instead they appear randomly, on a Tuesday night or following a big breakfast. I try for years to chart the triggers, plot out my weaknesses like data points on a graph. If I haven't exercised or slept enough the episodes are more severe. Night shift is bad. Alcohol is bad. Hot shower is good. *Breathe, Sokol.*

I desperately want to blame my anxiety on work, because "paramedic with trauma" is way more culturally respected than "white girl with too many feelings." My background is otherwise unimpressive. I was raised by loving parents in an interesting city. I haven't overcome anything dramatic enough to justify any real mental health problems. But there's got to be something about this work, right? Wedged in the ambulance cab, night after night, the radio zapping us with adrenaline like a Taser: *bzzt, bzzt, bzzt,* every time the tones go off. Shivering with the relief of a call getting cancelled, or clenching your jaw when a patient three times your size balls his fists at you. Or that moment at the end of an exhausting shift thinking you might finally go home and then feeling your whole body tighten when the radio says no, we don't have coverage, you're taking another call, one more backache tonight, one more tragedy.

Maybe it's from stifling all the anger over the years at waiting in line at hospitals, again and again. Having to tell your elderly patient that you understand how much it hurts but they are going to have to wait a little while longer. Having to say no, again and again and again, we can't help you, I can't do anything for you. I'm sorry, I'm so sorry. There's nothing I can do. Staring at my protocols and knowing that in another place I might be able to help, I might have the right drug or the right tool, but here I can't because the booklet says I can't, because our medical director doesn't trust paramedics, because my city doesn't have the resources, because my country's health care is a mess. So I look my patient in the eye and say, "I'm sorry, let's wait until you get to the hospital. Hopefully they can help you there." And seeing that look of betrayal when the hospital tosses them in a waiting room.

Maybe this is just who I am. If I had worked in an office, or a school, or a sporting goods store, would I still have spent hours huddled in the bathroom, shaking, breathing, willing the floor to stay in one place? Maybe that's just my chemistry and it would have followed me down any path. Maybe I don't get to blame my bullshit on my cool-sounding job.

An old teacher of mine once told me that your shadows never disappear, that if you don't bring them up and confront them they will hide further and further inside of you until you risk a violent explosion when you least expect it. I've always pictured an eel in a dark ocean reef, slithering deeper into the coral to wait for its moment. Maybe these attacks were there all along, hiding beneath the surface, tucked against cold wet rocks below midnight waves.

After five years on an ambulance my body starts to break down. Anecdotally speaking, this seems about average. I played rough in my twenties, so I'm not sure exactly how much of my pain I can blame on work versus old sports injuries, but cramming them into night after night of lifting, loading, crunching, sitting, pushing, pulling, tweaking, and leaning doesn't seem to have helped. In the summer of 2018 I schedule two surgeries, both delayed repair jobs on old injuries, thinking maybe I can ruin one summer and minimize the amount of time away from work. The plan is to get my ankle done first, in June, and as soon as I'm off the crutches we'll fix my shoulder. Then I'll limp around for a few months, watch some movies, and be all tuned up and good as new by winter. It almost works.

My recovery starts out okay. I watch a lot of TV; I spend a lot of time with the dog. She sniffs my cast and then curls up next to my injured leg, ready to protect me while I heal. We lay out in the yard at the Anchorage House, watching the grass dry out and brown. I build a small castle out of pillows every night to support everything at just the right angle and jam a sweatshirt under my neck folded up just so. I am out of work for five months total, which probably isn't enough time, because after a few weeks back I get a massive diarrheal infection. I ask the doc if it could have been caused by working on the ambulance or taking five different courses of antibiotics all summer. He raises his eyebrows but ducks the question.

The diarrhea clears, but then I get strep throat. I keep getting sick, and every time I get sick I have to take more antibiotics and then start to get more anxious about getting sick. The whole thing spirals. I'm fatigued, and on edge, and I start to dread going to work. I question my relationship with Kyle. I cry in the shower. I trudge through my day, running calls, getting along with my partner the best I can, just a little more tired and a little less quick to laugh.

In spring the dog dies. She was beginning to age, and it's a graceful death, but it comes suddenly and it hits me like a freight train. I get sick to my stomach again and start feeling shaky and anxious every time I eat. What had been sporadic panic attacks become a constant, low-grade fear. I stare at my food, wondering whether it will make me sick, wondering who handled it at the factory and what illnesses they might have had. I buy chicken at Safeway and then bring it home and throw it away.

I keep surfing and I keep going to the gym to try to put muscle onto my still-recovering bones. But every time I eat a meal, I end up shaking in the bathroom. I start to lose weight.

I make smoothies and eat peanut butter from the jar to keep calories on. Then I get scared that maybe you're supposed to refrigerate peanut butter, that it will go bad, and I put it in the fridge, but the fat congeals and it's too stiff to spread. I google "do you refrigerate peanut butter" but get a bunch of websites about food poisoning and organic peanuts and palm oil. I give up on the peanut butter and put protein powder in plain soy milk instead. My chest starts to sink in; the flesh between my ribs shrinks. I eat bananas since they come in their own rind. I sweat in the bathroom, wondering whether they will come back up. I eat tortillas with butter but stop halfway through when they taste off. My cheeks sink into my jawbone.

At work we take a guy from the top floor of the homeless shelter down to the ambulance and all five of us are crammed into a tiny elevator. The guy is high out of his mind on meth and being aggressive and mean. He tells us he has to shit and we tell him no problem, there's a bathroom just downstairs in the lobby. Then he pulls down his pants, bends over, jumps up and down, and sprays diarrhea water across the back wall of the elevator like machine gun fire. It arcs, it splatters. We all shout and cover our faces. He screams back at us and keeps shitting, twitching and jumping from the meth so that no corner of the tiny elevator is safe. I yell, "Fuck *you*, man," knowing full well I'm being recorded by the elevator's security camera. When the doors open everyone is furious and it feels like a little layer of diarrhea vapor is covering every surface. We throw him on the gurney. I make eye contact with a tired-looking janitor and tell him, "I'm sorry, dude, I'm so, so sorry" and point towards the elevator. I feel like I should help clean up, but mostly I just want to get this guy the hell out of this building. I look down at my shirt and don't see any visible fecal matter. A few years ago I would have laughed about the story as I ate my lunch an hour later, but now I know that for the next week every time I try to eat there's going to be a swarm of fecal-oral microorganisms clouding my mind, constantly forcing me to wonder if I've caught some bug from the incident, if I'm going to get whatever he had, if it's going to come out of me the same way it came out of him. I wonder how long you can go without eating at all; maybe just a few days won't kill me.

A guy at work says, "Jo, you're melting away." I know he means well but I start wearing sweatshirts all the time to hide.

The whole time, I know what's happening. I know that this is anxiety, that this is a psych issue, how obvious it is what kind of help I need. I stare at my food, willing myself to overcome the fear. *This is anxiety*, I tell myself, looking at a turkey sandwich. *This sandwich is fine. You have eaten sandwiches before. You will not get sick. It's all in your head. This is a psych issue.* I pick up the sandwich and stare at it. It looks gross. I look at my shrinking waistline, and then over at my truck. *If you want to be strong enough to surf today, you have to eat the sandwich.* I take a few bites. It feels slimy and off. Maybe the turkey's gone bad. Maybe the cheese has soured. I try to smell it but something's not right. Can't risk it. *This sandwich is fine. You just opened the turkey. You are wrong. Eat the fucking sandwich, Sokol.* Fuck it. It will be easier to be a little dizzy today than spend the next hour shaking in the bathroom wondering if the turkey was bad. I toss it in the trash. I can try again at dinner.

Kyle is a saint. I push food around on my plate, thinking if I shorten and flatten the pile of potatoes it will seem as though some are gone. I am using a toddler's strategy on a man with an engineer's attention to detail, but his facial expression remains passive. He asks softly if I'd like him to cook something else instead. I tell him I'm trying as hard as I can.

People start to ask if I'm okay and I tell them I've been getting stomach aches. They seem sympathetic and ask if I've been to a doctor, maybe it's celiac, maybe it's an allergy. "Totally," I say. "Yeah, I'm getting it looked at, hopefully figure it out soon. Thank you."

I've done therapy a few times in the past but never really stuck with it; it always seemed expensive and slow. But I step on the scale one day at the gym and it says 114. I started the summer at 150. I sit down, towel around my shoulders, and start googling "therapist Santa Cruz" in the locker room.

Her office is down by the harbor, so when you're waiting to go in you can see the water. I feel like I should be surfing instead of paying $140 to talk to a stranger, but I also don't want to see the number on the scale get any smaller and I still haven't made it through a whole sandwich, so clearly whatever I'm doing isn't working. I listen to the seagulls and stare at my phone while I wait.

The therapist is nice enough and we talk through a lot. She specializes in first responders and trauma, whatever that means. We talk about work, surfing, food, and what excites me or makes me afraid. She asks what my source of comfort and peace is between all the adrenaline, and I tell her that's an easy one; it's about sixty pounds, four legs, covered in fur, butts her head into your knees when she wants attention. Wanted attention. Died a few months ago. "What have you been doing since then for comfort, when you need help?" I squint. "I don't know," I tell her. *Sweating a lot, I guess.*

She works with me on calming down. I start drinking kombucha and eating yogurt and taking probiotics. I manage to go a few months without severe injuries or illnesses, and upgrade from tortillas to soup. I discover a recipe for Irish soda bread and teach myself to bake it, watching the flour brown in the oven. I cut thick farm slices and cover them in butter and picture the carbs sticking straight to my bones.

Slowly the weight comes back. I still have to rush home from restaurants sometimes, and I spend so much time in the bathroom that I can get through a *New York Times* Wednesday crossword without any hints. But day by day I put myself back together. Work remains blurry. I run calls the whole time, with varying degrees of numbness. I have less patience than I used to, after watching the same problems plague the same streets over and over, year after year. The holdovers and the late calls never stop. The lines at the hospitals grow longer, three ambulances, then five, then six, waiting in a hallway for hours while nurses avoid eye contact. I try meditation, with little success. I surf more, and get back into rock climbing. I get bitchy with my supervisors, knowing there will be no consequences for my attitude. I call out sick more often, opting to spend the day at the beach or at home with a book instead of crammed into an ambulance listening to never-ending radio chatter. I think about leaving EMS, not knowing what I'd do instead. I still throw away a lot of food, if it's one day past its expiration or the color looks off or something about it doesn't feel quite right, but I manage to eat bigger meals and keep putting weight back on and my jawline softens again. I smile one day when my pants feel tight around my hips.

When COVID hits, all the adrenaline that had been choking me out in bathrooms the last couple years finally has somewhere to go. It feels like all of the pain and terror and sweat and uncertainty that has been trapped inside my gut for the last three years has a purpose. I can breathe for the first time. I catch some great waves. Everyone who calls 911 is jacked out of their minds, terrified of the boogieman, and I revel in my ability to soothe their concerns. I have spent the last two years washing my hands raw and shitting my brains out, terrified of every public surface, and COVID sweeps all that preparation into the ultimate performance art for me: it's a perfect large-scale conceptual satire of my own mental illness. At work I am a beacon of peaceful courage. I am a dollar-store Buddha statue. I am a flower.

The excitement of that first month wears off pretty quickly and we settle back into the grind. Only now the rest of the world is shut down. I am required to go to work but not allowed at the gym or swimming pool, which I have come to rely on in order to keep my injuries in check. I buy hand weights and a stationary bike but it's not the same. The whole time the gyms are closed I try to keep up my physical therapy strengthening for my shoulder, ankle, and back, but without the machines I can't get in the right exercises. I'm furious at a world that would make me continue to work full-time but not allow me access to the equipment I need to physically be able to do the work. We have a small weight room at work, and I find out I'm not the only medic in this mindset when a supervisor tries to shut it three separate times but returns to work each day to find the "Closed" sign torn down and the tape on the door ripped off. More than a few of us would rather take the vague threat of potential future respiratory illness to the certainty of debilitating pain right now, today. We are trapped in the tiny front cab of an ambulance together for twelve hours per day. We share bathrooms and locker rooms. It's not like we're not going to infect each other if one more of the rooms in our station is closed. But the weight room at work is still not really enough to keep me fully in shape.

Without the gym, my body breaks down. Maybe it was just my time, maybe it would have happened anyway, but I will never really forgive the universe for pushing me out of my exercise routine right when I needed it the most. My shoulder starts to disintegrate again. My back goes out a couple of times.

The frequency of back injuries in paramedics is usually blamed on lifting and carrying patients into and out of the ambulance and hiking heavy bags up the stairs. This makes our sacrifice sound noble and heroic—the paperwork even includes sexy military phrases like *injured in the line of duty*. The truth, as usual, is more obvious and more depressing. Poor working conditions are just more profitable for companies. In the early 1980s an economist named Jack Stout reimagined EMS from the perspective of, well, an economist. He wrote papers on maximizing productivity and profits, and EMS as a "public utility model" emphasizing performance metrics and profitability over patient or employee welfare. His equations heavily emphasized response times as a measure of the success of an ambulance service, rather than patient outcomes.

One of his most lasting changes was the introduction of "system status management," or SSM, a clean, corporate-sounding phrase that may or may not have ruined my long-term ability to sit upright. The idea was that rather than waiting for calls at a station or quarters, ambulances would drive around the city and sit on street corners closer to where calls might arise. A dispatching algorithm could use factors like time of day, day of the week, and weather patterns to predict where the next call might come from. Ambulances would be posted closer to the areas that might need them, and could be moved around in real time by the dispatch algorithm like chess pieces waiting for their next move. Sounds cool, right? It was the type of idea that makes accountants and capitalists drool.

What it meant in reality was that paramedics lost the ability to stretch or rest or move around or use the bathroom between calls.

Rather than heading back to a station house for a break to wait for the next adrenaline rush, we stuff ourselves into the front cab of a van and drive endlessly around the city. We park on street corners for a few minutes but can be paged halfway across the city to cover a different zone if the dispatcher's computer says that a call might pop there. We drive across town at 2:00 a.m. only to get a call in the neighborhood we just left, swing the van around, and drive right back. We spend whole shifts driving, criss-crossing the city, circling neighborhoods, sometimes without ever stopping or even running a call. And the whole time we are sitting, crouched, in the poorly ventilated front cab of a blinking, beeping, grumbling mobile clinic on wheels. The seats only go back a couple of inches, and most of the leg room is taken up by mechanical modifications. I listen to news radio conversations about climate change and CO_2 emissions while I drive a ten-year-old ambulance back and forth along the same streets a hundred miles a day. My chief once told me over lunch that the whole concept was actually invented as a union-busting strategy, to prevent paramedics from being able to gather at stations and discuss their work conditions. I have never been able to find a source backing him up on this, but it's not as though Mr. Stout would have included that in his promotional literature.

To management, the idea sounded amazing on paper. And companies would no longer have to pay rent on rooms for their medics to rest in. The idea seemed so good, in fact, that very little was done to research its effects. It was widely implemented within the next decade. Although some rural departments continue to maintain quarters, street posting has become the norm for busier areas in the United States.

Though little formal research has been done into the effects of system status management, what has been published has been damning. In a 2003 article for *EMS World*, Dr. Bryan Bledsoe quotes studies showing a 46 percent increase in ambulance maintenance costs and a 71 percent increase in overall back pain. He describes a Canadian study in which 93 percent of paramedics surveyed reported back pain or discomfort from sitting in the ambulance all shift. And what's it all for? One of the first major studies took place in 1986 in Tulsa, Oklahoma, and relayed that system status management was found to have saved an average of, wait for it: thirty-seven seconds per call. A "non-clinically significant" amount of time.

I have read a number of essays in the last few years defending system status management. They explain the difference between SSM and "dynamic deployment," an equally confusing phrase that refers to a different strategy for optimizing ambulance response times. They also beg me not to blame Jack Stout for overworking providers and contributing to burnout and poor patient outcomes. They tell me that these are the fault of the increased call volume, or the poor staffing, or the hospitals for creating lengthy wait times. Basically: Don't hate the player, hate the game. And when all else fails, pin it on the hospitals.

I'll admit I have a very biased, very emotional reaction when I read this research. I don't travel much anymore, as plane trips and long car rides are a challenge. I do physical therapy. I go to the gym. All the pain, all the disability—it would be worth it if I had given up my back in the righteous struggle to save human lives. If I had stepped on a land mine while rescuing a child, I like to imagine I could carry my limp with some dignity. Everyone has their injuries. I have mine; I can live with it. But to learn that I have this much largely preventable pain, this much frustration, so that I could save some economist thirty-seven seconds? That stings.

In spring of 2024, I meet several times with retired supervisor Dan Quinto to collect his thoughts for several sections of this book. Quinto worked in the 911 service for almost fifty years, thirty-seven of them in Santa Cruz. He sat on every advisory board and committee, constantly advocating for better coverage, better protocols, and a higher standard of care. Although I only worked in the county for a short time, I have fossilized a particular image of Quinto in my brain: disgruntled, awake at 2:00 a.m. for something stupid, looking every inch the tired father. Taking a deep breath, rubbing his forehead, and then fixing the fax machine, or sorting out the schedule, or, in one instance, calling the gas station to apologize for driving off with their hose still dangling out of our rig. (Sorry again about that one, Dan.)

When I first mention that my book will discuss some of the challenges facing modern ambulance work, he sighs. Before I even get to my question, he dives into the money-saving changes that EMS management has forced on their workers in the last two decades. Santa Cruz County was actually one of the last systems in the state to implement some of these changes: no more two-paramedic cars, for example; now the rigs carry one paramedic and one EMT. And instead of twenty-four-hour shifts with stations and kitchens available, the ambulances spend their twelves driving in circles. The company still rents a couple of rooms throughout the county, called *substations* or *posts*, where crews can theoretically stop to use the bathroom or microwave. But the crews are usually kept too busy to take advantage, and many employees suspect that they too will soon be phased out.

In Santa Cruz County, ambulances are managed by a privately owned company rather than the fire department. This company, called American Medical Response, is the largest ambulance provider in the United States. You may have seen the letters *AMR* painted across the side of a red-and-white van in your hometown.

EMTs and paramedics call AMR the Walmart of ambulance companies. They are massive, everywhere, and economically powerful enough to influence the business practices of everyone else in the industry. But the corporate structure of AMR, like most American health-care businesses, has changed in recent years. AMR is now owned by Global Medical Response, the largest medical transportation company in the world. And Global Medical Response is in turn owned by Kohlberg Kravis Roberts & Company, a multinational investment firm run by, as my dad put it, "the same ten fuckwads who own everything in this economy."

Quinto tells me that one of the original founders of AMR, a man named Paul Shirley, was known in the county as a good dude. He explains that Shirley's original idea was to find ambulance companies that were doing well, beloved by their communities, and treated their employees right. He would then buy them up and remain relatively hands off. The model proved successful. Maybe too successful. The company grew far larger than Shirley's original vision and was eventually purchased by a bus transportation group that parted ways with Shirley. After the bus corporation, a series of mergers and purchases slowly turned AMR into, as Quinto said with a shake of his head, ". . . what it is today."

It's easy for me to pick on AMR. The truth is that many of the smaller "mom and pop" ambulance companies treat their employees just as badly, if not worse, than the big corporations. And the fire department is far from perfect. But AMR is the biggest and the loudest player in the game. They have used their power to set the standard for pay and schedules for EMTs and paramedics everywhere, and to change the laws regulating ambulance work itself. And more than one AMR employee has told me that every time the company was sold, management looked for new ways to cut costs. Each of these cuts—get rid of stations, split up units, stretch staffing even thinner—made working conditions worse.

Quinto tells me that he believes the economic streamlining of modern EMS has brought true ugliness into the industry. He cites increased call volume, a dumbing down of our educational standards, and a focus on increasing profits. He says that the change from twenty-four-hour shifts to twelves "ruined the ambulance business." My own experience with twenty-fours was so sleep-deprived that I felt like I was driving the ambulance drunk, but Quinto explains that back when staffing was kept at safe levels the medics loved the round-the-clock schedule. I believe him, because I have seen how much my firefighter friends value working twenty-fours and even forty-eights. When there is enough time during the day for food, hydration, and rest, the culture of emergency work is completely different.

He tells me how Stout and his cohort emphasized a metric called the UHU: the unit hour utilization. If an ambulance did not run enough calls per hour, it was determined to be unproductive and removed from the system. Quinto explains, "They took away accountability for your zone, and the comradery of having everyone together as a cohesive group." He goes on to describe how having a feeling of responsibility for a certain geographical area for a full twenty-four hours emphasizes the team aspect of the job, and the connection to the community. "When you move to twelve-hour shifts, with no station houses, and everyone moving around constantly, the idea of what they're doing gets lost. Now everyone is just trying to get to the end of their shift. It's like you're putting together boxes on the assembly line. It's not tolerable for a lot of people now."

——

As exhausting as ambulance work is, when I am with the SFFD I can't imagine doing anything else for a living. After spending a year on a Street Crisis unit following COVID, I return to the ambulance at the first chance I get. The day I get back onto my old rig I come into the work with an enthusiasm I haven't had since my first year. The work is exciting to me again, and joyful. I sit on scene with patients, explaining their conditions to them, helping them, laughing with them. My partner is a thoughtful new EMT who plays word games with me late into the night. I'm old, I'm tired, my joints are crunchy, but at least I'm running calls. My first day back I take an elderly man with a urinary tract infection to the hospital, smiling the whole time at such a straightforward medical issue with a realistic cure. *I'm helping*, I think, delighted to be back where I belong.

Within about a month I feel a shooting pain up my right wrist. It happens when I lift the gurney, and then again when I pick up the monitor. I ignore it for a few weeks. Every time I grab the backpack or the cardiac monitor it's a little bit worse; twenty, thirty, fifty times a day. It shoots up my wrist into my elbow, pulling at the joint at a strange angle whenever I turn my hand. It starts to throb even when I'm not using it. I stare at myself in the mirror, thinking about how far I've come only to fail again. I've never seen a movie about a ball player who, sick of injury after injury, eventually takes a desk job and gets into gardening. I want my righteous comeback tournament. After about five weeks of pain my fingers start to tingle and I sigh and head back to the supervisor's office. As I fill out the same injury paperwork I've completed so many times before, I'm no longer upset. I'm not scared, or anxious. I'm just tired. I don't know what's coming next in my life, but it occurs to me that I may have run my last call on an ambulance.

It turns out I have a bone condition called ulnar impaction syndrome, which sounds much more impressive than it is. Basically, one of my forearm bones is a little longer than it should be. It's a degenerative disorder, aggravated by years of using my right wrist to compensate for my aching left shoulder and back. Every gurney lift, every time I grabbed the cardiac monitor and threw it into or out of the ambulance, every time I heaved the red backpack over my shoulder to hike upstairs. A thousand paper cuts over a decade of work.

I feel like a wuss. I can think of a dozen guys who have been doing the job longer than me and haven't given up. Mikey has worked more overtime in a busier system than me for twice as long. Kyle points out that Mikey's built like a dump truck and didn't spend half his twenties throwing himself off cornices on boards and bikes. *Yeah, but still.* I finally look up at Kyle slowly and sigh. *It's the girl thing.* He nods. He knows this conversation by heart. I'll never really not have something to prove, even after ten years. If I injure out and give up it's because I wasn't strong enough, because girls aren't strong enough, because they never should have let us in. *Emily Dunning Barringer, forgive me. I wasn't up to the task.*

I am placed on "light duty," a department euphemism for any number of office jobs given to injured paramedics—clean this, file this, answer these phones. I sit at a desk for a few weeks doing data entry and chatting with the other broken toys. The guy behind me is the type of medic who always makes me feel inferior—he picks up more shifts, works harder, complains less. He's in here because his back blew out so badly that he hasn't been able to pick up his own baby in a year and a half. He's finally healed enough to be able to walk, and he comes in for four hours a day until the pain gets too much and then waddles home. I also run into two ACL surgeries (both female), two more low backs (one male, one female), and a shoulder (male). One of the low backs is coming from a fire engine; the other five of us are all ambulance.

It's well known that the ambulance hurts you over time. We knew what we were getting into, or thought we did. When Emily Dunning Barringer worked her first shift in 1903 the ambulance was already known as a dirty, dangerous place to work.

And there are jobs much, much more physically demanding than ours. I have friends in plumbing, HVAC, and construction who see my hot water bottle and ibuprofen and shrug. Most blue-collar jobs degrade the body over time. God forbid a roofer is reading these words; they would strain their eye muscles from rolling them so hard. When I worked as an EMT in Watsonville, every morning I would drive past fields full of fruit and vegetable pickers, bent over in the sun. They wore long sleeves, masks, and gloves to protect their bodies from pesticides. Even on the hottest days of the summer, they were covered in thick clothing. Some of the kids I went to EMT school with are the children of these farmworkers, excited to have a much more stable and easy life than their parents. And they will. It's a good life; a hard job but a good life. But there is a statute of limitations. Most of us are lucky to get five years on the box, maybe seven. I got almost ten.

In 2018, AMR spent $22 million funding a California state ballot measure to avoid having to give EMTs and paramedics lunch breaks. The issue came up because a Supreme Court ruling two years earlier held that private security guards must be allowed a rest period, during their shift, in which they are "relieved of all duties." That is: for a few minutes every twelve or twenty-four hours, employees must be allowed to turn their radios off and stop responding to calls. When it became clear that the law would also apply to emergency health-care workers, the California EMS community was plunged into a frenzy of legal proceedings. The state Legislative Analyst's office estimated the new law would cost ambulance companies roughly $100 million in staffing increases alone. On top of that, AMR was hit with multiple lawsuits for rest break and wage violations, including a class-action suit attempting to represent workers in more than fifteen counties. I followed the updates with excitement at first. Although none of these changes would directly affect my job at the fire department, I thought it would be cool to see some parts of EMS be forced to improve their hiring practices and response times.

For the record, no one was suggesting that paramedics would kick up our feet and ignore emergency calls during a blizzard or a busy summer weekend. To me personally, thirty minutes here or there didn't actually seem like that big of a deal. I just loved the idea that our bosses might be required to build some padding into our schedules. It would mean more of us available to help our cities when things went really sideways, and it would be nice to take turns breaking each other out to eat a meal or take a poop. But it was never going to happen.

AMR appeared to waste no time in their efforts. They created the ballot measure exempting themselves (and other ambulance companies) from the new ruling. They ran an advertising blitz. They lobbied lawmakers. It was a very American strategy: dedicating $22 million to political action when faced with over $100 million in potential labor costs. As union director Jason Bollini pointed out in an interview for Mission Local, "That's a four-to-one return on investment."

As the political fight gained traction, my friends and I grew disgusted. We felt as though we were witnessing the company buy their way out of the law in real time. The measure passed. Private ambulance providers would be excluded from the new law.

As for the lawsuits, the court denied the class-action nature of the largest suit, stating instead that workers would have to sue individually. At least one of those cases appears to have been settled, and the outcome of the rest of the legal action is unclear.

The way I see it, there are several ways in which modern EMS is deeply, deeply broken. Poverty, social welfare, and the brutality of the American health-care industry will always be a battle for our profession. But the labor issues that plague our ambulances—the fix for this seems impossible in its simplicity. Treat your employees better. Hire enough of us to do the job safely. Pay us more, staff us higher, stop making us work forty-eight hours in a row without sleep or bathroom breaks or seats that recline. Just stop it. Better-rested paramedics in less pain—this is so easy, so obvious—will produce better outcomes for patients.

Of course, for this to happen, corporations would have to stop rewriting the law to squeeze every last penny of productivity out of their employees, no matter who dies waiting for an ambulance. And lawmakers would have to stop letting them get away with it. The owners of $40 billion private-equity firms would have to stop their yachts for three seconds and think about the mile-high pyramid of human suffering upon which their fortunes are built. Counties would have to demand better staffing, higher pay, and shifts that end when they are supposed to. Hospitals would have to upstaff their nurses and doctors, instead of bullying ambulance companies into sitting on their patients in the triage area for half the day. Treating many of the problems faced by today's ambulances requires nothing less or more than pressure against the heavy grinding wheel of American capitalism. I personally believe this is achievable, but that might be the Oakland in me talking.

———

My buddies that cross over to firefighting say that after a year away from the ambulance, health issues they didn't even realize they had start to clear up. Their injuries heal. They sleep better. They put on muscle mass and lose fat. After a few weeks on light duty, I apply for a six-month unpaid leave to pursue my education. It's an idea I've been toying with for years, and the timing suddenly feels unavoidable. I take some classes at a local community college, read lots of books, and start my own writing. I go for long walks and sleep eight hours a night.

My stomach starts to feel a little bit better and my back gives me less trouble. I pay a physical therapist eighty-five dollars a week to work on my shoulder and hit the gym religiously. I go to a doctor's appointment and learn that my blood pressure has dropped twelve points. One day about two months into my leave I realize I've eaten an entire burrito without a stomach ache and I stare at the crumpled tin foil and start to cry.

I'm sitting in my Tacoma at the time, parked in front of a taqueria near my house. Their front facade is painted bright purple with yellow flowers and the awning throws a gentle shadow over their stems. Across the street is Central Fire Station 3, where I did my first EMT ride-along fourteen years ago. I was twenty-two then, hair still purple, no idea where I was going with all of this. I still smoked so much pot that producing clean urine for a job application was a legitimate concern. We ran three calls that day, although for the life of me I can only remember one—a seizure in the park. We showed up once she was done seizing, so by the time we arrived she was fairly calm. Still, standing between the three firefighters, the two paramedics, the flashing lights, the woman, her family, and all the other park-goers, I felt completely lost. One of the firefighters grunted something about a ride-along and pushed me to the front of the crowd, where a medic handed me a blood pressure cuff. I tried a couple of times but couldn't hear anything over the commotion and told him as much, embarrassed. The medic smiled and took the cuff back. Then they loaded her up and she was gone.

I look back down at my tin foil. My whole afternoon—the burrito, the firehouse, the flood of memories—it feels like some grand metaphor, but I can't quite make the pieces fit. Fourteen years have passed since that day. I have no regrets about choosing this line of work, but I'm not sure that I have what it takes to continue. I will return to the field when my educational leave ends, but I know it's time to start looking for a way out. I know guys who last ten or twenty years on the bus. They have much stronger backs than I do, and probably a stronger heart. I always wanted to be tough enough to be one of those guys.

I hope that in the future, if my injuries heal, maybe I can come back and work part time somewhere. Pick up a couple shifts a month, just to stay in the game. But I know my full-time days will soon be in the past. Still, I did what I could, and I gave what I had. For now I suppose that will have to be enough.

"DEFINE 'SAVED'"

MICHAEL HAMILTON, PARAMEDIC/RN;
TWENTY-FOUR YEARS IN EMS
RENO, NEVADA

But the job is still fun! The job is still fun. You're doing the craziest shit. You walk into situations that no other human being gets to walk into, and then you start calling the shots. You're driving around the city in a freaking Sprinter van with your best friend, blasting heavy metal and drinking coffee. It's an absolute freaking blast.

You never truly know what you're walking into. Dispatch gives you a little bit of information, but until you pull up in front of the house, your boots are on the ground, or you get off the elevator in the casino, you don't truly know. And maybe you have the training and the knowledge and the skill set to handle it, and maybe you don't. You take that chance, every single time. EMS offers you insane highs and insane lows. It's an experience unlike any other. Most people that I know that do not do this kind of work live in somewhat of a bubble. Academics hang out with academics, and then they go work at a college. Hard hats go to the job site. But as a paramedic, I treated a heart attack on a homeless guy crawling out of an alley downtown, and then our next call was in the multi-million-dollar mansion of a local celebrity.

You go into broken homes. You go onto the reservation. You go into the college, and into the dorms. You go into fancy restaurants and into the dive bars. You see everything, you interact with everybody. You don't have a choice. You see all different sides of ethnicity and human culture and experience. It's wild. I feel like not a lot of jobs offer that. And once you've had a taste, man, it's hard to give up.

And the other part of it is, I *do* feel like I make a difference. Maybe not every day, and maybe not to everyone. Maybe they are few and far between. But they are there.

I was in a rough patch a couple of years ago. I was so burnt out, and I was so depressed, and I just wanted it to stop. I was ready to end my life. I talked to a friend that I knew I could trust, and he helped me through a lot of it. One of the things he said to me was "You know, you've been doing this job a long time. How many lives do you think you've saved?"

My first thought was *Okay, define "saved."*

But then I stopped and thought about it. Let's say myself and my crew, under my direction, intervened at a time where had we not done the things that we did, this person would have died. Instead, because we intervened, they went on to live. I guessed at a number and told him.

"Holy shit, Mike, do you even hear what you're saying?"

I've thought about that conversation for a couple of years now. There are people walking around Reno right now that are alive because of me, and my co-workers, and my colleagues. Because we did this job that we are hired, trained, and paid to do.

I worked a cardiac arrest one time a few years ago. We had a rash of overdoses due to counterfeit Percocets containing carfentanyl. These young kids at parties were just dropping like flies. We were at a hotel and this twenty-one-year-old kid dies. Security got there first and started CPR, and then Reno PD arrived and took over and continued. We arrived, and we got pulses back. By the time we dropped him off at the hospital he was confused but awake, looking around, and pulling at the mask on his face.

Fast-forward about a year, maybe a year and a half later. I'm working a night shift and I run a motor vehicle accident, a minor fender-bender. This lady got hit by a pickup truck that drove away. She ended up refusing care from us. She was saying, "I'm okay, my neck's a little sore, but I was wearing my seatbelt. I'm okay."

We're doing our refusal process, telling her, "Okay, well, if you need us, you just call us back and we'll come see you. We don't mind."

She says, "Oh, if I need you, I'll call you, don't worry. You guys are my angels. You saved my son's life."

She says that last year, her son was at a hotel room party, and she told us the name of the hotel. She said he overdosed, the paramedics came in, and they saved his life.

I said, "Ma'am, what was your son's name?"

And she tells me. And I say, "Oh my god. Ma'am. I'm the medic. That was me and my crew. That was us. I was there. I ran that call." And she starts crying; she throws her arms around me. She asks if I want to talk to him. I say, "He's here?"

"Yeah, he's in the back of my car right now! You want to go say hi?"

It was during COVID, so we were wearing masks. I walk up to the rear driver's-side window of the car and decide I'm going to fuck with him a little bit. I motion to roll down the window, and the kid goes, "Can I help you?"

I say, "Do you remember me?"

"No?"

Then I pull down the mask and say, "How about now?"

And his eyes got as big as saucers. He recognized me. He said, "Holy shit, it's you."

I said, "Yeah, man. It's you. How are you?"

He gets out of the car and gives me a big, meaty, bro hug. He says, "I got out of the hospital, I was there for a week, my kidneys were really messed up." He tells me he came home and moved back in with his mom and got rid of all those people he was hanging out with. He says he's focusing on school now, trying to get a degree so he can help support his mom and his family.

That's a real thing that happened.

I try to write fiction. I'm not good at it. I mean, I'm trying to write a campaign for Dungeons & Dragons right now, and it's fucking hard! And it's about elves, and orcs, and shit. But that story really happened. Hand of God, I will go to my grave. So if you ask me, why do I still do this? Even through all the burnout, all the pain? Because I have some knowledge and some skills and I have some experience and I can help more than I've harmed. Because the world is a hard place, and it can be a sick, sad place, but it is also very beautiful. And when we do work like this, it helps it be more beautiful for more people. And that feels good.

"I LOVED MY JOB"

DAN QUINTO, RETIRED EMS SUPERVISOR;
FORTY-SEVEN YEARS IN EMS
SANTA CRUZ, CALIFORNIA

Nance and I met in junior high. She sat in front of me. She left for college a year before I did, because she was so smart and focused, and we corresponded for the year writing letters. That sounds crazy nowadays, but it's what we did. When she came back from school, we dated, even though we'd known each other forever. We got married when we were nineteen.

I went to work at White's Ambulance Service, in Azusa, California, down in the San Gabriel Valley. We covered two little cities, Glendora and Covina, in a '68 Pontiac Bonneville. It had two rotating gumball lights on the top; we loved that. And it had the old bullet-shaped growler sirens on the fender. They looked like jet engines on the inside. You would push a button on the floor, and when it wound up you could see it torque and all the lights would dim. Then the noise would just blow your ears out. When you got to the call, you had to press a different button to make it stop. They were chrome, of course, and if even if everything else was dirty you kept that siren shiny.

Later, when we got a van, that was hot shit.

White's was a funeral home and an ambulance service, so our ambulance quarters were inside the funeral home. We slept upstairs.

During the day we had to do linens, and help the morticians if they needed it. We did our own sheets for the ambulances in commercial washers, and we had to fold them all with these big roller steamers. My shift was Monday, Tuesday, Wednesday, and I got off Thursday afternoon at four o'clock. I only got paid for fourteen hours a day, unless we ran more than three calls after 10:00 p.m. I made minimum wage, $2.60 an hour. Even after they passed federal minimum wage laws, they tried to get it to not apply to us. And for a long time, they didn't. We didn't get paid for the time we were at work. We would have to wait around and hope for calls.

Eventually Nance and I made it back to Santa Cruz. Nance loved Santa Cruz. She was an actual, real live hippie. She never wore shoes; she didn't shave. She had really long hair that she kept in braids. We were married forty-eight years. It was in 2017 when she started to have some short-term memory loss. The diagnosis didn't come until later; it's called primary progressive aphasia. Her condition is degenerative. It's not that fast, but it's normally faster than Alzheimer's. All my plans for the rest of my life are . . . I don't know. I'm not ready.

There's a lot of stuff that people say Winston Churchill said that he never actually said, so I looked this one up. He really said this one. It's a quote I heard years and years ago, and it's been one of my mantras. During World War II, he said, "When you're going through hell, keep going."

I worked here in this county for thirty-seven years. And generally speaking, I loved every minute of it. I loved my job. I taught paramedic school for almost fifteen years. I trained a whole generation of people that came through here.

Why did I last so much longer than most paramedics? I loved it. I loved my job.

"TAKE MY PAIN AWAY"

"When did you get pink mascara, hon?"

It's running down Krista's face and up her forehead in a sloppy neon river. Her hair was bleached a couple of months ago and the roots shine with grease.

"I gotta lay down," she says. She tells us she has had chronic pain all over her body for the last year and feels cold. She's had some beers and a few shots. At first she's crying and crying but once the heater warms up the back of the ambulance she settles down. Her right hand is in a sling and both arms are filled with bracelets. In her purse is some trash, some toiletries, an empty pint of vodka, and an inhaler of albuterol.

I try to get a blood pressure a few times but we've had such a long day and I can't figure out why it won't take. I fix her shirtsleeve, smooth out the cuff. After the third failed attempt I realize the machine is unplugged.

She's cranky. She wants more from us than we have. She keep telling us she feels "like crap," but won't give us any more specifics. I ask if she has a shelter bed anywhere and she says she needs one. She has a tent down by the beach but she wants somewhere indoors.

When we arrive at the hospital, the nurse recognizes her and sighs. She kneels down at our patient's level and takes her hand.

"So you've been to the ER twenty-five times for this, ma'am? Twenty-five times. What can we do for you that we haven't already done?"

Krista takes her hand back, folds her arms defiantly and squints. She spits out, "More than you've been doing."

The nurse stands up. "Okay. Give me one second."

I lean down and talk to Krista about her past. I tell her I know she's uncomfortable, and I genuinely would like to help. But what exactly would you like them to do for you at the ER? Why did we bring you here for the twenty-sixth time?

She unfolds her arms and looks at me.

"I want them to take my pain away."

LAST DAY

My last day at the SFFD, we throw a big dinner. Charlie cooks pot roast and mashed potatoes and cuts up a watermelon. Maggie and I bring cookies from every bakery we drove past all week.

We toast with Martinelli's as radios crackle on and off. I ask the guys what they would want to see in a book about EMS, what would make them keep reading instead of rolling their eyes. Everyone looks uncomfortable for a minute before Charlie says, "An entire book of Caleb Jackson stories."

Oh my god.

The table busts up. Everyone interrupts each other relaying their favorite tale of one of the most notorious medics to work in our unit. He got in a fender-bender once, and called in his own trauma ring-down on the radio. Charlie launches into an imitation: "The patient is a forty-one year old male, struck by—"

Taylor breaks in to say, "No, twice!! It was twice!! He did it in Oakland too! He's on the radio like, 'My pain is a six, aww, no, it's a ten!' So they fucking code two'd him to Highland, to give him the ol' Highland handshake!" Taylor holds up a first finger crooked into a C to mimic the digital rectal exam given to an incoming trauma to check for bleeding.

Charlie is still talking: "He's saying, 'I have taken c-spine precautions, I am confused, I have a GCS level of fourteen.'"

"He reported his *own* GCS as fourteen?" The *GCS* is a three-part scoring system; Maggie wants to know if he had really done the math to report himself as neurologically disoriented.

"Swear to god."

"You guys remember his license plate?"

"Deez nuts!!"

"Dude, I'm in the middle of a call one time in East Oakland, assessing this little old grandma for chest pain, trying to do a twelve lead, and this guy is just elbowing his way in, like, 'Hey! Hey! You guys know Caleb Jackson?' I'm like, who the fuck did he piss off, ah, shit, getting ready to fucking fight, and this guy gets all in my face and is like, 'You tell him Littlebones says what's up!' and then just leaves. Like, that's it?"

"Were any of you there for the South County bathroom thing?"

Everyone groans in unison.

The new guy is bewildered, soaking it all in. I skip the body of the story but tell him the punchline—Caleb marching purposefully out of the bathroom of South County Hospital, placing a five-dollar bill on the nurse's station and saying, "My condolences to the janitor."

I don't know what I had been hoping for when I asked the dinner table for their thoughts. Some insight into what to write, how to find my voice, how to possibly approach the task of speaking for an entire group of the most cynical people in the world. It seems that no one took my request seriously. But the thing is that they did.

Earlier that night the police had identified the body of one of our favorite regular patients, brutally murdered and left in public, and each of us carried that pain somewhere in our hearts and our guts at that dinner. No one wants me to write about our losses, our grief. They want me to tell stories of our love and our resilience and our silliness. Of Caleb and car accidents and destroyed bathrooms and screw-ups and pranks and late nights hammering Red Bulls and talking shit. I have wished for years that I was a better writer of humor, because I still believe that the only way to truly capture our job is with dark absurdist comedy, told as deadpan as it felt at the time. On my left at the dinner is Robbie White, a guy I've worked with for years. During a lull in conversation, he leans towards me and says, quietly, "Tell them some of the lighthearted side, about hanging out at station and the jokes and the banter." I think what he means is tell them about the medics. Everyone knows how messed up the world is. Tell them about the people who go out there every day and manage to face it all with humor and love. Tell them about *us*, Jo.

I promise him I'll try my best.

AFTERWORD: SPEAKING UP

When I interviewed my friend Jamie for this manuscript, I asked what she would want to see in a book about EMTs and paramedics—what she would choose to put out into the world if we could control the narrative instead of letting Hollywood make caricatures out of us. Jamie thought for a moment. She told me she wanted my book to capture feelings and emotions that would help her feel like she wasn't insane. She spoke about compassion fatigue, curbside prejudice, and the dehumanization that all health-care workers face over time. She thought that maybe if other EMTs and paramedics could find themselves in my stories, it would help them to feel like they are not monsters.

As I spoke with Jamie, I began to understand my central struggle in developing this book. When I swung too far into gritty cynicism and darkness, I lost my message. But when I added too much love and compassion, I felt like I was lying. It seemed a betrayal when I made our patients too sympathetic and our responses too kind. I didn't want to cater too fully to the hero archetype. As sociologist Matthew Desmond once wrote, "There are two ways to dehumanize: the first is to strip people of all virtue; the second is to cleanse them of all sin." In this book I have tried my best to find a middle ground. To explain to you the realities of the work without veering too far into bitterness or exploitation.

Though several excellent memoirs have been written about our line of work, we are still largely excluded from larger conversations about health care and public safety. In 2023, California governor Gavin Newsom signed into law a new state bill mandating a twenty-five-dollar minimum wage for all health-care workers. Well, almost all. While legislators thought to include janitorial staff, laundry workers, food service staff, and billing departments for nursing homes and dialysis clinics, they specifically excluded EMTs and paramedics. We were classified as "outside workers," along with delivery contractors and waste management.

So there you have it. Our outsider status has now been legislatively codified into California state policy. How very punk rock. I will not pretend to understand the political machinations that carved us out of that particular bill, but it comes to mind when I think about my own point of view. I have sought to find language that would speak not only to my co-workers and peers but that could also be taken seriously by the academics, politicians, and string-pullers of our society. I hope that someone louder and more politically connected than I am can find some small piece of humanity in my writing and advocate for us to be allowed to sit at the table next time.

I want to describe how impossible it seems to maintain hope underneath the never-ending crush of heartbreak and corruption and how somehow, my patients and co-workers manage to do it anyway. I hope that I have conveyed that our work can be boring, frustrating, and exhausting, but also punctuated with tremendous humanity and joy. I do not have a simple answer to the problems that plague the ambulance. I distrust any sentence that includes the phrase, "they just need to…" But I do think small improvements are possible. I like to imagine a future where paramedics are allowed to leave work at the end of their scheduled shifts, instead of being held over for hours with no advance notice. One where we receive regular feedback about our patient outcomes and participate in developing and improving our own protocols. I'd love to see the day when efficient patient hand-offs at emergency rooms are prioritized, so that hospitals aren't allowed to pull ambulances off the street for half a day to compensate for their own staffing deficiencies.

And I want the world to hear our stories. First responders can retreat sometimes into a members-only club, which is understandable due to the nature of our work. The things we go through can make us feel separate from the civilian world, and we will often double down on that division in an act of self-preservation. But I think that there is value in pulling back the curtain. In speaking out.

I did the best I could all these years, both in my writing and in the work itself. I can only hope that the people who worked alongside me think I showed up for enough shifts to have earned the right to talk about our world. As Dan Quinto told me over coffee, "I hope that I walked the walk."

ACKNOWLEDGEMENTS

To Haley: thank you for being my friend in the cold, wet, Pacific Northwest. Thank you for being interesting and hilarious and brilliant and always up for an adventure. For crawling around the back of a dirty van searching for spare change to buy donuts in the rain, for facing off against poison spiders in a tent in the jungle, for holding my hand through a break-up, for picking up the phone when I couldn't breathe. For nudging and coaching me through the first two essays and thinking I had a book in me when I had no idea how to move forward. You are the best editor and the best family in the world. Come visit soon.

To the rest of the team at Penguin Random House Canada, thank you for taking a chance on me. Hannah, thank you for the insightful read and comments. Linda Pruessen, thank you for the clarity and intelligence of your copy edits and the Herculean efforts with my source list. To Tonia Addison, Shona Cook, Aruna Dahanayake, Bree Duwyn, Jordan Ginsberg, Sarah Howland, Kimberlee Kemp, Danielle LeSage, Adeeba Noor, Rebecca Rocillo, Kate Sinclair, Stephanie Sinclair, and Sean Tai: thank you for all of your work.

Thank you to Kris Hurst and Gary Niblock, my very first EMT teachers: you saw a hyperactive, purple-haired stoner in the back of their class and thought I had what it took to do this job. The day I sat down in that classroom was the first day that my life started to make any sense.

Thank you to all of my mentors, partners, and family in EMS, who are far too many to list. Terry, every day I still try to suck less. Sam, thank you for bullying me into applying for the SFFD. You were right about everything. To the whole CP crew, boy were we in the shit of it. To all of Station 49: you guys are my heroes. Give 'em hell.

Jamie and Jody and A.K., thank you for letting me use your voices in this story. Your experiences add an immeasurable amount of legitimacy and meaning to this project and I am deeply grateful for your openness and your time. I was incredibly humbled by your candor and your strength. Chief Perryman, thank you so much for your hospitality and generosity. You guys are fighting the good fight.

To Stephanie Griest, my deepest gratitude for the encouragement and the eleventh-hour edits. You are a force. Sam Quinones, thank you for picking up the phone, for lunch, for your advice and your open heart and your genuine interest my story. Beth Macy, I cannot describe what it meant to me to have an 'atta girl' from such a heavy hitter so early in the process. Your support and energy has meant the world to me. Meli, you have taught me so much about life and perspective and art and justice and what it means to collaborate as a team. I am so grateful to be in your orbit. Gemma, thank you for being an amazing partner and friend and support, and for so many long walks full of ranting and anxiety. You are both a grounding force in my life and an inspiration to me. To Ali: Thank you for being on the other end of the phone all year and listening to so, so, so much crazy; you have helped me through this process more than you know. Sean, thank you for the last-minute reads and all of the support and notes on the manuscript. Let's hang out soon.

Dan Quinto, I was nervous to call up and ask for an audience with such a local legend, but you have been an incredible mentor and friend. I am so, so lucky to have been able to spend the time with you that we have and I look forward to many more coffees and movie nights. Thank you for all of the work that you have done for our people over the years, and for spending the time with me to get through this chapter. Your advice, your ear, and your stories have given me so much confidence in my own voice. I appreciate every minute that we have spent together.

Mikey, thank you for being my brother and my mentor and my friend. You and Rosie are an incredible team and I am lucky to have you as my family. You have been a guiding force in my career, my life, and this project. Thank you for letting me tell parts of your story, which really deserves its own book. Maybe two.

To Aaron and Josie, thank you for opening your home to me to make the career move to SF possible in the first place. Thank you for your love and support, for making this job and this book a reality for me. Aaron, thank you for telling me that I could do anything the boys could do, for never noticing or caring that I was a girl instead. Thank you for teaching me to tie my shoes and for putting a banana on my head when I was seasick. To this day when I am scared, I hear you telling me that all I have to do is jump.

Mom and Dad, I truly lucked out in the parents department. You guys are so full of love and support it is just bonkers. In everything that I do, I am hoping to figure out ways to make you proud. I am grateful every day to have a family like ours.

To Kyle: You are the light of my life. With you, for the first time, I am excited to plan for my future. Which is good, because you are always three steps ahead. For as long as you will let us, Louie and I will do our best to keep up with your plots and schemes. Oh, and there's a cookie for you on the counter.

———

To every single working EMT and paramedic in the world right now: thank you for doing what you do. Thank you for showing up, for making horrifying jokes under your breath, for eating cold leftovers with one hand and leaning on the airhorn with the other on your way to a call. Thank you for lending me your badge and helmet when I forgot mine, for listening to my rants, for calling me on my bullshit, and for sharing your last protein bar even when I just said something rude. I hope your shift is filled with kind patients and interesting medical complaints, I hope you have time to pee and eat, and I hope your favorite supervisor is on the schedule. May you never run another late call. I love you all.

WORKS CITED AND
RECOMMENDED READING

Abbey, E. *The Monkey Wrench Gang.* New York: HarperCollins, 2000.

Alexander, M. *The New Jim Crow: Mass Incarceration in the Age of Colorblindness.*
New York: New Press, 2012.

Almojera, A. *Riding the Lightning: A Year in the Life of a New York City Paramedic.*
New York: HarperCollins, 2022.

"Ambulance Service Planned by City." *New York Times,* December 28, 1929.

"American Medical Response, Inc." International Directory of Company Histories.
Encyclopedia.com (September 11, 2024). https://www.encyclopedia.com
/books/politics-and-business-magazines/american-medical-response-inc.

"AMR to Pay $162,500 to Settle EEOC Pregnancy Discrimination Lawsuit."
U.S. Equal Employment Opportunity Commission, December 19, 2020.
https://www.eeoc.gov/newsroom/amr-pay-162500-settle-eeoc-pregnancy
-discrimination-lawsuit.

Asbury, H. *The Barbary Coast: An Informal History of the San Francisco
Underworld.* New York: Basic Books, 1933.

Barkley, K.T. *The Ambulance: The Story of Emergency Transportation of Sick and
Wounded Through the Centuries.* N.p.: Load N Go Press, 1990.

Barringer, E.D. *Bowery to Bellevue: The Story of New York's First Woman Ambulance
Surgeon.* New York: W.W. Norton, 1950.

Barry, S. "AMR Defends Response Times, Laments Lack of Union Support to
Recent Wage Hike Offer." EMS1, October 19, 2019.

"Bartoni v. American Medical Response West." Justia US Law, 2017. https://law
.justia.com/cases/california/court-of-appeal/2017/a143784.html.

Bass, R.R. "History of EMS," In *Emergency Medical Services: Clinical Practice and Systems Oversight*, edited by D.C. Cone, J.H. Brice, T.R. Delbridge, and J.B. Myers, 1–16. Edison, NJ: Wiley & Sons, 2015.

Bell, R.C. *The Ambulance: A History.* Jefferson, NC: McFarland, 2008.

Bishnoi, R. "Six Minutes to Live or Die." *USA Today*, July 30, 2003.

Blackwell, T.H., and J.S. Kaufman. "Response Time Effectiveness: Comparison of Response Time and Survival in an Urban Emergency Medical Services System." *Academic Emergency Medicine* 9, no. 4 (April 2002): 288–95.

Bledsoe, B. "EMS Myth #7: System Status Management (SSM) Lowers Response Times and Enhances Patient Care." *Emergency Medical Services* 32, no. 9 (September 2003): 158–9.

Bloor, A.J. *Letters from the Army of the Potomac: Written during the Month of May, 1864.* N.p.: Leopold Classic Library, n.d.

Bollag, S. "California Will Launch Care Court Program to Get Severely Mentally Ill People into Treatment." *San Francisco Chronicle*, November 29, 2022. https://www.sfchronicle.com/politics/article/California-will-launch-Care -Court-program-to-get-17410964.php.

Booth, M. *Opium: A History.* New York: St. Martin's Press, 1996.

Booth, T. *You Called an Ambulance for What?* Sydney: Macmillan, 2023.

Bosnyak, M.V. "Dynamic Deployment Models for High-Performance Emergency Medical Services." *Canadian Journal of Emergency Management/ Revue canadienne de gestion des urgences* 3, no. 1 (2022): 8–41.

Brown, J.F., et al. "Frequent Users of 9-1-1 Emergency Medical Services: Sign of Success or Symptom of Impending Failure?" *Prehospital Emergency Care* 23. no. 1 (2019): 94–96.

Brundage, J. "Deciphering the Paradox: Why Consolidation of Fire and EMS Organizations Does Not Yield Expected Economies of Scale." *Medium*, June 13, 2023. https://jbrundage.medium.com/deciphering-the-paradox

-why-consolidation-of-fire-and-ems-organizations-does-not-yield-expected
-23120ddb1f06.

Bucher, J., and H.Q. Zaidi. "A Brief History of Emergency Medical Services in the United States." EMRA, n.d. https://www.emra.org/about-emra/history /ems-history.

Campbell, N.D., and A.M. Lovell. "The History of the Development of Buprenorphine as an Addiction Therapeutic." *Annals of the New York Academy of Sciences* 1248 (2012): 124–39.

Careless, J. "The Ugly Battle Behind California's Prop 11." *EMS World*, February 1, 2019.

"Caring for the Sick: Some Facts about the Ambulance System of New York." *Los Angeles Herald*, October 16, 1892.

Carlisle, R.J. *An Account of Bellevue Hospital, with a Catalogue of the Medical and Surgical Staff from 1736–1894.* New York: Forgotten Books, 2012. Originally published in 1893.

Carmen J. and L. Charbonneau. "New Law (SB 525) Sets Higher Minimum Wages for Certain Healthcare Employees." LCW, January 26, 2024. https:// www.lcwlegal.com/news/new-law-sb-525-sets-higher-minimum-wages-for -certain-health-care-employees/.

Cheesman, W.S. "With an Ambulance." *Hospital Review* XXIII, no. 8 (March 15, 1887): 126–28.

Chief of Department. "General Order 21 A-02: Street Crisis Response Team H3L2 Positions." San Francisco Fire Department. January 5, 2021.

Christopher, S. "The Effects of System Status Management (SSM) and the Eight Minute Response Target on the Health and Well-Being of Ambulance Personnel and Patients: A Review of the Literature (Part 1)." *Ambulance UK* 20, no. 6 (December 2005): 415–20.

Cinader, R. and H.J. Bloom, creators. *"Emergency!"* Universal Studios (1972–77).

Conlon, E. *Blue Blood.* New York: Penguin, 2004.

Connelly, J. *Bringing Out the Dead*. New York: Random House, 1999.

"Cost Is Chief Factor," *New York Times*, December 31, 1929.

"Coverage and Reimbursement for Emergency Medical Services Care Delivery Models and Uncompensated Services" (Reports Required under Senate Bill 682). Baltimore, MD: Maryland Healthcare Commission and Maryland Institute for Emergency Medical Services Systems, 2019.

Davis, R. "Six Minutes to Live or Die, Part 1." *USA Today*, July 28, 2003.

———. "Six Minutes to Live or Die, Part 2." *USA Today*, July 29, 2003.

Desmond, M. *Evicted: Poverty and Profit in the American City*. New York: Broadway Books, 2016.

Doughty, C. *Smoke Gets in Your Eyes: And Other Lessons from the Crematory*. New York: W.W. Norton, 2014.

"Drug Overdose Mortality by State." CDC National Center for Health Statistics, 2022. https://www.cdc.gov/nchs/pressroom/sosmap/drug_poisoning _mortality/drug_poisoning.htm.

Edgerly, D. "Birth of EMS: The History of the Paramedic." *JEMS*, October 13, 2023.

"EEOC Sues Global Medical Response and American Medical Response for Religious and Disability Discrimination." U.S. Equal Employment Opportunity Commission, October 26, 2022. https://www.eeoc.gov /newsroom/eeoc-sues-global-medical-response-and-american-medical -response-religious-and-disability.

Eisenberg, M.S. *Life in the Balance: Emergency Medicine and the Quest to Reverse Sudden Death*. New York: Oxford University Press, 1997.

"Emerging Infectious Disease (EID) Response Plan" (CAAS Standard 202.02.01). Regional Medical Services Authority, Health and Safety Division, Reno, NV. Revised October 1 2014.

EMS Agenda 2050: Envision the Future. Washington, D.C.: National Highway Traffic Safety Administration, 2019.

"EMS-6." San Francisco Fire Department, July 2024. https://sf-fire.org /community-paramedicine/ems-6.

Eng, M. "First Responder: Why Do Fire Trucks Often Arrive Before Ambulances for Medical Emergencies?" WBEZ Chicago, April 2, 2017.

"Envision Healthcare to Sell American Medical Response." KKR, August 8, 2017. https://media.kkr.com/news-details/?news_id=a2cdf104-0986-4b35 -aac9-59fa2c2f2274&type=1.

"Experience in Ambulance Was Scarcely Joy Ride." *Los Angeles Herald*, August 6, 1909. https://chroniclingamerica.loc.gov/lccn/sn85042462/1909-08-06 /ed-1/seq-16/#date1=1908&index=0&rows=20&words=ambulance+joy -riding&searchType=basic&sequence=0&state=&date2=1910&proxtext =ambulance+joyride&y=0&x=0&dateFilterType=yearRange&page=1.

Fahy, R.F. "U.S. Fire Service Fatalities at Structure Fires: 1977–2018." National Fire Protection Agency, Research (Quincy, MA), 2020.

Faloyin, D. *Africa Is Not a Country: Notes on a Bright Continent*. New York: W.W. Norton & Company, 2022.

Fanon, F. *The Wretched of the Earth*. New York: Grove Press, 1963.

"Final Offer of Employment—H-3 Level 1 EMT." Email from Jessica Bushong (FIR) to Joanna Sokol, April 7, 2016.

"Fire Department Calls." National Fire Protection Association, n.d. https:// www.nfpa.org/News-and-Research/Data-research-and-tools/Emergency -Responders/Fire-department-calls.

"Fire Department Overall Run Profile as Reported to the National Fire Incident Reporting System." *FEMA Topical Fire Report Series* 17, no. 8 (January 2017): 1–8.

Fitzharris, L. *The Butchering Art: Joseph Lister's Quest to Transform the Grisly World of Victorian Medicine*. New York: Farrar, Straus and Giroux, 2018.

Gawande, A. *Being Mortal: Medicine and What Matters in the End*. New York: Henry Holt and Company, 2014.

Gehweiler, R. *Pop a Smoke: Memoir of a Marine Helicopter Pilot in Vietnam.* Jefferson, NC: McFarland, 2022.

"Governor Newsome Signs Historical Bill Setting 25-Hour Statewide Healthcare Worker Minimum Wage to Address Staffing Shortages, Improve Patient Care." United Healthcare Workers West, October 13, 2023. https://www.seiu-uhw.org/press/governor-newsom-signs-historic-bill-setting-25-hour-statewide-healthcare-worker-minimum-wage/.

Greenspan, J. "The Charge of the Light Brigade, 160 Years Ago." History.com, October 28, 2019. https://www.history.com/news/the-charge-of-the-light-brigade-160-years-ago.

Griest, S.E. *All the Agents and Saints: Dispatches from the U.S. Borderlands.* Chapel Hill: University of North Carolina Press. 2017.

Grote, M. "Six Minutes to Live or Die (Part 3)." *USA Today*, July 30, 2003.

Groth, P. *Living Downtown: The History of Residential Hotels in the United States.* Berkeley: University of California Press, 1994.

Guzman, D. de. "SF Fire Station Says They're Being Asked to Get Rid of Their Beloved Cat. But They Want Her to Stay." *SFGate*, February 12, 2019.

Habegger, B. "System Is Burdened with Non-Emergency Calls. Sacramento Metro Fire Is Piloting a Solution." ABC 10 News, October 9, 2023.

Hall, K.M. "EMS-STARS: Emergency Medical Services "Superuser" Transport Associations: An Adult Retrospective Study." *Prehospital Emergency Care* 19, no. 1 (2015): 61–67.

Hall, S. "Home Structure Fires." National Fire Protection Agency (NFPA) Research, April 1, 2023.

Hammerl, T. "To the Rescue: SFFD Marks 20 Years of Providing Paramedic Care." *Hoodline*, July 5, 2017. https://hoodline.com/2017/07/to-the-rescue-sffd-marks-20-years-of-providing-paramedic-care/.

Hart, H.W. "The Conveyance of Patients to and from Hospital, 1720–1850. *Medical History* 22 (1978): 397–407.

Hazzard, K. *A Thousand Naked Strangers: A Paramedic's Wild Ride to the Edge and Back*. New York: Simon and Schuster, 2016.

———— *American Sirens: The Incredible Story of the Black Men Who Became America's First Paramedics*. New York: Hachette, 2022.

Heightman, A.J. "Staff Systems with More EMTs and Fewer Paramedics." *Journal of Emergency Medical Services* 40, no. 4 (April 6, 2015).

Herr, M. *Dispatches*. New York: Random House, 1991.

Herring, C. "Complaint-Oriented 'Services': Shelters as Tools for Criminalizing Homelessness." *Annals of the American Academy of Political and Social Science* (January 2021): 264–83.

Junger, S. *Tribe: On Homecoming and Belonging*. London, UK: HarperCollins, 2016.

Kamiya, G. *Cool Gray City of Love: 49 Views of San Francisco*. New York: Bloomsbury, 2013.

Kamiya, G., and P. Madonna. *Spirits of San Francisco: Voyages Through an Unknown City*. New York: Bloomsbury, 2022.

Keisling, P. "Why We Need to Take the 'Fire' Out of 'Fire Department.'" *Governing*, June 26, 2015. https://www.governing.com/archive/col-fire-departments-rethink-delivery-emergency-medical-services.html.

Kilgore, J. *Understanding Mass Incarceration: A People's Guide to the Key Civil Rights Struggle of Our Time*. New York: New Press, 2015.

"KKR Net Worth 2010–2024." Macrotrends, July 5, 2024. https://www.macrotrends.net/stocks/charts/KKR/kkr/net-worth

Kolk, B.V. *The Body Keeps the Score: Brain, Mind, and Body in the Healing of Trauma*. New York: Penguin Random House, 2014.

Landry, D.W. "The Vocation of a Doctor." *Linacre Quarterly* 79, no. 1 (February 2012): 14–18.

Leahy, G. "Homeless People Account for 25% of Ambulance Rides in San Francisco." *SF Standard*, November 10, 2023. https://sfstandard.com/2023/11/10/san-francisco-homeless-patients-ambulance-rides/.

Lelchuk, I. "Merger with S.F. Fire Dept. Is Rocky." *SFGate*, June 27, 2001. https://www.sfgate.com/politics/article/Merger-with-S-F-Fire-Dept-is-rocky -2905414.php.

LeSaint, K.T., J.C. Montoy, E.C Silverman, M.C. Raven, S.L. Schow, P.O. Coffin, J.F. Brown, and M.P. Mercer. "Implementation of a Leave-behind Naloxone Program in San Francisco: A One-year Experience." *Western Journal of Emergency Medicine* 23, no. 6 (November 2022): 952–57.

Lewin, W. *For the Love of Physics: From the End of the Rainbow to the Edge of Time: A Journey Through the Wonders of Physics.* New York: Free Press, 2011.

Lieberman, J. *Shrinks: The Untold Story of Psychiatry.* New York: Little, Brown, 2015.

Lulla, A., and B. Svancarek. *EMS USA Emergency Medical Treatment and Active Labor Act.* Treasure Island, FL: StatPearls Publishing [updated October 17, 2022]. https://www.ncbi.nlm.nih.gov/books/NBK539798/.

Maccarone, B. "AMR Facing FLSA Lawsuit over Misclassifying EMTs and Paramedics as Independent Contractors." FirefighterOvertime.org, July 30, 2023. https://www.firefighterovertime.org/2023/07/30/amr-flsa-suit/.

Macy, B. *Dopesick: Dealers, Doctors, and the Drug Company That Addicted America.* New York: Hachette, 2018.

———. *Raising Lazarus: Hope, Justice, and the Future of America's Overdose Crisis.* New York: Hachette, 2022.

Maté, G. (2008). *In the Realm of Hungry Ghosts: Close Encounters with Addiction.* Berkeley, CA: Random House, 2008.

Matthews, A.L. "Voters to Settle Dispute over Ambulance Employee Break Times." *California Healthline*, August 15, 2018. https://californiahealthline .org/news/voters-to-settle-dispute-over-ambulance-employee-break-times/.

McBurney, C., and L.A. Stimson. Letter to the Editor. *New York Times*, March 26, 1892.

McCall, W.M. *The American Ambulance: 1900–2002.* Hudson, WI: Iconografix, 2002.

McNeal, S. "This Beloved 'Fire Cat' Was Kicked Out of Its Station after an Anonymous Complaint." BuzzFeed News, February 12, 2019.

Meier, B. *Pain Killer: An Empire of Deceit and the Origin of America's Opioid Epidemic.* New York: Penguin Random House, 2018.

"Mrs. Woodworth-Etter and Her Faith Curing Establishement." *Rock Island Argus*, December, 1, 1902.

Mukherjee, S. *The Emperor of All Maladies: A Biography of Cancer.* New York: Simon & Schuster, 2010.

Murphy, E. "Prop. 11: Ambulance Company Has Spent Nearly $22M on State Ballot Measure That Could Shield It From Lawsuites, Save It Millions." *Mission Local*, October 10, 2018.

National Academy of Sciences (US) and National Research Council (US) Committee on Shock. "Accidental Death and Disability: The Neglected Disease of Modern Society." Washington, D.C.: National Academy of Sciences National Research Council, 1966.

National EMS Advisory Council. "EMS System Performance-based Funding and Reimbursement Model: Final Advisory." NEMSAC Advisory, September 2019.

"New Law Is Wanted for 'Suicide Bluffs,'" *Times Americus Reporter*, July 25, 1922.

Norman, S.B., and S. Maguen. "Moral Injury." National Center for PTSD, n.d. https://www.ptsd.va.gov/professional/treat/cooccurring/moral_injury.asp.

O'Brien, K. "Fire Dept. Defends Using Trucks for Medical Calls." Boston.com, January 23, 2009.

Ohler, N. *Blitzed: Drugs in the Third Reich.* Cologne, Germany: Verlag Kiepenheuer & Witsch, 2016.

"Overview: A Global Medical Response Solution." AMR, 2024. https://www.amr.net/about/overview.

"Owner Given First Jaunt in Ambulance." *Imperial Valley Express*, May 6, 1936.

Page, J.O. *The Paramedics*. Morristown, NJ: Backdraft Publications, 1979.

"Patient Dies as Hospital Crew Delay for Meal." *Imperial Valley Press*, January 30, 1924.

Perry, B.D. and M. Szalavitz. *The Boy Who Was Raised as a Dog*. New York: Hachette, 2006.

Pitt, D. "Joseph Lister: Father of Modern Surgery." *Canadian Surgical Journal* 55, no. 5 (October 2012): E8–E9.

Platt, S.R. *Imperial Twilight: The Opium War and the End of China's Last Golden Age*. New York: Penguin Random House, 2018.

"Policy 4050: Death in the Field." Policies and Protocols for Emergency Medical Services, San Francisco, CA, 2018. https://portal.acidremap.com/sites /SanFrancisco/.

Pollak, A.N., A. Benney, K. Hjermstad, and M. Wilcox. *Community Health Paramedicine*. Burlington, MA: Jones & Bartlett, 2018.

"Proposition 11: Requires Private-Sector Emergency Ambulance Employees to Remain on Call During Work Breaks. Changes Other Conditions of Employment. Initiative Statute." Legislative Analyst's Office, CA, 2018.

Quammen, D. *Ebola: The Natural and Human History of a Deadly Virus*. New York: W.W. Norton, 2014.

———. *Spillover: Animal Infections and the Next Human Pandemic*. New York: W.W. Norton, 2012.

Quinones, S. "'I Don't Know That I Would Even Call It Meth Anymore.'" *The Atlantic*, October 18, 2021. https://www.theatlantic.com/magazine/archive /2021/11/the-new-meth/620174/.

———. *The Least of Us: True Tales of America and Hope in the Time of Fentanyl and Meth*. New York: Bloomsbury, 2021.

Quinto, D. (AMR Clinical Supervisor, EMT-P). Interviews with author, May–October 2024.

Randall, D. *Black Death at the Golden Gate: The Race to Save America from the Bubonic Plague*. New York: W.W. Norton, 2019.

Reding, N. *Methland: The Death and Life of an American Small Town.* New York: Bloomsbury, 2009.

Reinke, K. "Study Finds Denver's STAR Program Is Reducing Crime." 9News, June 9, 2022. http://www.9news.com/article/news/local/star-program -reducing-crime.

Rogers, H. *Ambulances: Rescue Machines at Work.* Eden Prairie, MN: Child's World, 2000.

Rosenthal, E. "Think the E.R. Is Expensive? Look at How Much It Costs to Get There." *New York Times,* December 4, 2013.

Safar, P. *Advances in Cardiopulmonary Resuscitation.* Pittsburgh: Springer-Verlag, 1977.

San Francisco Fire Department Deputy Chief. "Operations Memorandum (CD2-19-01)." February 11, 2019.

"San Francisco Firefighters Ask Public for Help to Keep Cat." CBS News, February 11, 2019.

San Francisco Homeless Count and Survey: Comprehensive Report. San Francisco: Department of Homelessness and Supportive Housing, 2019.

Sernoffsky, E. "Woman in Stolen SF Ambulance Crashes on Treasure Island." *SFGate,* June 7, 2016. https://www.sfgate.com/news/article/Thief-steals-SF -ambulance-leads-cops-on-chase-to-7968029.php.

"SFPD Narcan Kits Continue to Save Lives." San Francisco Police Department, September 12, 2016. https://www.sanfranciscopolice.org/news/sfpd-narcan -kits-continue-save-lives.

Shah, M.N. "The Formation of the Emergency Medical Services System." *American Journal of Public Health* 96, no. 3 (March 2006): 414–23.

Sheff, N. *Tweak: Growing Up on Methamphetamines.* New York: Simon & Schuster, 2008.

Shelley, M. *Frankenstein (unabridged).* New York: Dover, 1994.

Shilts, R. *And the Band Played On: Politics, People, and the AIDS Epidemic.* New York: St. Martin's Griffin, 1987.

A Short History of the San Francisco Fire Department. San Francisco: SFFD Local 798, 2015.

Sivils, A., P. Lyell, J.Q. Want, and X.-P Chu. (2022, October 28). "Suboxone: History, Controversy, and Open Questions. *Frontiers in Psychiatry* (October 28, 2022): 1–16.

Smith, S. "California First Responders Say 'No on Prop 11.'" IATSE Local 728, September 10, 2018.

Snider, M. "Mobile Integrated Health Advances." *Carmichael Times*, June 11, 2024.

Spillane, R. "One Dry Month." *Arizona Republican*, August 10, 1919.

Starr, P. *The Social Transformation of American Medicine.* New York: Basic Books, 1982.

Steinbeck, J. *Cannery Row.* New York: Penguin, 1994.

Stevenson, B. *Just Mercy: A Story of Justice and Redemption.* New York: Spiegel & Grau, 2015.

Stout, J. "System Status Management: The Fact Is, It's Everywhere." *JEMS* (April 1989): 65–71.

———. "System Status Management: The Strategy of Ambulance Placement." *JEMS* (May 1983): 22–32.

Supples, M.W., and A.N. Baraki. "Back Pain in EMS, Part 1." *EMS World*, April 2021.

Suratos, P., L. Fernandez, and S. Murphy. "Woman Steals San Francisco Department Ambulance, Crashes on Treasure Island." NBC Bay Area, June 7, 2016. https://www.nbcbayarea.com/news/local/san-francisco-fire -truck-stolen-crashed-on-treasure-island/74022/.

Swor, R.A. "Funding." In *Prehospital Systems and Medical Oversight*, edited by M.M. Alexander Kuehl, 132–38. National Association of EMS Physicians, Mosby-Year Book, 2002.

Talbot, D. *Season of the Witch.* New York: Simon & Schuster, 2012.

Tangherlini, N., M.J. Pletcher, M.A. Covec, and J.F. Brown. "Frequent Use of

Emergency Medical Services by the Elderly: A Case-Control Study Using Paramedic Records." *Prehospital and Disaster Medicine* 25, no. 3 (June 2, 2010): 258–64.

Tangherlini, N., J. Villar, J. Brown, R.M. Rodriguez, C. Yeh, B. Friedman, and P. Wada. (2016, December). "The HOME Team: Evaluating the Effect of an EMS-based Outreach Team to Decrease the Frequency of 911 Use Among High Utilizers of EMS." *Prehospital and Disaster Medicine* 31, no. 6 (December 2016): 603–7.

Terkel, S. *Working: People Talk About What They Do All Day and How They Feel About What They Do.* New York: Ballantine, 1974.

Thadani, T. "SF Could Compel More Severely Mentally Ill People into Treatment Under Law." *San Francisco Chronicle*, October 3, 2019. https://www.sfchronicle.com/politics/article/SF-may-compel-more-severely-mentally-ill-people-14487044.php.

———. "'They've been getting sicker': Inside SF's Effort to Help the Toughest Homeless Cases." *San Francisco Chronicle*, July 13, 2020.

Tong, S. "SFFD: EMS and Community Paramedicine." Fire Commission Report, January 2023.

———. "SFFD: EMS and Community Paramedicine." Fire Commission Report, September 2023, 1–18.

Tseng, A., and C.H. Collins. "How Does Involuntary Mental-Health Treatment Work, and What Rights Do Patients Have?" *Los Angeles Times*, October 4, 2021.

"Unique Hospital Van: First Contagious Fever Ambulance in Use in America." *Sacramento Daily Record-Union*, November 20, 1896.

Vargas, T. "The Harm Caused by D.C.'s Broken 911 System Goes Beyond Deaths." *Washington Post*, October 7, 2023.

Wagner, G., to D. Bernal, "Re: DPH Proposed Budget, FY 2020-2021 and FY 2021-2022" (memorandum), July 31, 2020. City and County of San Francisco Department of Public Health., San Francisco, CA. https://www.sfdph

.org/dph/files/budget/files/FY_20-22_HC_Memo_and_Details_Fourth _Meeting.pdf.

Wainaina, B. "How to Write About Africa." *Granta* 92 (May 2, 2019).

Ward, M. "The Resilience of Fire-Based EMS 'Wicked Problems.'" *Company Commander*, April 11, 2023. https://companycommander.com/2023/04/11 /the-resilience-of-fire-based-ems-wicked-problems/.

Watson, E. "Multnomah County Fines AMR $513,650 for 1 Month of Late Ambulance Responses." KGW8 News, November 14, 2023. https://www .kgw.com/article/news/investigations/multnomah-county-fines-amr-late -ambulance-responses/283-da1caafc-8a1b-4843-b648-5b5017d4550d.

Wayt, T. "Medical First Responsders Say They're Underpaid and Overworked. Will Anything Change?" NBC News, December 30, 2019.

"What Does the HIPAA Privacy Rule Do?" U.S. Department of Health and Human Services, December 19, 2002. https://www.hhs.gov/hipaa/for -individuals/faq/187/what-does-the-hipaa-privacy-rule-do/index.html.

"Why Do Fire Trucks Respond to EMS Calls?" *The Link* (Columbia Southern University), November 13, 2020. http://www.columbiasouthern.edu/blog /blog-articles/2020/november/why-do-fire-trucks-respond-to-ems-calls/.

"Why Does a Fire Engine Come with an Ambulance." Cosumne Community Services District, n.d. https://www.cosumnescsd.gov/537/Why-Does-a-Fire -Engine-Come-With-an-Ambu.

"Why Does a Fire Truck Come When You Call for an Ambulance?" Town of Stevensville Fire Department, n.d. http://www.townofstevensville.com/fire /faq/why-does-fire-truck-come-when-you-call-ambulance.

Yoo, I.-S. "Six Minutes to Live or Die (Part 3)." *USA Today*, July 30, 2003.

Yuen, J.K., M.C. Reid, and M.D Fetters. "Hospital Do-Not-Resuscitate Orders: Why They Have Failed and How to Fix Them." *Journal of General Internal Medicine* 26, no. 7 (July 2011): 791–97.

Ziwe. *Black Friend: Essays.* New York: Abrams Image, 2023.

CHAPTER NOTES

MOSTLY ADRENALINE

p. 23   **In fact, as a paramedic I am not even allowed to *recommend* that the patient visit an urgent care:** There are places in which a particularly brave medical director has instituted what is often called a *provider-initiated refusal protocol*, which is a fancy way of saying that their paramedics are actually allowed to say no. After a thorough medical assessment, and usually a phone call with a base hospital, the ambulance is allowed to refuse transport and leave the patient at the scene. These protocols are extremely controversial, and are usually opposed by doctors, nurses, and lawyers. They were a very hot topic during the COVID-19 pandemic, when many jurisdictions were looking into drastic measures to cut down on hospital use. There are also laws on the books preventing so-called 911 abuse, although personally I have never actually seen them enforced. I did see a police officer try, once, on a man who used to call us six or seven times a day with a chief complaint of "loneliness." The cop wrote down my name and unit number and took some notes on the call, but I am not sure of the outcome.

THE POO SHOW

p. 52   **Large municipal hospitals shut down their programs:** A detailed history of ambulance development can be found in Ryan Corbett Bell's *The Ambulance: A History* (Jefferson, NC: McFarland, 2013). For a shorter and wonderfully readable summary, see chapter eight of Kevin Hazzard's *American Sirens: The Incredible Story of the Black Men Who Became America's First Paramedics* (New York: Hachette, 2022), pages 46–57. Other sources include Dennis Edgerly, "Birth of EMS: The History of the Paramedic," *JEMS* 13 (October 2013); Manish Shah, "The Formation of the Emergency Medical System," *American Journal of Public Health* 96, no. 3 (2006): 414–23; and Robert Carlisle, *An Account of Bellevue Hospital, with a Catalogue of the Medical and Surgical Staff from 1736–1894* (New York: Forgotten Books, 2012).

p. 52   **In the 1960s everything changed:** R.R. Bass, "History of EMS," in *Emergency Medical Services: Clinical Practice and Systems Oversight*, ed. D.C Cone et al. (Edison, NJ: John Wiley & Sons, 2015), 1–16; Hazzard, *American Sirens*; and National EMS Advisory Council, "EMS System Performance-based Funding and Reimbursement Model" (National EMS Advisory Council, 2012, rev. 2019).

p. 53   **One night in San Francisco I am paging through *Living Downtown*:** P. Groth, *Living Downtown: The History of Residential Hotels in the United States* (Berkeley: University of California Press, 1994).

p. 54   **Virtually no one passing on Broadway:** Groth, *Living Downtown*.

p. 54   **About two blocks from here:** G. Kamiya, *Cool Gray City of Love* (New York: Bloomsbury, 2013).

p. 58   **There is a big fight going on in California:** S. Bollag, "California Will Launch Care Court Program to Get Severely Mentally Ill People into Treatment," *San Francisco Chronicle*, November 29, 2022; T. Thadani, "SF Could Compel More Severely Mentally Ill People into Treatment Under Law," *San Francisco Chronicle*, October 3, 2019; and T. Thadani, "'They've been getting sicker': Inside SF's Effort to Help the Toughest Homeless Cases," *San Francisco Chronicle*, July 13, 2020.

DEATH

p. 75   **They bent bodies over shipping barrels . . . "hearts too good to die.":** M.S. Eisenberg, *Life in the Balance: Emergency Medicine and the Quest to Reverse Sudden Death* (New York: Oxford University Press, 1997).

p. 81   **The rules in San Francisco:** "Policy 4050: Death in the Field," Policies and Protocols for Emergency Medical Services, San Francisco, CA, 2018.

p. 82   **"Resuscitation applied without judgment and compassion":** P. Safar, *Advances in Cardiopulmonary Resuscitation* (Pittsburgh: Springer-Verlag, 1977).

p. 82   **A "moral injury":** S.B. Norman and S. Maguen, "Moral Injury," National Center for PTSD, n.d.

p. 87   **"We are all just future corpses" . . . "a culture that denies death":** C. Doughty, *Smoke Gets in Your Eyes: And Other Lessons from the Crematory* (New York: W.W. Norton, 2014), pages 164–68, 228–32.

p. 88   *Hopkins,* **he rasped:** The name of this hospital was changed for privacy reasons, but the institution that he did mention was equally famous for research and medical innovation.

SAN FRANCISCO: SCARY NARNIA

p. 126   **A flaming, sideways ambulance, jammed ass-first over the median:** P. Suratos, L. Fernandez, and S. Murphy, "Woman Steals San Francisco Department Ambulance, Crashes on Treasure Island," NBC Bay Area, June 7, 2016; and E. Sernoffsky, "Woman in Stolen SF Ambulance Crashes on Treasure Island," *SFGate*, June 7, 2016.

p. 127   **I learned later that this gravitational hole is actually an echo of the city:** Groth, *Living Downtown.*

p. 128   **According to a 2023 count, roughly a quarter of San Francisco's 911 calls were for homeless people:** G. Leahy, "Homeless People Account for 25% of Ambulance Rides in San Francisco," *SF Standard*, November 10, 2023.

p. 128   The fire department was organized into two divisions: fire suppression and EMS: When I joined the SFFD, there were two divisions. Several years later, the department created a third division for the rapidly growing community paramedicine program, which had previously been run out of the EMS side. As of 2024, the department continues to contain three separate divisions: fire suppression, EMS, and community paramedicine.

p. 128   Until the late 1990s, emergency medical transport in San Francisco had been handled by a combination of private companies and a government ambulance service: T. Hammerl, "To the Rescue: SFFD Marks 20 Years of Providing Paramedic Care," *Hoodline*, July 5, 2017; and I. Lelchuk, "Merger with S.F. Fire Dept. Is Rocky," *SFGate*, June 27, 2001.

p. 129   Some of the first successful rescue breathing techniques were pioneered by fire departments during the early 1900s: Eisenberg. *Life in the Balance*; and Bell, *The Ambulance*.

p. 130   The population-based rate of home fires and home-fire-related deaths: R. Fahy, "U.S. Fire Service Fatalities at Structure Fires: 1977–2018," National Fire Protection Agency, Research (Quincy, MA), 2020; S. Hall, "Home Structure Fires," National Fire Protection Agency (NFPA) Research, April 1, 2023; and "Fire Department Calls," National Fire Protection Association, n.d.

p. 130   A lot more work, actually: nationally, medical calls represent 71.8 percent of fire department calls: "Fire Department Overall Run Profile as Reported to the National Fire Incident Reporting System," *FEMA Topical Fire Report Series* 17. no. 8 (January 2017): 1–8.

In researching the ambulance-versus-fire-truck debate, I found several amusing articles on local government websites answering the same question: *Why does a fire engine arrive when I call an ambulance?* Apparently enough people have questioned this tradition that several small towns saw fit to post the answer on their website. See, for example: "Why Do Fire Trucks Respond to EMS Calls?" *The Link* (Columbia Southern University), November 13, 2020; "Why Does a Fire Engine Come With an Ambulance?" Cosumne Community Services District, n.d.; and "Why Does a Fire Truck Come When You Call for an Ambulance?" Town of Stevensville Fire Department, n.d.

p. 132 **Unlike the New York Fire Department (FDNY):** A. Almojera, *Riding the Lightning: A Year in the Life of a New York City Paramedic* (New York: HarperCollins, 2022).

p. 134 **From its inception back in the horse-and-buggy days:** Bell, *The Ambulance.*

p. 135 **famously burned to the ground six times in eighteen months:** *A Short History of the San Francisco Fire Department* (San Francisco: SFFD Local 798, 2015).

p. 137 **It's not the first or the last time an intoxicated patient will stumble out of the doors:** Okay, some backstory is indicated here. Legally, if a hospital ER releases a patient who is so intoxicated that they can't walk safely, and this individual teeters out in front of oncoming traffic and gets smoked by a bus, the hospital can get in trouble. But it is widely accepted in our industry that this kind of thing happens all the time. I have also personally witnessed hundreds, if not thousands of patients in various states of chemical and medical distress kicked out of every hospital in San Francisco. Semi-conscious, unable to walk or speak, clothing soiled or torn or not present at all. I'm not going to name the hospital that kicked out Tom's guy, or the developmentally disabled girl in "When Elephants Fight," or any of the rest. One reason is that I understand why these things happen. Every emergency room must make difficult decisions about what constitutes a truly life-threatening emergency and what their resources and capabilities are in each moment. The other reason is that I simply do not feel like violating patient privacy laws or defending myself against a libel lawsuit. So you will have to take my word for it.

p. 137   **It is while working in San Francisco that I first read Matthew Desmond:**
M. Desmond, *Evicted: Poverty and Profit in the American City* (New York: Broadway Books, 2016.)

If you are interested in reading more on the great fire-versus-EMA debate, the following suggestions are a good place to start (see "Works Cited and Recommended Reading" for full bibliographic details). I would especially recommend Anthony Almojera.

Almojera, A. *Riding the Lightning.*

Blackwell, T.H. and J.S. Kaufman, "Response Time Effectiveness."

Brundage, J. "Deciphering the Paradox."

Eng, M. "First Responder."

Fahy, R.F. "U.S. Fire Service Fatalities at Structure Fires: 1977–2018."

Heightman, A.J. "Staff Systems with More EMTs and Fewer Paramedics."

Keisling, P. "Why We Need to Take the 'Fire' Out of 'Fire Department.'"

"Fire Department Calls." National Fire Protection Association.

O'Brien, K. "Fire Dept. Defends Using Trucks for Medical Calls."

Rosenthal, E. "Think the E.R. Is Expensive? Look at How Much It Costs to Get There."

Tong, S. "SFFD: EMS and Community Paramedicine" (January 2023).

Ward, M. "The Resilience of Fire-Based EMS 'Wicked Problems.'"

Wayt, T. "Medical First Responsders Say They're Underpaid and Overworked. Will Anything Change?"

THE PAST IS THE PRESENT, THE OLD IS THE NEW, AND OUR PAIN IS NOT OURS ALONE

This history is detailed thoroughly in Bell's *The Ambulance* and Hazzard's *American Sirens*. A good summary of ambulance revenue and government financing attempts can be found in Robert A. Swor,

"Funding" (in *Prehospital Systems and Medical Oversight*, M.M. Alexander Kuehl, ed., 132–38 [National Association of EMS Physicians, Mosby-Year Book, 2002]).

Another interesting resource is the U.S. Library of Congress website. There are many newspaper and magazine articles detailing ambulances struggling with funding or call volume for the last hundred years. Here is a brief selection (see "Works Cited and Recommended Reading" for full bibliographic details):

"Ambulance Service Planned by City."

"Caring for the Sick: Some Facts About the Ambulance System of New York."

Hart, H.W. "The Conveyance of Patients to and from Hospital, 1720–1850."

McBurney, E. and L.A. Stimson, Letter to the Editor.

"Mrs. Woodworth-Etter and Her Faith Curing Establishement."

"New Law Is Wanted for 'Suicide Bluffs.'"

"Patient Dies as Hospital Crew Delay for Meal."

"Unique Hospital Van: First Contagious Fever Ambulance in Use in America."

"With an Ambulance."

p. 158   **Cloth stretchers, sedan chairs:** K.T. Barkley, *The Ambulance: The Story of Emergency Transportation of Sick and Wounded Through the Centuries* (N.p.: Load N Go Press, 1990).

p. 158   **The word *ambulancia* first appeared in a military context . . . By the 1950s, American ambulances were run by a hodgepodge of private companies:** Bell, *The Ambulance.*

p. 159   **Ambulances were never profitable:** See list of sources above, also Bell, *The Ambulance.*

p. 162   **The federal government noticed . . . "a public health problem second only to the ravages of ancient plagues or world wars":** National

Academy of Sciences (US) and National Research Council (US) Committee on Shock, "Accidental Death and Disability: The Neglected Disease of Modern Society" (Washington, DC: National Academies Press, 1966).

p. 162 **Several government acts set aside funding for ambulances:** Swor, "Funding"; Bell, *The Ambulance*; and D. Quinto (AMR Clinical Supervisor, EMT-P), interviews with author, May–June 2024.

p. 162 **Then, on top of all of these changes:** Bell, *The Ambulance*; and J.O. Page, *The Paramedics* (Morristown, NJ: Backdraft Publications, 1979). The *Emergency!* plot points referenced here are from season one, episode 2, episode 4, and episode 5.

p. 165 **But when the federal money ran out, the local governments:** Swor, "Funding."

p. 166 **memoir by an Australian paramedic:** T. Booth, *You Called an Ambulance for What?* (Sydney: Macmillan, 2023).

p. 166 **New York Fire Department lieutenant Anthony Almojera:** Almojera, *Riding the Lightning*.

p. 168 **Bellevue hospital commissioners fighting with the police department:** Bell, *The Ambulance*.

p. 168 **"Its inhabitants are, as the man once said, 'whores, pimps, gamblers, and sons of bitches'":** J. Steinbeck, *Cannery Row* (New York: Penguin, 1994).

Other sources used for background information and context in terms of ambulance history for this chapter and throughout the book (see "Works Cited and Recommended Reading" for full bibliographic details):

"Ambulance Service Planned by City."

Barkley, K.T. *The Ambulance*.

Barringer, E.D. *Bowery to Bellevue*.

Bass, R.R. "History of EMS."

Bishnoi, R. "Six Minutes to Live or Die."

Bloor, A.J. *Letters from the Army of the Potomac.*

Brown, J.F., et al. "Frequent Users of 9-1-1 Emergency Medical Services."

Bucher J. and H.Q. Zaidi. "A Brief History of Emergency Medical Services in the United States."

"Caring for the Sick: Some Facts About the Ambulance System of New York."

Carlisle, R.J. *An Account of Bellevue Hospital.*

Connelly, J. *Bringing Out the Dead.*

"Cost Is Chief Factor."

"Coverage and Reimbursement for Emergency Medical Services Care Delivery Models and Uncompensated Services."

Davis, R. "Six Minutes to Live or Die (Part 1)."

———. "Six Minutes to Live or Die (Part 2)."

Edgerly, D. "Birth of EMS: The History of the Paramedic."

EMS Agenda 2050: Envision the Future.

Grote, M. "Six Minutes to Live or Die (Part 3)."

Groth, P. *Living Downtown.*

Hart, H.W. "The Conveyance of Patients to and from Hospital, 1720-1850."

Hazzard, K. *A Thousand Naked Strangers.*

———. *American Sirens.*

Keisling, P. "Why We Need to Take the 'Fire' Out of 'Fire Department.'"

Landry, D.W. "The Vocation of a Doctor."

McCall, W.M. *The American Ambulance.*

National Academy of Sciences (US) and National Research Council (US) Committee on Shock, "Accidental Death and Disability: The Neglected Disease of Modern Society."

National EMS Advisory Council. "EMS System Performance-based
  Funding and Reimbursement Model." Final Advisory. 2012, 2019.

"Patient Dies as Hospital Crew Delay for Meal."

Page, J.O. *The Paramedics.*

Pitt, D. "Joseph Lister: Father of Modern Surgery."

Rogers, H. *Ambulances.*

Rosenthal, E. "Think the E.R. Is Expensive? Look at How Much It
  Costs to Get There."

Safar, P. *Advances in Cardiopulmonary Resuscitation.*

Shah, M.N. "The Formation of the Emergency Medical System."

Starr, P. *The Social Transformation of American Medicine.*

"Unique Hospital Van: First Contagious Fever Ambulance in Use in
  America."

Wayt, T. "Medical First Responsders Say They're Underpaid and
  Overworked. Will Anything Change?"

Yoo, I.-S. "Six Minutes to Live or Die (Part 3)."

COVID

p. 169   **Every winter, we stood around a windy courtyard:** While researching
this book, I found myself cleaning and reorganizing shelves full of work
notebooks, old memorabilia, and memories. I found a crumpled hand-
out stuffed in the bottom of an old backpack and audibly gasped when
I realized what I was looking at. After watching the COVID-19 pandemic explode and then settle back down over the last four years, I had
stumbled upon a souvenir from almost a decade earlier, describing
exactly what we were heading into. When I was done shaking my head
and chuckling, I set about rewriting the top of the COVID chapter.
("Emerging Infectious Disease (EID) Response Plan" [CAAS Standard
202.02.01], Regional Medical Services Authority, Health and Safety
Division [Reno, NV], revised October 1 2014.)

p. 185 The hospital we are standing in now housed the very first ward dedicated to caring for AIDS patients . . . I picture Selma Dr. Dritz—the clinician in the STD clinic in the Castro in 1983: R. Shilts, *And the Band Played On: Politics, People, and the AIDS Epidemic* (New York: St. Martin's Griffin, 1987).

p. 199 **During a bubonic plague outbreak in London in 1665 . . . Back in 1866 as cholera ravaged Northern Europe:** Bell, *The Ambulance*.

p. 211 **There is a quote in David Quammen's *Spillover*:** D. Quammen, *Spillover: Animal Infections and the Next Human Pandemic* (New York: W.W. Norton, 2012).

FREEDOM HOUSE

This essay relies heavily Kevin Hazzard's *American Sirens*. It is a wonderfully researched book, and I strongly recommend it to anyone who has an interest in paramedicine, racial justice, urban history, or humanity in general (unless otherwise noted below, this can be assumed to be the source citation for facts that appear in this essay). There is also a short but thorough write-up of Freedom House Enterprises found in Bell's *The Ambulance*, and a rather whitewashed version in Page's *The Paramedics*.

p. 218 **This was the same Safar who had arrived from Austria, revolutionized rescue breathing and CPR:** Eisenberg, *Life in the Balance*.

p. 219 **The new standard set by FHE:** Bell, *The Ambulance*.

SAVE EDNA

p. 225 **The website *SFGate* picks up the story:** D. de Guzman, "SF Fire Station Says They're Being Asked to Get Rid of Their Beloved Cat. But They Want Her to Stay," *SFGate*, February 12, 2019.

p. 225 **Then #saveEdna goes viral on Twitter . . . Our cat is retweeted by @FDNY in solidarity:** "San Francisco Firefighters Ask Public for Help to Keep Cat," CBS News, February 11, 2019; and S. McNeal, "This Beloved 'Fire Cat' Was Kicked Out of Its Station after an Anonymous Complaint," BuzzFeed News, February 12, 2019.

Note: Unfortunately, partially due to the transition from Twitter to X, I am no longer able to find these exact tweets. The BuzzFeed article does reference an Instagram post by FDNY Station 57, and a quick Google search for "Fire Cat Edna" will confirm her status as an international social media darling.

p. 226 **Edna has functioned for years as a de facto station therapy cat:** de Guzman, "SF Fire Station Says."

p. 226 **We receive a memo from operations reminding us:** San Francisco Fire Department Deputy Chief, "Operations Memorandum (CD2-19-01)," February 11, 2019.

BLACK WREATHS

The technique for this story was heavily inspired by both Kevin Hazzard's *A Thousand Naked Strangers* ("The Summons," pp. 241–45), and Ziwe's *Black Friend: Essays.*

REMY

p. 260 *February, peeved at Paris, pours a gloomy torrent*: Charles Baudelaire, "Spleen," tr. Richard Howard, 1982.

MAGIC ERASER JUICE

There has been a ton of literature in the last ten years about the "opiate crisis," as it seems to have been dubbed. I gravitated towards Beth Macy and Sam Quinones, as I found their voices to be particularly authentic and readable. Stephen Platt and Martin Booth gave me a fascinating historical perspective about humanity's complicated and ancient relationship with the poppy flower. The current fentanyl crisis in the United States has overwhelmed us so breathtakingly that one could be forgiven for thinking that this issue began out of nowhere just a few years ago.

During both the writing of this book and in my work as a paramedic and community paramedic, I read a fair amount about fentanyl, methamphetamine, addiction, economics, and trauma. It is impossible to overstate how interconnected all of these issues are.

Fun fact: it was actually Peter Safar, of CPR and Freedom House fame, who first introduced Narcan to the streets. It had been used in operating rooms for some time to reverse anesthesia, but a heroin epidemic in Pittsburgh caused Safar to give the drug to his paramedics to use in the field. Yet another medical advancement we owe to Freedom House Enterprises.

p. 262 **fentanyl overdose deaths have skyrocketed not only in San Francisco but around the country:** B. Macy, *Raising Lazarus: Hope, Justice, and the Future of America's Overdose Crisis* (New York: Hachette, 2022); and "Drug Overdose Mortality by State," CDC National Center for Health Statistics, 2022.

p. 264 **Police carry them, social workers, other drug users:** "SFPD Narcan Kits Continue to Save Lives," San Francisco Police Department, September 12, 2016; and K.T. LeSaint et al., "Implementation of a Leave-behind Naloxone Program in San Francisco: A One-year Experience," *Western Journal of Emergency Medicine* 23, no. 6 (November 2022): 952–57.

p. 267 **A lot of people blame the Sackler family:** B. Macy, *Dopesick: Dealers, Doctors, and the Drug Company That Addicted America* (New York: Hachette, 2018); B. Meier, *Pain Killer: An Empire of Deceit and the Origin of America's Opioid Epidemic* (New York: Penguin Random House, 2018); and S. Quinones, *The Least of Us: True Tales of America and Hope in the Time of Fentanyl and Meth* (New York: Bloomsbury, 2021).

p. 267   The soul of the poppy flower: M Booth, *Opium: A History* (New York: St. Martin's Press, 1996).

p. 267   Purdue Pharma, owned by the Sacklers, marketed the drug so heavily: Macy, *Dopesick.*

p. 267   So did the first doctor to inject morphine with a syringe: Booth, *Opium.*

p. 267   Purdue Pharma bought lunches and dinners and weekends on yachts: Macy, *Dopesick.*

p. 268   Long before the Sacklers: S.R. Platt, *Imperial Twilight: The Opium War and the End of China's Last Golden Age* (New York: Penguin Random House, 2018).

WHEN ELEPHANTS FIGHT

p. 277   The flyer is vague: Chief of Department, "General Order 21 A-02: Street Crisis Response Team H3L2 Positions," San Francisco. January 5, 2021.

p. 283   In 1995, a rural area in New Mexico with a desperate need for primary care doctors: A. Pollak et al., *Community Health Paramedicine* (Burlington, MA: Jones & Bartlett, 2018). For this section I also referenced personal notes taken during lectures in my community medicine training course, which took place in February and March 2021.

p. 283   Back in the 1990s, an EMS captain in San Francisco helped author a series of studies: The studies referenced for this section are as follows (see "Works Cited and Recommended Reading" for full bibliographic details):

Brown, J.F. et al. "Frequent Users of 9-1-1 Emergency Medical Services: Sign of Success or Symptom of Impending Failure?"

Hall, K.M., et al. "EMS-STARS: Emergency Medical Services 'Superuser' Transport Associations: An Adult Retrospective Study."

Tangherlini, N., et al. "Frequent Use of Emergency Medical Services by the Elderly: A Case-Control Study Using Paramedic Records."

————. "The HOME Team: Evaluating the Effect of an EMS-based Outreach Team to Decrease the Frequency of 911 Use Among High Utilizers of EMS."

p. 284   **The media-friendly description of the goals of the program: "EMS-6."** San Francisco Fire Department, July 2024.

p. 284   **By the numbers:** The department's analysis shows that many frequent 911 users have decreased their utilization of city services following EMS-6 contacts. But I have also personally witnessed the successes of this program over my time with the SFFD. A couple of statistics can be found in: N. Tangherlini et al., "The HOME Team: Evaluating the Effect of an EMS-based Outreach Team to Decrease the Frequency of 911 Use Among High Utilizers of EMS," *Prehospital and Disaster Medicine* 31, no. 6 (December 2016): 603–7; and S. Tong, "SFFD: EMS and Community Paramedicine," Fire Commission Report, January 2023.

p. 284   **We had callers with annual counts in the four hundreds:** To my knowledge, the SFFD has not published these numbers for individual 911. But I have personally witnessed this dramatic of a call reduction with several patients who are familiar to me, and have confirmed through many conversations with EMS-6 captains over the years that it has happened more than once.

p. 289   **The budget of the San Francisco Department of Public Health this year is just shy of $3 billion:** G. Wagner to D. Bernal, "Re: DPH Proposed Budget, FY 2020-2021 and FY 2021-2022" (memorandum), July 31, 2020. City and County of San Francisco Department of Public Health., San Francisco, CA.

p. 292   **The journalist, Sam Quinones, describes a profound change in the American drug trade over the last couple of decades:** S. Quinones,

"'I Don't Know That I Would Even Call It Meth Anymore,'" *The Atlantic*, October 18, 2021.

p. 292 **For most of its history methamphetamine was synthesized from the ephedra plant:** Quinones, "'I Don't Know That I Would Even Call It Meth Anymore.'"

p. 293 **He asks me if I've seen the influence of methamphetamine in my work on the ambulance:** Personal conversations with S. Quinones, 2022.

p. 294 **In it, he quotes Dr. Rachel Solotaroff . . . Jennie Jobe, the leader of a Tennessee drug court:** Quinones, *The Least of Us.*

p. 295 **For many decades it was the drug of choice of the American working class:** N. Reding, *The Death and Life of an American Small Town* (New York: Bloomsbury, 2009).

p. 297 **As Sofia and I debate how to break the fewest number of rules, Jaya lies down on the sidewalk:** I worked closely with Jaya during the development of this entire chapter, and when I shared this part of the story she filled me in on her version of that day. I had actually not remembered her interaction with the patient at all, as at the time I was focused on the logistics of the call and distracted by my own emotions about the situation. Our conversation after the fact was a good reminder of what an incident can look like from different perspectives. I was also blown away yet again by just how many times per day a care worker performs some emotionally exhausting and unseen miracle that will never be recognized formally. Jaya had not intubated the patient or gotten a return of pulses; her achievement on this call would not be recorded into the annals of academia or published in a journal. The patient herself probably wouldn't even remember the interaction. But Jaya had gotten down onto the sidewalk and given of herself to this work in a way that helped in the moment. If that's not medicine I don't know what is.

Jaya also remembered transporting this patient to the hospital, and speaking with the ER social worker on our arrival. In her recollection, we learned that our patient had actually already been legally conserved, and had been illegally dumped from or allowed to leave her care home. This would of course make the first emergency room's behavior even more egregious. Although Jaya is fairly confident in her memory, we decided that with no way to confirm the story, we would leave this part out of the formal text. I personally cannot remember the details of our conversation with the social worker, and can only remember the emotions I felt: anger, disappointment, disillusionment, bitterness, and the desire to get out of the room before the full tragedy of the situation wormed its way into my psyche.

p. 298 **Usually this would be a ridiculous request:** A. Lulla and B. Svancarek, *EMS USA Emergency Medical Treatment and Active Labor Act* (Treasure Island, FL: StatPearls Publishing [updated October 17, 2022].)

p. 299 **one detail from early in Starr's book keeps jumping out at me:** P. Starr, *The Social Transformation of American Medicine* (New York: Basic Books, 1982).

p. 309 **I visit the Sacramento Metropolitan Fire Department:** From an in-person ride-along in 2023.

p. 309 **One local reporter says the number of frequent 911 callers dropped by 43 percent over two years:** B. Habegger, "System Is Burdened with Non-Emergency Calls. Sacramento Metro Fire Is Piloting a Solution," ABC 10 News, October 9, 2023.

p. 309 **Another estimates that the program has saved the county over $2.4 million in only one year:** M. Snider, "Mobile Integrated Health Advances," *Carmichael Times*, June 11, 2024.

p. 310 **There has been modest success for opiate users with methadone and Suboxone:** N.D. Campbell and A.M. Lovell, "The History of the

Development of Buprenorphine as an Addiction Therapeutic," *Annals of the New York Academy of Sciences* 1248 (2012): 124–39.

p. 310   **What hope can I find in writing involuntary psych holds on the same clients, over and over again, dozens of times:** Technically, most paramedics do not write involuntary psychiatric holds. Instead, we assess the patient to determine whether we believe they possess the mental capacity to make their own medical decisions. If we believe that the patient is too confused to understand the risks of refusing medical care, we are required to physically restrain and transport the patient so that a doctor can make the official determination. In California, the entities that can write legal holds include police, social workers, and many mental health professionals. In all of these cases, the paramedics are called to transport the patient and are handed a piece of paper indicating that we are to "bring them in." During my time on the Street Crisis team, I was trained and authorized to write involuntary holds as a community paramedic.

The initial field paperwork is a suggestion—it does not guarantee that the patient will be held for seventy-two hours. It simply allows the hospital to hold the patient until he or she can be properly evaluated by a physician, which must take place within three days at maximum. I absolutely cannot count the number of times I have struggled to restrain a deeply altered patient and transported them to a hospital only to see them walking away while I am still cleaning my gurney. I once saw an ER doc read a police hold, roll his eyes, physically rip the hold in half and throw it on the floor, and then release my patient.

Another call that for some reason particularly affected me took place deep in the heart of the Black Lives Matter protests. A young police officer, white guy, was with me helping to talk to a woman who was well known to both of us. He described how he had been running calls on her for weeks, struggling to gain rapport, and finally decided to place her on a psychiatric hold. Her legs, covered in wounds and infected, were rotting into her wheelchair. He told me he spent hours with her that day attempting to convince her to accept help and getting to know the details of her current situation. He told me, "When I finally wrote the hold, I tried *so hard.* I wrote everything down that I had done, I explained it all. I redid the paperwork three times to make sure it was good. I crossed all my *t*'s and dotted all my *i*'s, I swear." I pictured this young twenty-something, bent over in the front seat of his patrol car, filling out a handwritten form again and again until he got the wording right. He said that he explained the situation to the patient, called an ambulance, and followed them to the hospital, feeling as though he had made a difficult but ultimately correct decision. I winced, hoping I was wrong about the outcome, knowing that stories like these are how police officers turn into the people that everyone loves to hate. "When I got back down the hill to her spot, she was already there!! I mean, she *beat me* back here!! I was only gone like an hour! How did she even get back that fast?!" The cop—blond hair, blue eyes—blinked back actual tears as he told me the story. He said he had written many more holds in his career, on her and others, but since that day had never tried quite so hard to be thorough.

p. 310 **In the first twenty years after surgeons invented anesthesia, surgical outcomes worsened:** L. Fitzharris, *The Butchering Art: Joseph Lister's Quest to Transform the Grisly World of Victorian Medicine* (New York: Farrar, Straus and Giroux, 2018).

p. 310 **As modern medicine prevents more and more heart attacks and strokes, cancer rates go up:** S. Mukherjee, *The Emperor of All Maladies: A Biography of Cancer* (New York: Simon & Schuster, 2010).

p. 313 *Theirs not to reason why/theirs but to do or die*: J. Greenspan, "The Charge of the Light Brigade, 160 Years Ago," History.com, October 28, 2019.

All references and quotes in this piece are from Emily Dunning Barringer, *Bowery to Bellevue: The Story of New York's First Woman Ambulance Surgeon* (New York: W.W. Norton, 1950).

SIDE EFFECTS

p. 356 **Most paramedics injure their backs sooner or later:** Okay, most *humans* experience back pain at some point in their lives. But back injuries in EMS professionals are approximately three times the average for other health-care professionals. Notably, EMS professionals also experience the highest rate of injury of all public safety professions (see M.W. Supples and A.N. Baraki, "Back Pain in EMS, Part 1," *EMS World*, April 2021).

p. 369 **In the early 1980s an economist named Jack Stout reimagined EMS:** J.L. Stout, "System Status Management: The Fact Is, It's Everywhere." *JEMS* (April 1989): 65–71.

p. 370 **A 71 percent increase in overall back pain:** S. Christopher, "The Effects of System Status Management (SSM) and the Eight Minute Response Target on the Health and Well-Being of Ambulance Personnel and Patients: A Review of the Literature (Part 1)," *Ambulance UK* 20, no. 6 (December 2005): 415–20.

p. 370 **One of the first major studies took place in 1986:** B.E. Bledsoe, "EMS Myth #7: System Status Management (SSM) Lowers Response Times and Enhances Patient Care," *Emergency Medical Services* 32, no. 9 (September 2003): 158–9. Note: a more recent study based in Toronto compares a "dynamic deployment" model favorably to a static system in terms of increased call volume and response times. However, in this study, "static" versus "dynamic" refers not to the use of base stations, but to the shift start times. The study compares a traditional 0700/1900 shift flop to a model with staggered start times to promote coverage during times of peak 911 usage. In fact, both systems utilize substations for their ambulances to rest at between calls, recommending a "hub and spoke" model for physical locations of deployment centers and substations (see M.V. Bosnyak, "Dynamic Deployment Models for High-Performance Emergency Medical Services," *Canadian Journal of Emergency Management/Revue canadienne de gestion des urgences* 3, no. 1 (2022): 8–41).

p. 372   **The company grew far larger than Shirley's original vision:** "American Medical Response, Inc." International Directory of Company Histories, Encylopedia.com (September 11, 2024).

p. 376   **In 2018, AMR spent $22 million funding a California state ballot measure to avoid having to give EMTs and paramedics lunch breaks:** A.L. Matthews, "Voters to Settle Dispute over Ambulance Employee Break Times," *California Healthline*, August 15, 2018; E. Murphy, "Prop. 11: Ambulance Company Has Spent Nearly $22M on State Ballot Measure That Could Shield It From Lawsuits, Save It Millions," *Mission Local*, October 10, 2018; and S. Smith, "California First Responders Say 'No on Prop 11.'" IATSE Local 728, September 10, 2018.

p. 377   **The state Legislative Analyst's office estimated the new law would cost roughly $100 million in staffing increases alone:** Careless, J. "The Ugly Battle Behind California's Prop 11." *EMS World*, February 1, 2019; and "Proposition 11: Requires Private-Sector Emergency Ambulance Employees to Remain on Call During Work Breaks. Changes Other Conditions of Employment. Initiative Statute." Legislative Analyst's Office, CA, 2018.

p. 377   **On top of that, AMR was hit with multiple lawsuits:** Careless, J. "The Ugly Battle Behind California's Prop 11." *EMS World*, February 1, 2019; and "Bartoni v. American Medical Response West." Justia US Law, 2017.

p. 377   **As union director Jason Bollini pointed out:** Murphy, E. "Prop. 11:
         Ambulance Company Has Spent Nearly $22M on State Ballot Measure
         That Could Shield It from Lawsuits, Save It Millions." *Mission Local*,
         October 10, 2018.

p. 378   **As for the lawsuits, the court denied the class-action nature of the
         largest suit:** "Bartoni v. American Medical Response West." Justia US
         Law, 2017.

p. 378   **But the labor issues that plague our ambulances:** Just for fun, here
         is some more reading about AMR facing legal action over various
         labor violations (see "Works Cited" list for full details):
         "AMR to Pay $162,500 to Settle EEOC Pregnancy Discrimination
             Lawsuit."
         Barry, S. "AMR Defends Response Times, Laments Lack of Union
             Support to Recent Wage Hike Offer."
         "EEOC Sues Global Medical Response and American Medical
             Response for Religious and Disability Discrimination."
         Maccarone, B. "AMR Facing FLSA Lawsuit over Misclassifying EMTs
             and Paramedics as Independent Contractors."
         Watson, E. "Multnomah County Fines AMR $513,650 for 1 Month
             of Late Ambulance Responses."

p. 378   **The owners of $40 billion private-equity firms would have to stop
         their yachts for three seconds:** "Envision Healthcare to Sell American
         Medical Response," KKR, August 8, 2017; "KKR Net Worth 2010–
         2024," Macrotrends, July 5, 2024; and "Overview: A Global Medical
         Response Solution," AMR, 2024.

AFTERWORD: SPEAKING OUT

p. 395   **"There are two ways to dehumanize":** Desmond, *Evicted*.

p. 396   **In 2023, California governor Gavin Newsom signed into law:** "Gov.
         Newsom Signs Historic Bill Setting $25/hour Healthcare Worker

Minimum Wage to Address Staffing Shortages, Improve Patient Care."
United Healthcare Workers West, October 13, 2023.

p. 396 **they specifically excluded EMTs and paramedics. We were classified as "outside workers":** J. Carman and L.S. Charbonneau, "New Law (SB 525) Sets Higher Minimum Wages for Certain Health Care Employees." *California Public Agency Labor & Employment Blog,* Liebert Cassidy Whitmore, January 16, 2024.

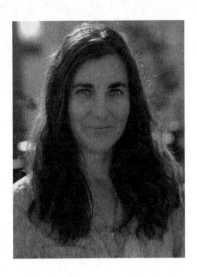

JOANNA SOKOL has worked on a 911 ambulance for ten years: along the beach in Santa Cruz, in the high desert of Reno, and on the steep streets of San Francisco. Before that, she spent time as a ski patroller, wilderness EMT, and medical stand by for raves and music festivals. She holds a paramedic license and a Bachelor's degree in Biological Sciences from the University of California at Santa Cruz. During her time at the San Francisco Fire Department, she received an award for Clinical Excellence and served as a member of the Street Crisis Response team. Her literary work has appeared in *Reader's Digest*, *Epoca*, and Hazlitt, and she received a Sidney Award in 2019. Born and raised in Oakland, California, Sokol currently lives in Santa Cruz with her boyfriend and a very stubborn dog.